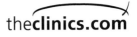

VETERINARY CLINICS

CLINICS

OF NORTH AMERICA

Small Animal Practice

Dietary Management and Nutrition

GUEST EDITORS
Claudia A. Kirk, DVM, PhD
Joseph W. Bartges, DVM, PhD

November 2006 • Volume 36 • Number 6

SAUNDERS

An Imprint of Elsevier, Inc.
PHILADELPHIA   LONDON   TORONTO   MONTREAL   SYDNEY   TOKYO

W.B. SAUNDERS COMPANY
A Division of Elsevier Inc.

Elsevier, Inc., 1600 John F. Kennedy Blvd., Suite 1800, Philadelphia, PA 19103-2899

http://www.vetsmall.theclinics.com

VETERINARY CLINICS OF NORTH AMERICA:	**Volume 36, Number 6**
SMALL ANIMAL PRACTICE	**ISSN 0195-5616**
November 2006	**ISBN 1-4160-3829-9**

Editor: John Vassallo; j.vassallo@elsevier.com

The ideas and opinions expressed in *Veterinary Clinics of North America: Small Animal Practice* do not necessarily reflect those of the Publisher. The Publisher does not assume any responsibility for any injury and/or damage to persons or property arising out of or related to any use of the material contained in this periodical. The reader is advised to check the appropriate medical literature and the product information currently provided by the manufacturer of each drug to be administered to verify the dosage, the method and duration of administration, or contraindications. It is the responsibility of the treating physician or other health care professional, relying on independent experience and knowledge of the patient, to determine drug dosages and the best treatment for the patient. Mention of any product in this issue should not be construed as endorsement by the contributors, editors, or the Publisher of the product or manufacturers' claims.

Veterinary Clinics of North America: Small Animal Practice (ISSN 0195-5616) is published bimonthly (For Post Office use only: volume 36 issue 5 of 6) by Elsevier Inc., 360 Park Avenue South, New York, NY 10010-1710. Months of issue are January, March, May, July, September, and November. Business and Editorial offices: 1600 John F. Kennedy Blvd., Suite 1800, Philadelphia, PA 19103-2899. Customer Service Office: 6277 Sea Harbor Drive, Orlando, FL 32887-4800. Periodicals postage paid at New York, NY and additional mailing offices. Subscription prices are $187.00 per year for US individuals, $297.00 per year for US institutions, $94.00 per year for US students and residents, $248.00 per year for Canadian individuals, $373.00 per year for Canadian institutions, $259.00 per year for international individuals, $373.00 per year for international institutions and $127.00 per year for Canadian and foreign students/residents. To receive student/resident rate, orders must be accompanied by name of affiliated institution, date of term, and the *signature* of program/residency coordinator on institution letterhead. Orders will be billed at individual rate until proof of status is received. Foreign air speed delivery is included in all *Clinics* subscription prices. All prices are subject to change without notice. **POSTMASTER**: Send address changes to *Veterinary Clinics of North America: Small Animal Practice*, Elsevier Periodicals Customer Service, 6277 Sea Harbor Drive, Orlando, FL 32887-4800, USA; phone: 1-800-654-2452 [toll free number for US customers], or (+1)(407) 345-4000 [customers outside US]; fax: (+1)(407) 363-1354; email: usjcs@elsevier.com.

Veterinary Clinics of North America: Small Animal Practice is also published in Japanese by Inter Zoo Publishing Co., Ltd., Aoyama Crystal-Bldg 5F, 3-5-12 Kitaaoyama, Minato-ku, Tokyo 107-0061, Japan.

Reprints: For copies of 100 or more, of articles in this publication, please contact the Commercial Reprints Department, Elsevier Inc., 360 Park Avenue South, New York, New York 10010-1710. Tel. (212) 633-3813 Fax: (212) 462-1935, email: reprints@elsevier.com

Veterinary Clinics of North America: Small Animal Practice is covered in *Current Contents/Agriculture, Biology and Environmental Sciences, Science Citation Index, ASCA, Index Medicus, Excerpta Medica,* and *BIOSIS*.

Printed in the United States of America.

VETERINARY CLINICS
SMALL ANIMAL PRACTICE

ELSEVIER
SAUNDERS

Dietary Management and Nutrition

GUEST EDITORS

CLAUDIA A. KIRK, DVM, PhD, Diplomate, American College of Veterinary Internal Medicine; Diplomate, American College of Veterinary Nutrition; Associate Professor of Medicine and Nutrition, Department of Small Animal Clinical Sciences, Veterinary Teaching Hospital, College of Veterinary Medicine, The University of Tennessee, Knoxville, Tennessee

JOSEPH W. BARTGES, DVM, PhD, Diplomate, American College of Veterinary Internal Medicine; Diplomate, American College of Veterinary Nutrition; Professor of Medicine and Nutrition, The Acree Endowed Chair of Small Animal Research, Veterinary Teaching Hospital, College of Veterinary Medicine, The University of Tennessee, Knoxville, Tennessee

CONTRIBUTORS

JOSEPH W. BARTGES, DVM, PhD, Diplomate, American College of Veterinary Internal Medicine; Diplomate, American College of Veterinary Nutrition; Professor of Medicine and Nutrition, The Acree Endowed Chair of Small Animal Research, Veterinary Teaching Hospital, College of Veterinary Medicine, The University of Tennessee, Knoxville, Tennessee

STEVEN C. BUDSBERG, DVM, MS, Diplomate, American College of Veterinary Surgeons, Professor of Surgery, Department of Small Animal Medicine and Surgery and Director of Clinical Research, Office of Associate Dean for Research and Graduate Affairs, University of Georgia, Athens, Georgia

NICHOLAS J. CAVE, BVSc, MVSc, MACVSc, Diplomate, American College of Veterinary Nutrition; Senior Lecturer in Small Animal Medicine and Nutrition, Institute of Veterinary, Animal, and Biomedical Sciences, Massey University, Palmerston North, New Zealand

DANIEL L. CHAN, DVM, MRCVS, Diplomate, American College of Veterinary Nutrition, Lecturer in Veterinary Emergency and Critical Care, Clinical Nutritionist, Department of Veterinary Clinical Sciences, The Royal Veterinary College, University of London, United Kingdom

SEAN J. DELANEY, DVM, MS, Diplomate, American College of Veterinary Nutrition; Founding Consultant, Davis Veterinary Medical Consulting, PC, Davis, California; Associate Veterinarian-Assistant Clinical Professor, Department of Molecular Biosciences, School of Veterinary Medicine, University of California-Davis, Davis, California

DENISE A. ELLIOTT, BVSc(HONS), PhD, Diplomate, American College of Veterinary Internal Medicine; Diplomate, American College of Veterinary Nutrition; Director of Scientific Affairs, Royal Canin USA, St. Charles, Missouri

LISA M. FREEMAN, DVM, PhD, Diplomate, American College of Veterinary Nutrition; Associate Professor, Department of Clinical Sciences, Cummings School of Veterinary Medicine at Tufts University, North Grafton, Massachusetts

DENNIS E. JEWELL, PhD, Diplomate, American College of Animal Nutrition; Fellow, Nutrition Science, Hill's Pet Nutrition, Topeka, Kansas

CLAUDIA A. KIRK, DVM, PhD, Diplomate, American College of Veterinary Internal Medicine; Diplomate, American College of Veterinary Nutrition; Associate Professor of Medicine and Nutrition, Department of Small Animal Clinical Sciences, Veterinary Teaching Hospital, College of Veterinary Medicine, The University of Tennessee, Knoxville, Tennessee

DOTTIE P. LAFLAMME, DVM, PhD, Diplomate, American College of Veterinary Nutrition; Nestle Purina PetCare Research, St. Louis, Missouri

SUSAN D. LAUTEN, PhD, Postdoctoral Research Associate, Department of Small Animal Clinical Sciences, Veterinary Teaching Hospital, University of Tennessee, Knoxville, Tennessee

ELLEN I. LOGAN, DVM, PhD, Manager, Veterinary Marketing Communications, Hill's Pet Nutrition, Topeka, Kansas; Adjunct Assistant Clinical Professor, Department of Clinical Sciences, Kansas State University, Manhattan, Kansas

KATHRYN E. MICHEL, DVM, MS, Diplomate, American College of Veterinary Nutrition; Associate Professor of Nutrition, Department of Clinical Sciences, School of Veterinary Medicine, University of Pennsylvania, Philadelphia, Pennsylvania

KORINN E. SAKER, MS, DVM, PhD, Diplomate, American College of Veterinary Nutrition; Associate Professor, Clinical Nutritionist, Department of Large Animal Clinical Sciences, Virginia-Maryland Regional College of Veterinary Medicine, Blacksburg, Virginia

SHERRY LYNN SANDERSON, DVM, PhD, Diplomate, American College of Veterinary Nutrition; Associate Professor of Medicine, Department of Physiology and Pharmacology, University of Georgia, College of Veterinary Medicine, Athens, Georgia

KAREN J. WEDEKIND, PhD, Principal Nutritionist, Hill's Pet Nutrition, Topeka, Kansas

STEVEN C. ZICKER, DVM, PhD, Diplomate, American College of Veterinary Internal Medicine; Diplomate, American College of Veterinary Nutrition; Principal Nutritionist, Hill's Pet Nutrition, Topeka; Adjunct Faculty Member, Department of Clinical Sciences, School of Veterinary Medicine, Kansas State University, Manhattan, Kansas

VETERINARY CLINICS
SMALL ANIMAL PRACTICE

Dietary Management and Nutrition

CONTENTS

VOLUME 36 • NUMBER 6 • NOVEMBER 2006

an important therapeutic intervention in the care of critically ill patients. The current focus of veterinary critical care nutrition, and the major focus of this article, is on carefully selecting the patients most likely to benefit from nutritional support, deciding when to intervene, and optimizing nutritional support to individual patients.

Management of Anorexia in Dogs and Cats 1243
Sean J. Delaney

The management of anorexia should center first on the urgent and emergent medical management of the patient and be followed by feeding of a highly palatable food in a low-stress environment and manner. Diet palatability can potentially be improved by increasing dietary moisture, fat, or protein, and, in the dog, by adding sugar or salt as well as by using a variety of fresh, pleasantly aromatic, and uncommon foods. Caution should be used when increasing or adding nutrients that may be harmful to patients with specific diseases. Concurrent drug therapy that may reduce appetite should be minimized, and physical barriers to eating should be removed. Patients that consume less than their resting energy requirement for longer than 3 to 5 days with no trend toward improving should receive parenteral or enteral nutrition.

Hydrolyzed Protein Diets for Dogs and Cats 1251
Nicholas J. Cave

The primary aim of a hydrolyzed protein diet is to disrupt the proteins within the diet sufficiently to remove existing allergens. Published assessment of hydrolyzed protein diets includes physicochemical and immunologic assays as well as nutritional and clinical feeding trials. Potential problems include poor palatability, hyperosmotic diarrhea, and a reduced nutritional value, although persistent allergenicity is the most significant. The primary indications for a hydrolyzed protein diet are use in elimination trials for the diagnosis of adverse food reactions, and the initial management of inflammatory bowel disease. Initial studies of hydrolyzed diet efficacy are encouraging. Consideration of the source ingredients should still be given when using hydrolyzed protein diets in elimination feeding trials because antigenic sites may not be fully destroyed.

Unconventional Diets for Dogs and Cats 1269
Kathryn E. Michel

Food plays a far more complex role in daily life than simply serving as sustenance. Social and cultural factors along with individual beliefs govern people's eating behaviors, and it is likely that these same factors influence their choice of diet and feeding practices for their pets. Some people seek alternatives to conventional commercial pet foods, including commercially available "natural" diets, raw food diets, and vegetarian diets, in addition to a variety of home-prepared diets. Exploring a person's knowledge and beliefs about feeding pets can aid in understanding her or his motives for seeking an alternative and may help in changing those practices when it is in the best interest of the pet to do so.

Understanding and Managing Obesity in Dogs and Cats   1283
Dottie P. Laflamme

Obesity is the most common form of malnutrition in pets, affecting more than one third of adult dogs and cats in developed countries. Obesity may be considered a disease itself because it is an inflammatory condition as well as a significant risk factor for other diseases. Diagnosis in pets is made earlier via routine use of a body condition scoring system. Management involves decreasing calorie intake and increasing calorie expenditure. Nutrient-modified diets can help when fed appropriately. Prevention and management of obesity involve early and frequent client counseling regarding suitable feeding management.

Feline Diabetes Mellitus: Low Carbohydrates Versus High Fiber?   1297
Claudia A. Kirk

Treatment of diabetes mellitus (DM) in the cat relies primarily on adequate insulin therapy and controlled dietary intake. The goals of managing DM in the cat have changed from attaining glycemic control to achieving diabetic remission (transient diabetes) in a large proportion of cases. Remission rates of up to 68% have been published. The use of low-carbohydrate foods for cats improves the odds of achieving diabetic remission by fourfold. Nonetheless, some cats show an improved response to high-fiber food. Clinical judgment, trial, and personal preference currently dictate which diet to offer an individual animal.

Nutrition and Osteoarthritis in Dogs: Does It Help?   1307
Steven C. Budsberg and Joseph W. Bartges

Osteoarthritis (OA) is a common disease, and nutrition has become an integral part of management. This article focuses on the role of nutrition and dietary ingredients in OA, evaluating current evidence for obesity management, ω-3 fatty acids, and chondromodulating agents. Additionally, keeping an animal in optimal to slightly lean body condition has been shown to decrease the risk of development of OA and to aid in management of dogs with OA.

Taurine and Carnitine in Canine Cardiomyopathy   1325
Sherry Lynn Sanderson

Some newer more promising therapies for dogs with dilated cardiomyopathy (DCM) do not involve drugs but rather nutritional supplements. Two of the more common nutritional supplements administered to dogs with DCM are taurine and carnitine. Deficiencies of these nutrients have been shown to cause DCM in dogs, and some breeds of dogs have shown dramatic improvement in myocardial function after supplementation with one or both nutrients. Although most dogs diagnosed with DCM do not have a documented taurine or carnitine deficiency, they may still benefit from supplementation. These nutrients are safe to administer to dogs. For some owners, the high cost of carnitine is the only deterrent to giving their dogs supplements of both nutrients.

Distinctive risk factors for disease are identifiable throughout life stages of large- and giant-breed dogs. From weaning to maturity, improper nutrition is linked to developmental skeletal diseases. As large dogs mature, skeletal diseases and obesity can lead to osteoarthritis. Improper nutritional management can lead to obesity, which is also linked to osteoarthritis. These dogs are difficult to manage when orthopedic or osteoarthritic disease affects mobility and quality of life, thereby increasing the risk for early death. Gastric dilatation and volvulus is another disease that is a leading cause of death in large- and giant-breed dogs. Management of health, including proper nutrition, exercise, and weight control, provides the best opportunity for successful aging of large- and giant-breed dogs.

Lower urinary tract disease occurs commonly in cats and is often associated with crystal-related disease. Dietary modification is beneficial in managing some of these diseases, including idiopathic cystitis, urolithiasis, and urethral matrix-crystalline plugs. Altering dietary formulation may result in decreasing urinary concentrations of crystallogenic compounds, increasing urinary concentrations of crystallogenic inhibitors, and diluting urine composition.

Chronic renal disease is a leading cause of death in dogs and cats. Recent clinical studies show that nutrition plays a key role in improving quality of life and life expectancy of these patients. Typical nutritional interventions include modifying the protein, phosphorus, and lipid concentrations. Nutritional therapy, however, does not simply mean changing the diet; consideration must also be given to ensuring adequate caloric intake and to the method of feeding. Monitoring the effects of the dietary therapy is also crucial to ensure that patients are responding appropriately to the selected nutritional modifications. Nutritional management must be coordinated with medical management for long-term successful treatment.

A pet cannot be healthy without oral health. Periodontal disease is a significant disease that has local and systemic ramifications. It has been stated earlier that effective plaque control prevents gingivitis. In human beings, 90% of periodontitis occurs as the result of progression of gingivitis, and this type of periodontitis can be completely prevented by plaque control. It is reasonable that dogs and cats react similarly and that effective plaque control could prevent a large percentage of periodontitis cases. Proper nutrition and effective oral hygiene are necessary components of oral health and should be jointly promoted in the management of oral disease in dogs and cats.

VETERINARY CLINICS
SMALL ANIMAL PRACTICE

FORTHCOMING ISSUES

January 2007

Effective Communication in Veterinary Practice
Karen Cornell, DVM, PhD
Jennifer Brandt, LISW, PhD
Kathleen A. Bonvicini, MPH
Guest Editors

March 2007

Clinical Pathology and Diagnostic Techniques
Robin W. Allison, DVM, PhD
and James Meinkoth, DVM, PhD
Guest Editors

May 2007

Evidence-Based Veterinary Medicine
Peggy L. Schmidt, DVM, MS
Guest Editor

RECENT ISSUES

September 2006

Current Topics in Clinical Pharmacology and Therapeutics
Dawn Merton Boothe, DVM, PhD
Guest Editor

July 2006

Wound Management
Steven F. Swaim, DVM, MS
D.J. Krahwinkel, DVM, MS
Guest Editors

May 2006

Pediatrics
Autumn P. Davidson, DVM, MS
Guest Editor

Vet Clin Small Anim 36 (2006) xi–xiii

VETERINARY CLINICS
SMALL ANIMAL PRACTICE

ELSEVIER
SAUNDERS

Preface

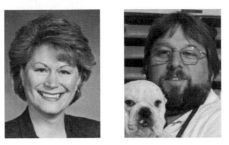

Claudia A. Kirk, DVM, PhD
Joseph W. Bartges, DVM, PhD
Guest Editors

The study of small animal veterinary nutrition initially defined essential nutrients and minimal requirements needed to meet the basic biological needs of companion animals. It was later recognized that health and vitality could be further improved by optimizing nutrient levels to the lifestage, lifestyle, and breed of an individual animal. In addition, the metabolic derangements associated with certain disease states could be corrected or controlled by adjusting levels of key nutrients. Early examples of foods designed for disease management include those used for pets with kidney, heart, and intestinal disease. A mounting number of therapeutic foods have become available for several medical disorders from diabetes mellitus to canine cognitive dysfunction. Although therapeutic foods have been widely applied in veterinary practice, they are often used with an attitude of uncertainty (eg, "It may help and probably won't hurt"). Previously, clinical nutrition was considered adjunctive therapy to common diseases, but in recent years it has emerged as a cornerstone of treatment based on the principles of grade 1 evidence-based medicine.

Recognition that veterinary clinical nutrition provides significant benefit to the treatment and management of disease is increasing. Improved nutrition has enhanced long-term health and increased longevity in our veterinary patients. Ongoing research and increased use of three key research methodologies has facilitated the understanding of clinical nutrition and its critical role in animal health and disease. These tools include broadened applications of (1) controlled clinical trials that test diet efficacy and put nutritional theory into practice; (2) epidemiological studies designed to detect nutritional associations to health and disease; and, more recently, (3) metabalomics and nutrigenomics, the study of nutritional influence on metabolism at the molecular and genomic level.

0195-5616/06/$ – see front matter
doi:10.1016/j.cvsm.2006.09.014

Several articles in this issue provide an overview of both basic and clinical research supporting recommendations for nutritional modification in the management of disease. Readers will note that remarkable clinical outcomes have been demonstrated following the nutritional treatment of disease. Studies of dietary modifications in renal disease have confirmed improved quality of life, slowed progression of disease, and increased survival compared with treatment with conventional medicine alone. Nutritional prevention of tartar and gingivitis, a contributor to systemic inflammation, is highlighted in the article on nutritional control of dental disease. Understanding the role of nutrition as both a cause and treatment of feline lower urinary tract disease has contributed to a reduction in the clinical recurrence of certain feline disorders, as well as having broad impact on the pet food industry. In addition, new nutritional strategies in the treatment of feline diabetes mellitus have resulted in high rates of disease remission and improved glucose control.

As described in this issue, several epidemiologic studies have identified association of certain diets, nutrients, or feeding practices with risk for disease. Several studies have highlighted health risks associated with obesity and the importance of weight control in our ever-growing population of overweight and obese pets. Risk factors associated with gastric dilation and volvulus, large breed growth disorders, and nutritional associations to canine cardiomyopathy have directed feeding recommendations and research leading to important nutritional discoveries. Taurine deficiency, once only a concern for cats, is now known to contribute to canine cardiomyopathy. Elucidation of foods and ingredient sources that reduce dietary taurine bioavailability or limit intake of precursor molecules is described within.

Advances in molecular biology have spawned new fields of study such as nutrigenomics, which defines how nutrients alter basic metabolic processes at the level of the genome. No longer are nutrients simple building blocks, cofactors, or enzymes, but instead regulators of cellular metabolism, gene transcription, or translation. New information continues to emerge on the molecular role of antioxidants in health, disease, and aging, as well as nutrient modification of inflammation and the immune response. The principles discussed in articles on antioxidants and immune function have a practical application in the control of pain and progression of osteoarthritis, use of protein hydrolysates in the management of adverse food reactions, and feeding animals under metabolic stress.

Nutritional advances continue to occur in all areas of veterinary medicine. Yet we are still faced with several very basic challenges. The ability to provide adequate nutrition to animals that are unwilling or unable to eat is often a major roadblock to optimal nutritional care. Conversely, the prevention and treatment of obesity is embroiled in numerous social and behavioral factors that sabotage owner and patient compliance, limiting long-term success. Finally, social attitudes concerning pets, nutrition, and food safety have prompted some pet owners to feed unconventional foods that may or may not be safe or nutritious.

To best serve the needs of patients and clientele, veterinarians must continue to stay abreast of nutritional advances in disease management and the pros and cons of nutritional controversies. Each author has contributed up-to-date scientific findings blended with practical recommendations that we hope will enhance the application of clinical nutrition in your daily practice. We sincerely thank the authors for sharing their time and expertise and look forward to new nutritional discoveries in the future.

Claudia A. Kirk, DVM, PhD
Joseph W. Bartges, DVM, PhD
Department of Small Animal Clinical Sciences
Veterinary Teaching Hospital
College of Veterinary Medicine
The University of Tennessee
Knoxville, TN 37996-4544, USA

E-mail addresses: cakirk@mail.ag.utk.edu
jbartges@utk.edu

Vet Clin Small Anim 36 (2006) 1183–1198

VETERINARY CLINICS
SMALL ANIMAL PRACTICE

Antioxidants in Veterinary Nutrition

Steven C. Zicker, DVM, PhD*, Karen J. Wedekind, PhD,
Dennis E. Jewell, PhD

Hill's Pet Nutrition, PO Box 1658, Topeka, KS 66601-1658, USA

Nutritional molecules with antioxidant properties have long been recognized, with vitamin E perhaps being the prototypical molecule in this class. The discovery of a fat-soluble factor, vitamin E, that supported reproduction in rats was first described in 1922 by Evans and Bishop [1]. Shortly thereafter, Olcott and Mattil [2] reported that this factor also possessed antioxidant properties. Evans coined the term *tocopherol* to describe the factor that comes from the Greek *tokos* (childbirth) and *pherein* (to bear).

Much like its name origin, the potential health benefits of tocopherol seem to have multiplied and may perhaps be unrivaled by any other nutritional molecule. Many of these claims have been birthed by scientific hypothesis, anecdotal reports, or, in some cases, sound scientific study. Whatever the origin of the purported benefit, intense debate often follows about the true scientific validity of the benefit.

Despite the intense debate surrounding benefits of vitamin E and other antioxidant-like molecules, significant scientific progress has been made in trying to define the complexities of nutritional antioxidants. It is the purpose of this article to try and define what a nutritional antioxidant is, how it functions in the body, and how to measure those benefits. Necessary to this discussion is a review of the free radical theory of aging because it directly interfaces with the proposed benefits of nutritional antioxidants. Finally, the scientific literature with specific application to dog and cat nutrition is reviewed.

DEFINITION OF ANTIOXIDANTS AND FREE RADICALS

Chemically speaking, antioxidants and free radicals derive their terminology from the field of electrochemistry. The loss of electrons from a substance is called oxidation, and the gain of electrons is referred to as reduction. An alternative terminology is to call a substance that donates electrons (it is being oxidized) to another substance a reducing agent and the acceptor of electrons (it is being reduced) an oxidizing agent. The oxidizing agent is always being reduced in a reaction, and the reducing agent is always being oxidized. When oxidation and reduction take place in the same chemical equation between two

---

*Corresponding author. E-mail address: steven_zicker@hillspet.com (S.C. Zicker).

0195-5616/06/$ – see front matter
doi:10.1016/j.cvsm.2006.08.002

substances, it is termed a *redox reaction*. The spontaneity of redox reactions is defined by physicochemical properties determined by thermodynamics, which can be quantitated by the Nernst equation. In general, the balance of this potential energy equation is a measure of how willing a molecule is to give up an electron as compared with its willingness to accept an electron in relation to the hydrogen half-cell.

One proposed definition of an antioxidant follows: an antioxidant is any substance, which when present in low concentrations compared with those of an oxidizable substrate, significantly delays or prevents oxidation of that substrate [3]. In serving this function, the antioxidant may preserve the structural integrity or function of a biologic molecule, and thus preserve its function in the cell. Nevertheless, this concept may be too simplistic, because it has been shown that some cellular signaling pathways seem to depend on redox chemistry to manifest their "normal" biologic function.

Free radicals are chemically unstable molecules that have an unpaired free electron. Most commonly, oxygen free radicals are used as examples, but other molecular species may also exist as free radicals. Oxygen free radicals are used as the prototypical molecule for the remainder of this discussion because they are perhaps the most biologically relevant.

The existence of an unpaired electron creates a thermodynamically unstable situation. As such, the molecule desires to gain (reduction) or to lose (oxidation) an electron to achieve a more thermodynamically stable state. Thus, a free radical may act as an oxidizing agent or a reducing agent depending on its thermodynamic propensity for stability. For example, superoxide is a normal byproduct of cellular respiration and is represented by the formula $O_2{}^{-}$. Superoxide is favored by thermodynamics to lose an electron to become oxygen, and eventually water, via a hydrogen peroxide intermediate. Conversely, hydroxyl radical, OH, has a strong preference to gain an electron (oxidize other molecules) to achieve an OH^- configuration. Thus, the chemistry of free radical reactions, with the reactant passing or gaining electrons, is complex. This chemistry depends not only on which species of free radical is generated in vivo but on where the generation of that molecule is located in the subcellular portion of the cell. For example, a highly reactive species produced in the mitochondria is unlikely to diffuse into the cytoplasm. Alternatively, a less reactive species, such as hydrogen peroxide, may diffuse into the cytoplasm before being chemically engaged in a redox reaction.

Redox and free radical chemistry reactions may occur via direct uncatalyzed means or may be catalyzed by other molecules and/or metals or proteins acting as enzymes. In addition, these systems may work in networks that are dependent on the proximity and species of redox coupling required. For example, superoxide is produced as a normal byproduct of cellular respiration in the mitochondria. Under normal cellular conditions, electrons "leak" from the electron transport chain, converting approximately 1% to 3% of oxygen molecules into superoxide. Cells have a multitude of mechanisms to detoxify free radicals, and in this case, they use a two-step enzymatic method. In the first step, superoxide free radical is simultaneously reduced and oxidized (dismutated) by superoxide dismutase to form hydrogen peroxide and oxygen (reaction 1). Although hydrogen peroxide is also a reactive oxygen species (ROS), it is much less reactive than superoxide to the point where it may diffuse out of the mitochondria before reacting with another molecule. In the second step, hydrogen peroxide is converted into water and oxygen by catalase enzymes (reaction 2). Ironically, the most mutagenic of the ROS, hydroxyl ($^{\cdot}$OH) free radical, is generated as a consequence of disabling superoxide to hydrogen peroxide. Termed *Fenton chemistry*, peroxide readily reacts with ferrous iron (Fe^{2+}) or other transition metal ions to produce hydroxyl radical (reaction 3). By the same token, ferric iron (Fe^{3+}) can accept an electron from superoxide, cycling it back to the ferrous state and making it available to react with another peroxide molecule (reaction 4). Thus, even trace amounts of iron ion can potentially catalyze the formation of large amounts of hydroxyl free radical:

$$2O_2^- + 2H^+ \xrightarrow{\text{superoxide dismutase}} H_2O_2 + O_2 \tag{1}$$

$$2\,H_2O_2 \xrightarrow{\text{catalase}} 2H_2O + O_2 \tag{2}$$

$$H_2O_2 + Fe^{2+} \longrightarrow {}^{\cdot}OH + OH^- + Fe^{3+} \tag{3}$$

$$O_2^- + Fe^{3+} \longrightarrow O_2 + Fe^{2+} \tag{4}$$

When these individual reactions are linked together in a biologic system, a more dynamic metabolic picture of potential pathways can be viewed (Fig. 1). From this more integrated picture, it can be seen that the production of free radicals is dependent on multiple pathways and the availability of detoxification mechanisms versus reactive materials. From this dynamic balance, some have referred to the relative overproduction of oxidative and/or reactive materials produced, as compared with the detoxification pathways, as oxidative stress.

The hydroxyl radical is highly reactive, oxidizing most organic compounds at almost diffusion controlled rates ($K > 10$ mol/L/s) [4]. Because of its high reactivity, it is indiscriminate, reacting with the first substrate available. It therefore has high destructive and mutagenic potential. Membranes of the mitochondria are particularly susceptible, because the radicals are formed in close proximity.

From this example, it is evident that redox reactions are quite complicated and may rely on a multiplicity of reactions to achieve an overall end result. It has been recently proposed that antioxidants may work in even more complex networks than the prior example, where several different steps or cellular components are required to achieve successful detoxification of an oxidizing agent. An example of this is given in Fig. 2, where an oxidant is produced and then detoxified by a series of stepwise reactions.

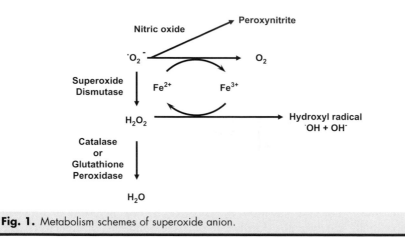

Fig. 1. Metabolism schemes of superoxide anion.

FREE RADICAL THEORY OF AGING

The free radical theory of aging was first proposed in 1956 by Harman [5]. The theory postulates that ROS produce cellular damage and that age-dependent pathologic changes may be a resultant cumulative response to these alterations. It is now generally accepted that the main source of ROS in mammals is from aerobic respiration byproducts in the mitochondria [6]. Accordingly, one interpretation of the free radical hypothesis of aging would predict that aging should be slowed, and possibly even reversed, by decreasing the effects of ROS.

This hypothesis has led to many strategies to try and mitigate the effects of ROS. One highly touted strategy is to increase the capacity to suppress ROS effects via antioxidants or antioxidant defense mechanisms through nutritional supplementation. The effectiveness of this seemingly simple strategy is dependent on a wide range of different biologic factors.

DETERMINANTS OF AN EFFECTIVE NUTRITIONAL ANTIOXIDANT

In consideration of the previous stated theory, it would seem straightforward to assume that the addition of antioxidants to a biologic system should result in positive effects in reducing the aging process. Many intervention studies have met with limited or contradictory results compared with this intended outcome, however. Many possibilities exist for why this may be true, and a few are discussed here.

Distribution and bioavailability of antioxidants are important determinants of biologic outcome and cannot be overlooked. It is important when evaluating potential antioxidant interventions to understand potential limitations to application. For example, several plant flavonoids and other polyphenols have limited solubility and absorption in the gut as compared with other water- or fat-soluble compounds [7]. Even antioxidants considered to be easily absorbed and distributed may have marked bioavailability depending on other

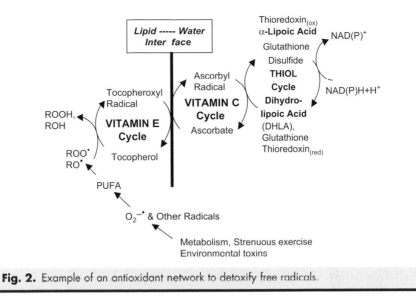

Fig. 2. Example of an antioxidant network to detoxify free radicals.

physiologic factors, such as food intake and composition [8,9]. This report showed that absorption of vitamin E was least effective from gel capsules given without a meal and variably effective when given with a meal. Application of vitamin E adsorbed onto a cereal provided consistently higher rates of bioavailability, however. This type of study highlights the importance of monitoring and extraneous factors that may affect bioavailability.

Metabolic transformation may alter the biologic activity or distribution of orally administered antioxidants differentially between species. For example, cats lack the enzyme, β-carotene 15,15′-dioxygenase, that cleaves β-carotene (provitamin A) into two molecules of retinal, whereas the activity of this enzyme is relatively high in herbivores [10]. Thus, carotenoids are more likely to be absorbed intact in cats, and possibly other carnivores, whereas they serve relatively more of a previtamin A function for herbivores. Another example is α-lipoic acid, which has been shown to have different rates of metabolic elimination in cats and other species. Cats metabolize and eliminate lipoic acid at a much slower rate than other species [11]. Finally, another functional consideration in this discussion is the effect of age itself. Although vitamin C is not considered essential for rats, it has been shown that as rats age, the metabolic enzymes responsible for recycling and transport of vitamin C in hepatocytes become impaired, which, if severe, may impart a state of conditional essential status for vitamin C to the aged rat [12,13].

NONCLASSIC MECHANISMS OF ACTION OF CLASSIC ANTIOXIDANTS

This discussion has focused on classic definitions and mechanisms of actions of antioxidants. Research in the past 10 years has revealed that many of these "antioxidant" molecules have other important physiologic functions. Some functions include but are not limited to antioxidants as regulators of second messengers, cell cycle signaling, and control of gene expression through a variety of mechanisms. These findings may be considered extensions of the classic antioxidant action, but it is clear from several lines of evidence that these aspects of redox status in the cell are well regulated and coordinated in such a manner that they probably are inherent in the design of cellular function and outcome rather than random in nature.

Resveratrol, a polyphenol from red grapes, has been shown to activate sirtuin 2, a member of the sirtuin family of nicotinamide adenine dinucleotide (NAD)+-dependent deacetylases, which mimics the effects of caloric restriction and results in prolongation of cell life [14]. Insulin signaling has been shown to be mimicked by hydrogen production, and it now recognized that this is a component of insulin signaling physiology [15]. Nuclear factor (NF)-κβ signaling of apoptosis has been shown to be activated by an alternative pathway via hydrogen peroxide, and specific mitochondrial-targeted antioxidants have been shown to alter this signaling pathway [16–18]. NF-κβ is not the only transcription factor considered to be redox sensitive, because several other factors have been characterized with these properties in the past several years [16,19]. As one can see from these few examples, the roles and physiology of antioxidant molecules are far reaching and go beyond classic chemistry understanding of previous years. It is also easy to see from these recent reports why effects of interventions have sometimes been contrary and difficult to interpret.

HOW TO MEASURE OUTCOMES OF STUDIES WITH ANTIOXIDANTS

Controversy and difficulty have developed in interpreting the vast number of studies with antioxidant supplements. As evidenced previously, the biologic effects of antioxidants may take place by way of multiple divergent or convergent pathways, thus making interpretation difficult. Also, because the effects of free radicals are supposed to be insidious and temporally delayed in taking effect, prediction of long-term outcomes from short-term experiments has proven to be a challenge. Finally, determining the outcome event of importance is also problematic, based on the variety of end point measures that have been developed to measure the effects of antioxidants. The advantages and disadvantages of some measurement outcomes are briefly discussed here so as to highlight some potential pitfalls of current methodology.

Increased Concentrations of Antioxidants in Foods and Tissues

Oral antioxidant administration as a supplement or in combination with a food does not ensure absorption and distribution into tissues. Some antioxidants are more readily absorbed than others and may display species differences in absorption, as discussed previously. Vitamin E is usually much easier to absorb than some water-insoluble plant phenols; yet, even vitamin E displays variable absorption and distribution depending on many factors. As discussed previously, the absorption of vitamin E was observed to be more efficient when administered with a meal [9]. In addition, vitamin E depletion and repletion seem to have different kinetic parameters depending on tissue type [20,21]. This highlights that the fact that absorption and distribution of oral antioxidants must be relevant to the target tissue and intended biologic outcome. Nonetheless, the variability in bioavailability and distribution has not limited the number of studies linking increased ingestion or increased serum values of antioxidants to a variety of health outcomes in various target tissues. If mere absorption and distribution do not prove causality, then what measurements are available to start developing mechanistic arguments for biologic efficacy?

Decreased Markers of Free Radical Damage

Free radicals are short lived and difficult to measure as to their native species. In lieu of measuring free radicals directly in target tissues, a variety of new laboratory methods have been developed that measure biologically stable molecules produced by free radical chemical reactions as markers of free radical production in a biologic system. If these markers increase in serum or tissue, it is presumed that there are more free radicals being produced, and thus more damage. If they decrease, it is presumed that the production of free radicals has been decreased. These markers are specific for different biomolecules, such as DNA (8-oxodeoxyguanosine), lipids (eg, alkenyls, malondialdehyde [MDA], thiobarbiturate reacting substances [TBARS]), prostaglandins (isoprostanes), protein (eg, nitrotyrosine, protein carbonyls), and advanced glycation end products (AGEs). The utility of these measurements has been debated because they are indirect measures of presumed free radical reactions, sometimes in distant tissues. As such, they are responses to oxidative events but do not provide direct mechanistic effects of antioxidant action in target tissues.

The next modality of investigation is to look directly at target tissue effects of orally administered antioxidants. Certainly, these studies can provide biochemical information on mechanisms in the tissue of interest as compared with the indirect measures discussed previously. This type of research has yielded interesting results with a variety of antioxidants. For example, aged rats, a vitamin C–independent mammal, have a decreased ability to recycle vitamin C in their hepatocytes, which may be restored by the administration of lipoic acid and acetyl-carnitine [12]. Aged rats had increased oxidative damage to their hepatic proteins, which imparted decreased enzymatic activity and more susceptibility to protein degradation [22]. Finally, it has been shown that oxidative damage increased in brains of aging Beagles and rats and that the damage was correlated with memory loss in the rats. [23,24]. Intervention with acetyl-carnitine and lipoic acid partially reversed the memory loss in the older rats [24].

Intervention Trial Outcomes of Antioxidant Interventions

These studies are much more difficult to perform, because the expense, length of time required for intervention, and ability to control the dietary intake of individuals is problematic. Use of animals with shorter life spans than human beings is useful in developing strategies that may be beneficial in characterizing these outcomes, however. It is presumed that the shorter life span models may show accelerated aging attributable to more rapid free radical damage; thus, interventions may be assessed more quickly [25]. In addition, specific genetic models, such as the senescent accelerated mouse that overproduces free radicals, and transgenic models are becoming more available and may lend some insight into the efficacy and modes of action of different dietary antioxidant supplement regimens.

APPLICATIONS TO VETERINARY NUTRITION

As one can see, the science of nutritional antioxidants has advanced over the past several years. Numerous studies have revealed new and important biologic benefits of supplementing foods or diets with oral antioxidants in a variety of species. The next question of interest is what is the body of evidence available to assess in the veterinary literature and what does it mean for the practitioner? In an effort to answer this, we examine the literature on mainstream antioxidants as they apply to canine and feline nutrition.

Vitamin E
Canine

Requirements for vitamin E in dogs and cats were suggested as early as 1939 and were modified based on selenium (Se) and polyunsaturated fatty acid (PUFA) content of foods in the 1960s [26–29]. From the published research, the National Research Council (NRC) states that the requirement for dogs should be met by vitamin E at a rate of 22 IU/kg of diet (based on a diet of Se at a rate of 0.1 ppm, not more than 1% linoleic acid, and metabolizable energy [ME] at a rate of 3670 kcal/kg). This results in a range roughly equivalent to 0.4 to 1.4 IU/kg of body weight for maintenance of pregnant and/or lactating dogs [30].

Effects of vitamin E on other biologic outcomes have been tested in dogs, and it has been found that levels higher than the requirement may confer targeted biologic benefits. Increasing the dietary intake of vitamin E up to 2010 mg/kg of diet (dry matter basis) in geriatric Beagles has been shown to improve immune function [31,32]. Increased intake of vitamin E in food is directly related to increased vitamin E content of skin, which may provide health benefits for targeted disease processes [33]. Vitamin E concentrations in blood decrease with exercise, and higher levels have been associated with improved performance [34,35]. Finally, vitamin E has been shown to provide protection from damage by ischemia in a variety of tissues [36–38]. There are no published toxicity data for vitamin E in dogs; however, concentrations exceeding 2000 IU/kg of dry matter of food have been fed for 17 weeks without observable negative reactions [31]. An upper limit of toxicity has not been documented; yet, a level of 1000 IU/kg of food (dry matter basis), or 45 IU/kg of body weight, has been suggested [27].

Feline

Foods for cats are often higher in fat and polyunsaturated fats, which may provide a different matrix reference for determining requirements. Nonetheless, several studies have shown that the amount of vitamin E needed to support growth and reproduction in cats is in the same general range as in dogs when adequate Se and excessive PUFAs are accounted for. Thus, vitamin E at a range of 0.5 to 1.7 mg/kg of body weight has been suggested by the NRC [39] for maintenance and pregnancy and/or lactation, respectively.

Vitamin E supplemented to food at 272 and 552 IU/kg of food (dry matter basis) resulted in improved immune function in aged cats [29]. Supplementation of D-α-tocopherol to cats at a dose of 1000 IU enhanced neurologic recovery in a model of spinal cord compression [26]. Supplementation of vitamin E at a dose of 800 IU/d via gel caps showed no difference from control in prevention of onion powder– or propylene glycol–induced Heinz body anemia [40]. Vitamin E and cysteine supplemented to food (vitamin E at a rate of 2200 U plus cysteine at a rate of 9.5 g/kg of food) showed protective effects on acetaminophen-induced oxidative production of methemoglobinemia [41]. Also, pretreatment of cats with a combination of vitamin E and Se (vitamin E at a rate of 200 IU plus Se at a rate of 50 μg) for 5 days delayed motor nerve degeneration in a model of axonal degeneration [42]. A presumed safe upper limit (SUF) for oral administration has not been established; however, administration of vitamin E parenterally at 100 mg/kg of body weight to kittens resulted in significant mortality [43].

Vitamin C
Dogs and cats
Dogs and cats are considered capable of synthesizing required amounts of vitamin C needed by de novo mechanisms [44,45]. Chatterjee and colleagues [46] showed that hepatic in vitro synthesis of vitamin C in dogs and cats was much less (10%–25%) than that in other mammals, leading to speculation that the ability to synthesize vitamin C may be limited; however, no follow up work has been performed. The pharmacokinetics of vitamin C administration in dogs showed that ascorbic acid and ester-C were rapidly absorbed and may possibly use an active transport mechanism in the gastrointestinal tract [47].

The subchronic intravenous toxicity of a median lethal dose (LD_{50}) has been reported to be greater than 500 mg/kg/d in cats and greater than 2000 mg/kg/d in dogs [48]. Supplementation of vitamin C (0, 200, 400, or 1000 mg/d) to cats resulted in a small progressive reduction in urine pH [49]. It has been noted in human beings that intake of ascorbate at the upper recommended limit of 2000 mg/d increased urine oxalate excretion and stone risk [50]. Moderate supplementation of vitamin C in healthy cats up to 193 mg/kg of food (dry matter basis), approximately 2 mg/kg of body weight, did not seem to increase the risk of oxalate stone formation in urine. However, because vitamin C may be converted to oxalate, higher levels may increase oxalate excretion in the urine [51]. Supplementation of vitamin C to rats at 1500 mg/kg of food (dry matter basis) may decrease erythrocyte fragility when vitamin E is near the requirement level in the diet [52]. Additionally, it has been reported that oral supplementation at 1 g/d may slow race times in Greyhounds [53].

β-Carotene and Other Carotenoids

Some work has been performed on the use of carotenoids, predominantly β-carotene, in canine and feline nutrition. As mentioned previously, β-carotene can serve as a precursor to vitamin A in the dog but not in the cat. Interestingly, although carotenoids possess antioxidant properties, most of the research in dogs and cats has focused on immunomodulatory benefits.

Supplementation with β-carotene has been shown to increase concentrations of β-carotene in the plasma and white blood cells of cats and dogs [54,55]. The concentrations reached in the plasma of cats are approximately 50-fold higher compared with those of dogs at the same approximate time and dose rate, however, indicating that most of the β-carotene administered to dogs is probably converted to vitamin A rather than absorbed directly as β-carotene (Table 1). Human beings convert approximately 60% to 75% of β-carotene into vitamin A and absorb approximately 15% intact. With this information, it is interesting to note that the mean concentration of β-carotene in serum from human beings is approximately 0.3 μmol/L, which is approximately 10-fold greater than concentrations observed in supplemented dogs. Nonetheless, supplementation of dogs with β-carotene has been reported to improve immune function in young and aged animals [56,57].

Supplementation of the carotenoid lutein has been shown to increase plasma and leukocyte concentrations of that ingredient in dogs and cats. In addition, improvement in the immune function of both species has been reported with lutein supplementation of the food [58,59]. A novel form of astaxanthin has been shown to provide cardioprotection from vascular occlusion in dogs [60].

Carotenoid safety, as β-carotene, has been evaluated in Beagles at extremely high doses from 50 to 250 mg/kg/d administered orally in the form of beadlets [61]. Although discoloration of the hair coat and liver vacuolization were noted at all levels, no consistent findings of toxicity were found. Carotenoid safety is not well evaluated in cats but could be presumed to be safe based on wide margins of safety in other mammals and lack of conversion to vitamin A. Nonetheless, canthaxanthin supplementation to cats for 6 months induced retinal pigment epithelial changes and some vacuolization but no functional electroretinogram changes [62].

Table 1
Concentration in blood of cats and dogs supplemented with β-carotene for at least 7 days

Species	Dose	Body weight	Peak plasma concentration
Cat	10 mg/d	3–3.5 kg	0.95 μmol/L at 7 days
Dog	25 mg/d	7–9 kg	~0.02 μmol/L at 7 days

Selenium

Se was first recognized as an essential nutrient in 1957 based on its ability to spare vitamin E in exudative diathesis in chicks [63]. The metabolic basis for its nutritional function remained unclear until it was discovered in 1973 [64] that Se was a component of glutathione peroxidase (GSHpx). Subsequent discoveries revealed several Se-dependent GSHpx isoforms (phospholipid, cytosolic, plasma, and gastrointestinal) as well as other selenoproteins (three iodothyronine 5'-deiodinases (types I, II and III), two thioredoxin reductases [TRs], and four other selenoproteins [in plasma (P), muscle (W), liver, and prostate]) [65].

The primary role for GSHpx is to defend against oxidative stress by catalyzing the reduction of H_2O_2 and organic hydroperoxides, which react with the selenol group of the active center of selenocysteine. The role of Se as a constituent of 5'-deiodinases (types I–III) is also of interest, because the thyroid gland produces quite large amounts of H_2O_2, which is used for the iodination of thyronine residues. The thyroid gland protects itself against oxidative damage by the activity of phospholipid and cytosolic GSHpx.

The peroxidase activity of GSHpx, together with the activity of TRs, is involved in a variety of key enzymes, transcription factors, and receptors. The discovery of the role of Se in TRs is of great interest because of the involvement of TRs in the modulation of redox-regulated signaling, including ribonucleotide reductase, prostaglandin and leukotriene synthesis, receptor-mediated phosphorylation cascades (ie, activation of NF-κβ), and even apoptosis [66,67].

The Se requirement of most animals is similar and is based on the maximization of GSHpx in plasma or red blood cells. Estimates of the Se requirement for kittens and adult cats [68,69] were determined to be 0.15 and 0.13 mg/kg, respectively, and for adult dogs [70], a diet containing Se at a rate of 0.10 mg/kg was recommended. Recommended allowances of Se in pet foods, which account for bioavailability, for dogs and cats are 0.35 and 0.40 mg/kg of diet, respectively [39].

Animal studies and clinical intervention trials with people have shown Se to be anticarcinogenic at intakes 5- to 10-fold greater than those recommended for recommended daily allowances or minimum requirements [65,67]. The following mechanisms have been proposed for the anticancer effects of Se: (1) antioxidant activity through GSHpx and TRs, (2) enhancement of immune functions, (3) alteration in the metabolism of carcinogens, (4) inhibition of tumor proliferation and enhancement of apoptosis, and (5) inhibition of angiogenesis [66].

Safe upper limits [SUL] for Se for most species are generally similar [71], approximately 2 mg/kg of food, although neither the Association of the American Feed Control Officials (AAFCO) [27] nor the NRC [39] has suggested an SUL of Se for the cat [68]. Compared with most other species, including dogs, cats display significantly higher Se concentrations in blood even when fed similar dietary Se intakes. It is unclear whether cats have a higher tolerance for Se, which may explain the inability to define an SUL, or whether other biomarkers or different forms of Se would have yielded more definitive limits. The AAFCO [27] suggests an SUL of Se of 2 mg/kg of diet for the dog [70].

Thiols: S-Adenosyl-L-Methionine, α-Lipoic Acid, and N-Acetylcysteine

Thiol metabolism has gained research momentum as the field of redox chemistry has matured. Thiols are capable of redox reactions similar to oxygen and have many metabolic correlates within the cell. Glutathione, S-adenosyl-L-methionine (SAMe), thioredoxin, and other sulfur-containing molecules have been shown to have important roles in metabolism and antioxidant defenses.

SAMe has been used successfully to treat acetaminophen toxicity in cats and dogs [72,73]. Administration of SAMe to clinically healthy cats has been shown to improve indices of redox status, as indicated by decreased red blood cell TBARS and increased hepatic glutathione disulfide (GSH) [74].

Lipoic acid is another thiol that may influence reduced glutathione content of cells. Administration of lipoic acid as a food additive resulted in increased ratios of white blood cells reduced to oxidized forms (GSH/GSSG) in dogs [75]. It has been shown that administration to cats has a prolonged elimination time compared with other species, however, and administration rates should be adjusted accordingly if used [11].

N-acetylcysteine has been shown to increase reduced glutathione in cats challenged by oral onion powder compared with controls [40]. N-acetylcysteine in combination with ascorbic acid has been shown to inhibit virus replication in feline immunodeficiency virus–infected cell lines [76]. Cysteine in combination with vitamin E was also shown to protect from acetaminophen-induced oxidative damage in cats [41].

Fruits and Vegetables

Fruits and vegetables are often rich in flavonoids, polyphenols, and anthocyanidins, ingredients that may all possess antioxidant properties. Exhaustive research of the effects of these ingredients in dogs and cats is not available, but a few studies have tried to evaluate some of the potential benefits of these additions to dietary regimens. Oral administration of a bioflavonoid complex reduced the amount of Heinz body anemia caused by acetaminophen administration in cats [77]. A combination of fruits and vegetables in a supplemented food was shown to increase selected flavonoids in the blood of aged dogs [78]. Although effective doses and safety are not well evaluated, it should be pointed out that administration of onion powder, which has purported antioxidant benefits in some species, to cats can result in Heinz body anemia, perhaps through increased oxidation [79].

Combination Therapies

In keeping with the idea that antioxidants work in networks, several studies have been designed to look at complex mixtures of antioxidants. Physiologic outcomes have varied; however, in general, positive results have been shown on immune function [80] and reduction in markers of antioxidant status or damage from oxidative stress [81–85]. In addition, long-term supplementation with a complex mixture of antioxidants has been shown to slow cognitive decline in aged dogs as well as to result in improved behavioral correlates in an in-home study [86]. It is unknown in any of these studies what each component contributes to the final results, and this remains an area of research that needs development in the future.

SUMMARY

In summary, nutritional antioxidant research has developed dramatically in the quality and quantity of publications over the past several years. Certainly, this overview indicates positive benefits as well as many questions still to be researched. Nonetheless, it is anticipated that antioxidant benefits are likely to remain in the forefront of adjunctive therapies over the next several years as more detail is learned about mechanisms, interactions, and target benefits.

References

[1] Evans HM, Bishop KS. On the existence of a hitherto unrecognized dietary factor essential for reproduction. Science 1922;56:650–1.

[2] Olcott HS, Mattil HA. The unsaponifiable lipids of lettuce. III. Antioxidant. J Biol Chem 1931;93:65–70.

[3] Halliwell B. Food derived antioxidants. In: Cadenas E, Packer L, editors. Handbook of antioxidants. 2nd edition. New York: Marcel Dekker; 2002. p. 1 46.

[4] Dorfman LM, Adams GE. Reactivity of the hydroxyl radical in aqueous solutions. National Standard Reference System. Monograph NSRDS-NBS 46. Washington (DC): National Bureau of Standards; 1973. p. 1–59.

[5] Harman D. Aging: a theory based on free radical and radiation chemistry. J Gerontol 1956;11:298–300.

[6] Beckman KB, Ames BN. The free radical theory of aging matures. Physiol Rev 1998;78: 547–81.

[7] Carbonaro M, Grant G. Absorption of quercetin and rutin in rat small intestine. Ann Nutr Metab 2005;49:178–82.

[8] Hacquebard M, Carpentier YA. Vitamin E: absorption, plasma transport and cell uptake. Curr Opin Clin Nutr Metab Care 2005;8:133–8.

[9] Leonard SW, Good CK, Gugger ET, et al. Vitamin E bioavailability from fortified breakfast cereal is greater than that from encapsulated supplements. Am J Clin Nutr 2004;79:86–92.

[10] Combs GF, Vitamin A. In: The vitamins: fundamental aspects in nutrition and health. 2nd edition. San Diego (CA): Academic Press, 1998. p. 107–53.

[11] Hill AS, Werner JA, Rogers QR, et al. Lipoic acid is 10 times more toxic in cats than reported in humans, dogs or rats. J Anim Physiol Anim Nutr (Berl) 2004;88:150–6.

[12] Lykkesfeldt J, Hagen TM, Vinarsky V, et al. Age-associated decline in ascorbic acid concentration, recycling, and biosynthesis in rat hepatocytes—reversal with (R)-alpha-lipoic acid supplementation. FASEB J 1998;12:1183–9.

[13] Michels AJ, Joisher N, Hagen TM. Age-related decline of sodium-dependent ascorbic acid transport in isolated rat hepatocytes. Arch Biochem Biophys 2003;410:112–20.

[14] Howitz KT, Bitterman KJ, Cohen HY, et al. Small molecule activators of sirtuins extend Saccharomyces cerevisiae lifespan. Nature 2003;425:191–6.

[15] Goldstein BJ, Mahadev K, Wu X, et al. Role of insulin-induced reactive oxygen species in the insulin signaling pathway. Antioxid Redox Signal 2005;7:1021–31.

[16] Haddad JJ. Antioxidant and prooxidant mechanisms in the regulation of redox(y)-sensitive transcription factors. Cell Signal 2002;14:879–97.

[17] Hughes G, Murphy MP, Ledgerwood EC. Mitochondrial reactive oxygen species regulate the temporal activation of nuclear factor kappaB to modulate tumour necrosis factor-induced apoptosis: evidence from mitochondria-targeted antioxidants. Biochem J 2005;389(Pt 1): 83–9.

[18] Kutuk O, Basaga H. Aspirin prevents apoptosis and NF-kappaB activation induced by H2O2 in HeLa cells. Free Radic Res 2003;37:1267–76.

[19] Azzi A, Gysin R, Kempná P, et al. Regulation of gene expression by α-tocopherol. Biol Chem 2004;385:585–91.

[20] Pillai SR, Traber MG, Steiss JE, et al. Depletion of adipose tissue and peripheral nerve alpha-tocopherol in adult dogs. Lipids 1993;28:1095–9.

[21] Pillai SR, Traber MG, Steiss JE, et al. Alpha-tocopherol concentrations of the nervous system and selected tissues of adult dogs fed three levels of vitamin E. Lipids 1993;28:1101–5.

[22] Starke-Reed PE, Oliver CN. Protein oxidation and proteolysis during aging and oxidative stress. Arch Biochem Biophys 1989;275:559–67.

[23] Head E, Liu J, Hagen TM, et al. Oxidative damage increases with age in a canine model of human brain aging. J Neurochem 2002;82:375–81.

[24] Liu J, Head E, Gharib AM, et al. Memory loss in old rats is associated with brain mitochondrial decay and RNA/DNA oxidation: partial reversal by feeding acetyl-L-carnitine and/or R-alpha-lipoic acid. Proc Natl Acad Sci USA 2002;99:2356–61.

[25] Magwere T, West M, Murphy MP, et al. The effects of exogenous antioxidants on lifespan and oxidative resistance in Drosophila melanogaster. Mech Ageing Dev 2006;127:356–70.

[26] Anderson DK, Waters TR, Means ED. Pretreatment with alpha tocopherol enhances neurologic recovery after experimental spinal cord compression injury. J Neurotrauma 1988;5:61–7.

[27] Association of the American Feed Control Officials (AAFCO) official publication. 2006

[28] Harris PL, Embree ND. Quantitative consideration of the effect of polyunsaturated fatty acid content of the diet upon the requirements for vitamin E. Am J Clin Nutr 1963;13:385–92.

[29] Hayes KC, Nielsen SW, Rousseau JE Jr. Vitamin E deficiency and fat stress in the dog. J Nutr 1969;99:196–209.

[30] Hayek MG, Massimino SP, Burr JR, et al. Dietary vitamin E improves immune function in cats. In: Reinhart GA, Carey DP, editors. Recent advances in canine and feline nutrition, vol. III. Wilmington (OH): Orange Frazer Press; 2000. p. 555–63.

[31] Hall JA, Tooley KA, Gradin JL, et al. Effects of dietary n-6 and n-3 fatty acids and vitamin E on the immune response of healthy geriatric dogs. Am J Vet Res 2003;64:762–72.

[32] Meydani SN, Hayek M, Wu D, et al. Vitamin E and immune response in aged dogs. In: Reinhart RA, Carey DP, editors. Recent advances in canine and feline nutrition, vol. II. Wilmington (OH): Orange Frazer Press; 1998. p. 295–303.

[33] Jewell DE, Yu S, Joshi DK. Effects of serum vitamin E levels on skin vitamin E levels in dogs and cats. Vet Ther 2002;3:235–43.

[34] Piercy RJ, Hinchcliff KW, Morley PS, et al. Association between vitamin E and enhanced athletic performance in sled dogs. Med Sci Sports Exerc 2001;33:826–33.

[35] Scott KC, Hill RC, Lewis DD, et al. Effect of alpha-tocopheryl acetate supplementation on vitamin E concentrations in Greyhounds before and after a race. Am J Vet Res 2001;62:1118–20.

[36] Fujimoto S, Mizoi K, Yoshimoto T, et al. The protective effect of vitamin E on cerebral ischemia. Surg Neurol 1984;22:449–54.

[37] Jorge PA, Osaki MR, de Almeida E, et al. Effects of vitamin E on endothelium-dependent coronary flow in hypercholesterolemic dogs. Atherosclerosis 1996;126:43–51.

[38] Sebbag L, Forrat R, Canet E, et al. Effects of dietary supplementation with alpha-tocopherol on myocardial infarct size and ventricular arrhythmias in a dog model of ischemia-reperfusion. J Am Coll Cardiol 1994;24:1580–5.

[39] National Research Council. Nutrient requirements of dogs and cats. Washington (DC): National Academy Press; 2006.

[40] Hill AS, O'Neill S, Rogers QR, et al. Antioxidant prevention of Heinz body formation and oxidative injury in cats. Am J Vet Res 2001;62:370–4.

[41] Hill AS, Rogers QR, O'Neill SL, et al. Effects of dietary antioxidant supplementation before and after oral acetaminophen challenge in cats. Am J Vet Res 2005;66: 196–204.

[42] Hall ED. Intensive anti-oxidant pretreatment retards motor nerve degeneration. Brain Res 1987;413:175–8.

[43] Phelps DL. Local and systemic reactions to the parenteral administration of vitamin E. Dev Pharmacol Ther 1981;2:156–71.

[44] Innes JRM. Vitamin C requirements of the dog. Attempts to produce experimental scurvy. 2nd report. Cambridge: Dir Camb Inst Anim Pathol; 1931. p. 143.

[45] Naismith DH. Ascorbic acid requirements of the dog. Proce Nutr Soc 1958;17:xlii–iii.

[46] Chatterjee IB, Majumder AK, Nandi BK, et al. Synthesis and some major functions of vitamin C in animals. Ann NY Acad Sci 1975;258:24–47.

[47] Wang S, Berge GE, Hoem NO, et al. Pharmacokinetics in dogs after oral administration of two different forms of ascorbic acid. Res Vet Sci 2001;71:27–32.

[48] Körner WF, Weber F. Tolerance for high dosages of ascorbic acid. Int J Vitam Nutr Res 1972;42:528–44.

[49] Kienzle E, Maiwald E. Effect of vitamin C on urine pH in cats. J Anim Physiol Anim Nutr (Berl) 1998;80:134–9.

[50] Massey LK, Liebman M, Kynast-Gales SA. Ascorbate increases human oxaluria and kidney stone risk. J Nutr 2005;135:1673–7.

[51] Yu S, Gross KL. Moderate dietary vitamin C supplement does not affect urinary oxalate concentration in cats. J Anim Physiol Anim Nutr (Berl) 2005;89:428–9.

[52] Chen LH. An increase in vitamin E requirements induced by high supplementation of vitamin C in rats. Am J Clin Nutr 1981;34:1036–41.

[53] Marshall RJ, Scott KC, Hill RC, et al. Supplemental vitamin C appears to slow racing greyhounds. J Nutr 2002;132(Suppl 6):1616S–21S.

[54] Chew BP, Park IS, Weng BC, et al. Dietary β-carotene is taken up by blood plasma and leukocytes in dogs. J Nutr 2000;130:1788–91.

[55] Chew BP, Park JS, Weng BC, et al. Dietary β-carotene absorption by blood plasma and leukocytes in domestic cats. J Nutr 2000;130:2322–5.

[56] Chew BP, Park JS, Wong TS, et al. Dietary beta-carotene stimulates cell-mediated and humoral immune response in dogs. J Nutr 2000;130:1910–3.

[57] Kearns RJ, Loos KM, Chew BP, et al. The effect of age and dietary β-carotene on immunological parameters in the dog. In: Reinhart GA, Carey DP, editors. Recent advances in canine and feline nutrition, vol. III. Wilmington (OH): Orange Frazer Press; 2000. p. 389–401.

[58] Kim HW, Chew BP, Wong TS, et al. Modulations of humoral and cell-mediated immune responses by dietary lutein in cats. Vet Immunol Immunopathol 2000;73:331–41.

[59] Kim HW, Chew BP, Wong TS et al. Dietary lutein stimulates immune response in the canine Vet Immunol Immunopathol 2000;74:315–27.

[60] Gross GJ, Lockwood SF. Acute and chronic administration of disodium disuccinate astaxanthin (Cardax) produces marked cardioprotection in dog hearts. Mol Cell Biochem 2005;272:221–7.

[61] Heywood R, Palmer AK, Gregson RL, et al. The toxicity of beta-carotene. Toxicology 1985;36:91–100.

[62] Scallon LJ, Burke JM, Mieler WF, et al. Canthaxanthin-induced retinal pigment epithelial changes in the cat. Curr Eye Res 1988;7:687–93.

[63] Schwarz K, Bieri JG, Briggs GM, et al. Prevention of exudative diathesis in chicks by factor 3 and selenium. Proc Soc Exp Biol Med 1957;95:621–5.

[64] Rotruck JT, Ganther HE, Swanson AB, et al. Selenium: biochemical role as a component of glutathione peroxidase. Science 1973;179:588–90.

[65] Combs GF. Impact of selenium and cancer-prevention findings on the nutrition-health paradigm. Nutr Cancer 2001;40:6–11.

[66] McKenzie RC, Rafferty TS, Beckett GJ. Selenium: an essential element for immune function. Immunol Today 1998;19:342–5.

[67] Neve J. Selenium as a 'nutraceutical': how to conciliate physiological and supra-nutritional effects for an essential trace element. Curr Opin Clin Nutr Metab Care 2002;5:659–63.

[68] Wedekind KJ, Howard KA, Backus RC, et al. Determination of the selenium requirement in kittens. J Anim Physiol Anim Nutr (Berl) 2003;87:315–23.

[69] Wedekind K, Kirk C, Yu S, et al. Defining safe lower and upper limits for selenium in adult cats [abstract]. J Anim Sci 2003;81(Suppl 1):90.

[70] Wedekind K, Kirk C, Yu S, et al. Defining the safe lower and upper limit for selenium in adult dogs [abstract]. FASEB J 2002;16:A992.

[71] Koller LD, Exon JH. The two faces of selenium—deficiency and toxicity—are similar in animals and man. Can J Vet Res 1986;50:297–306.

[72] Wallace KP, Center SA, Hickford FH, et al. S-adenosyl-L-methionine (SAMe) for the treatment of acetaminophen toxicity in a dog. J Am Anim Hosp Assoc 2002;38:246–54.

[73] Webb CB, Twedt DC, Fettman MJ, et al. S-adenosylmethionine (SAMe) in a feline acetaminophen model of oxidative injury. J Feline Med Surg 2003;5:69–75.

[74] Center SA, Randolph JF, Warner KL, et al. The effects of S-adenosylmethionine on clinical pathology and redox potential in the red blood cell, liver, and bile of clinically normal cats. J Vet Intern Med 2005;19:303–14.

[75] Zicker SC, Hagen TM, Joisher N, et al. Safety of long-term feeding of dl-α-lipoic acid and its effect on reduced glutathione:oxidized glutathione ratios in beagles. Vet Ther 2002;3: 167–76.

[76] Mortola E, Okuda M, Ohno K, et al. Inhibition of apoptosis and virus replication in feline immunodeficiency virus-infected cells by N-acetylcysteine and ascorbic acid. J Vet Med Sci 1998;60:1187–93.

[77] Allison RW, Lassen ED, Burkhard MJ, et al. Effect of bioflavonoid dietary supplement on acetaminophen-induced oxidative injury to feline erythrocytes. J Am Vet Med Assoc 2000;217: 1157–61.

[78] Zicker SC. Cognitive and behavioral assessment in dogs and per food market applications. Prog Neuropsychopharmacol Biol Psychiatry 2005;29:455–9.

[79] Robertson JE, Christopher MM, Rogers QR. Heinz body anemia in cats fed baby food containing onion powder. J Am Vet Med Assoc 1998;212:1260–6.

[80] Devlin P, Koelsch S, Heaton P, et al. The maintenance of a vaccine induced immune response in adult and senior dogs fed an antioxidant supplemented diet [abstract]. Compend Contin Educ Pract Vet 2001;23(Suppl):96.

[81] Baskin CR, Hinchcliff KW, DiSilvestro RA, et al. Effects of dietary antioxidant supplementation on oxidative damage and resistance to oxidative damage during prolonged exercise in sled dogs. Am J Vet Res 2000;61:886–91.

[82] Jewell DE, Toll PW, Wedekind KJ, et al. Effect of dietary antioxidants on concentrations of vitamin E and total alkenyls in serum of dogs and cats. Vet Ther 2000;1(4):264–72.

[83] Piercy RJ, Hinchcliff KW, DiSilvestro RA, et al. Effect of dietary supplements containing antioxidants on attenuation of muscle damage in exercising sled dogs. Am J Vet Res 2000;61: 1438–45.

[84] Wedekind KJ, Zicker S, Lowry S, et al. Antioxidant status of adult beagles is affected by dietary antioxidant intake. J Nutr 2002;132:1658S–60S.

[85] Yu S, Paetau-Robinson I. Dietary supplements of vitamin E and C and beta-carotene reduce oxidative stress in cats with renal insufficiency. Vet Res Commun 2006;30:403–13.

[86] Roudebush P, Zicker SC, Cotman CW, et al. Nutritional management of brain aging in dogs. J Am Vet Med Assoc 2005;227:722–8.

Vet Clin Small Anim 36 (2006) 1199–1224

VETERINARY CLINICS
SMALL ANIMAL PRACTICE

Nutrition and Immune Function

Korinn E. Saker, MS, DVM, PhD

Department of Large Animal Clinical Sciences, Virginia-Maryland Regional College of Veterinary Medicine, Blacksburg, VA 24061, USA

Illness is commonly associated with anorexia and altered nutrient requirements as a consequence of biochemical, metabolic, and pathologic abnormalities that influence nutrient use. This complicated cascade of events directly and indirectly involves immunocompetence. Several questions of importance to patient management should be considered. First, should the immune system be enhanced during disease and/or illness? If yes, how can nutrients enhance immunocompetence during disease and/or illness and which nutrients are efficacious immunomodulators? The complex workings of the immune system can be simplified to the fact that disease initiation and progression are correlated with a break in immunocompetence. Something in the system went awry, and the assumption is that nutritional intervention can potentially get the system back on track to help manage, resolve, and, in the future, prevent the disease process.

OVERVIEW OF THE IMMUNE SYSTEM

The immune system is part of the host's defense against destructive forces from outside the body, such as bacteria, viruses, and parasites, or from within, such as malignant cells or those that produce autoantibodies [1]. This system is composed of two components: the innate or nonspecific immune system and the adaptive or specific immune system.

The system of nonspecific immunity consists of anatomic barriers and a cellular component. The various barriers, including skin and mucous and gastrointestinal (GI) mucosa, are the true "first line of defense." Once compromised by microorganisms, endotoxins, or any substance considered to be foreign, the complement system may be activated. The complement system is a complex cascade of proteins that promote such functions as phagocytosis, viral neutralization, and destruction of virus-infected cells. Complement system defects are associated with increased susceptibility to bacterial infections. Inflammatory mediators, in addition to being products of cell membrane destruction, increase vascular permeability, causing the accumulation of acute-phase proteins and immune complexes that promote the cellular phase of acute inflammation [1].

The cellular phase of the nonspecific immune system includes circulating and "fixed" phagocytes. Initially, neutrophils bind to pathogenic microorganisms, phagocytose them, and kill them. Phagocytosis is facilitated by opsonization. Opsonins activate neutrophils, resulting in an oxidative burst that includes production of H_2O_2 and O_2^- free radicals. These substances kill the bacteria and the neutrophil with release of toxic waste products. Although this response is beneficial in moderation, prolongation of the inflammatory phase can be detrimental to the host. Monocytes and macrophages are also components of nonspecific immunity. They phagocytize antigens, process them through an oxidative burst reaction, and present antigen particles to T cells via major histocompatibility complex (MHC) class I or II receptors [2].

The specific immune system is composed of B and T cells, which are associated with humoral immunity and cell-mediated immunity. B lymphocytes mature in bone marrow and react to stimulation by certain antigens to differentiate into plasma cells, which synthesize and secrete antibodies commonly termed *immunoglobulins* (Table 1). Cell-mediated immunity, however, relies primarily on T lymphocytes derived from the thymus. Antigen-presenting cells, such as macrophages, are responsible for triggering the specific immune response. Interaction of an antigen and macrophage leads to production of interleukin (IL)-1 by means of arachidonic acid (AA) metabolism. The IL-1 produced by macrophages causes T cells to produce IL-2 and other lymphokines. Production of IL-2 helps to stimulate T and B cells to form clones that carry receptors specific to the sensitizing antigen. These clones form the long-lived memory cells, which proliferate and release lymphokines on re-exposure to the same antigen. These clones, in conjunction with macrophages, can destroy the antigen. Defects in cell-mediated immunity are associated with infections of bacteria, mycobacteria, viruses, fungi, and parasites [1,2].

T cells are not only responsible for mediating delayed hypersensitivity, graft rejection, destruction of pathogenic microorganisms, and destruction of malignant cells but also regulate responses of other immune cells. The subsets of T cells

Table 1
Immunoglobulins

Immunoglobulin	Type	Role and location
IgG	4	Coats microorganisms for uptake by other cells (opsonization); crosses placenta to affect passive immunity; enhances complement function; primarily present in serum
IgM	2	First to respond to antigens via agglutination and bacteriolysis; present in blood
IgA	1	Protects mucous membranes by preventing bacteria from attaching to mucosal surface; present in body fluids
IgE	1	Involved in hypersensitivity reactions and allergic responses; phagocytosis and other immunoglobulin activity; present in plasma and tissue and on surface membranes of basophils and mast cells
IgD	1	Involved in differentiation of B lymphocytes; present in serum and in plasma membrane of B lymphocytes

include helper-inducer T cells (CD4), which help plasma cells to produce antibodies and release lymphokines, which modulate the interaction between lymphocytes and other cells. Cytotoxic-suppressor T cells (CD8) may destroy target cells, inhibit antibody responses, or inhibit the inflammatory response [1,2].

NUTRIENT INFLUENCE ON SPECIFIC COMPONENTS OF THE IMMUNE SYSTEM

The small bowel contains an abundant amount of lymphoid tissue and is a primary component of innate immunity through its cellular component and protective barrier function. It is often considered to be the first line of defense to invasion by microbes into the systemic circulation. The physical barrier is created by the tight junctions between intact epithelial cells, gastric acid, digestive enzymes, mucus production, intestinal motility, and normal bacterial flora [3]. The gut-associated lymphoid tissue (GALT) or intestinal immune system consists of lymphocytes and macrophages situated throughout the intestinal wall. IgA is also secreted into the GI lumen to prevent adherence of microbes to the mucosa. By design, these two components prevent or minimize the spread of pathogens, or their products, across the intestinal wall into the systemic circulation, a process termed *translocation*. Multiple factors promote translocation, including luminal bacterial overgrowth, impaired host defense mechanisms, protein-calorie malnutrition (PCM), trauma, critical illness, interruption of the luminal nutrient stream, or any other process that leads to mucosal atrophy [4]. Fig. 1 depicts the potential life-threatening sequelae to bacterial translocation. Maintenance of an intact barrier and functioning GALT are imperative to preventing translocation. Certain nutrients, specifically glutamine (GLN), arginine, nucleotides, ω-3 fatty acids, and dietary fiber (a source of short-chain fatty acids), are necessary for growth and normal function of the mucosal epithelial cells and the lymphoid cells of the GALT intestinal barrier [3,5].

MOLECULAR ASPECTS OF NUTRITION AND IMMUNE FUNCTION

Basic Concepts

The structural complexity of mammalian cells has its basis in regulated expression of thousands of different proteins. Most of the information that defines these molecules and structures is contained in DNA sequences within the cell nucleus. The primary focus for the technology of molecular biology is DNA and the processes that translate the informational content of DNA into cellular structures and functions. Much of the informational content of DNA consists of regions of nucleotide or base sequences that define or code for the amino acid sequences of proteins. Steps involved in the information transfer from DNA to proteins are illustrated in Fig. 2. The DNA nucleotide sequence is transcribed into an mRNA nucleotide. The mRNA sequence is then translated into a protein. The proteins generated in this manner form cellular structures or function as enzymes or membrane transporters that dictate much of the overall structure and function of the cell [6].

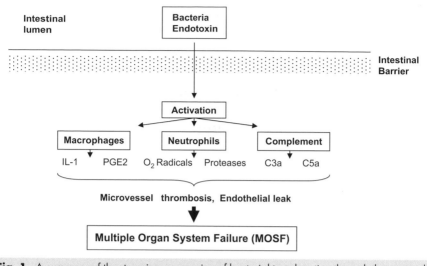

Fig. 1. A summary of the stepwise progression of bacterial translocation through the mucosal barrier resulting in multiple organ failure. PGE$_2$, prostaglandin E$_2$. (*Modified from* Rombeau JL. Enteral nutrition and critical illness. In: Borlase BC, Bell SJ, Blackburn GL, et al, editors. Enteral nutrition. New York: Chapman & Hall; 1994. p. 30; with permission.)

Practical Applications to Clinical Nutrition

Polysomes, the "preprotein" molecule sequence that builds on the mRNA backbone, can be isolated and quantified as a marker of nutrient intervention. GLN-supplemented total parenteral nutrition (TPN) versus a GLN-free control formula was given to patients for the first 3 days after abdominal surgery. Polysome content of the quadriceps femoris muscle obtained before and after day 3 after surgery showed a significant improvement in nitrogen balance and a sparing of free muscle GLN in the GLN-supplemented patients [7].

A second application involves DNA cloning (cDNA). A segment of DNA, or cDNA, that encodes for a specific protein of interest can be developed and used as a probe to assess expression of its corresponding mRNA in cells or tissues. Nutritionally relevant sequences derived from cDNA include proteins that function in carbohydrate (CHO; pyruvate kinase) and lipid (apolipoproteins) metabolism, growth control (growth hormone), and specific micronutrient actions (retinol-binding protein [RPB]). cDNA can be replicated multiple times over through host bacteria cultures. These recombinant proteins can be used to study normal and abnormal nutritionally important mechanisms of disease, including inflammation, cachexia, and oxidative stress, through such proteins as tumor necrosis factor and ILs [6].

Fig. 2 illustrates the process of creating and transferring a protein molecule from within the nucleus out to the cell cytoplasm. Examples of how the technologies associated with molecular biology can be used to monitor expression of nutrition-related molecules have been summarized. Interestingly, there seems to be a flip side of molecular nutrition, which involves the aspect of

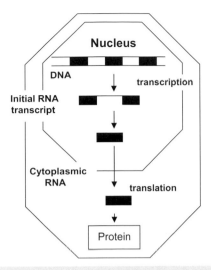

Fig. 2. Steps involved in the information transfer from DNA to protein. (*Modified from* Smith RJ. Molecular biology in nutrition. Nutr Clin Pract 1992;7:34; with permission from the American Society for Parenteral and Enteral Nutrition [ASPEN].)

uncovering the cellular mechanisms by which nutrients can influence gene expression. The transmission of signals from outside the cell into the nucleus can be profoundly influenced by nutrients. This area of technology is helping to identify how and which specific nutrients influence cell signal transduction and, ultimately, gene expression associated with immune function. Fig. 3 summarizes the complex relation between fatty acids, cell signal transduction cascades, apoptosis, and proliferation. This is one of numerous relations that are being clarified through nutrition research. The topic of nutrients as cell signals, although intriguing, is not meant to be a primary focus of this article. Several excellent reviews are available to develop this topic further. This level of nutritional science is likely to be extremely influential in optimizing patient management in the near future.

PATHOGENESIS OF ALTERED IMMUNOCOMPETENCE

Immunoimbalance is a systemic stress response to illness-induced anorexia or hypermetabolic food deprivation. It is associated with an increased metabolic rate, protein catabolism, and a release of multiple cell mediators, including cytokines, prostaglandins, and leukotrienes [8]. Oxidative (immune) cell function is escalated with the production of highly reactive radicals that damage cell constituents (membranes, proteins, lipids, and DNA), leading to cell death and multiple organ dysfunction. From a biologic perspective, stress is more accurately defined as oxidative stress, or the imbalance between production of damaging free radicals and antioxidant protection [9]. Oxidative stress plays a major role in many degenerative pathologic conditions, and free radical formation is considered to be a pathologic biochemical mechanism involved in the

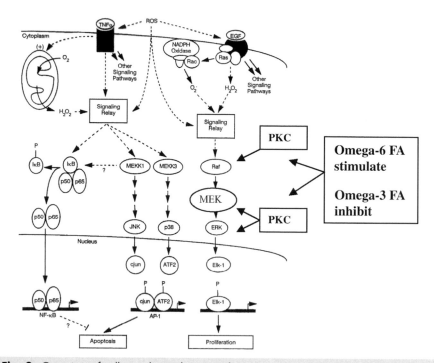

Fig. 3. Overview of cell signal transduction pathways suggesting points of signal enhancement or interruption via fatty acids (FA). AP-1, activator protein-1; EGF, epidermal growth factor; NF-κB, nuclear factor-κB; PKC, protein kinase C; ROS, reactive oxygen species; TNFα, tumor necrosis factor-α. (*Adapted from* Cowing BE, Saker KE. Polyunsaturated fatty acids and epidermal growth factor receptor/mitogen-activated protein kinase signaling in mammary cancer. J Nutr 2001;131:1127; with permission.)

initiation or progression phase of various diseases. These highly reactive radicals that can be so damaging if left unchecked are oxygen (reactive oxygen species [ROS]) and nitrogen (reactive nitrogen species [RNS]) based and are continuously and inescapably produced from the energy production cycle (mitochondrial electron transport chain), the detoxifying process via cytochrome P450 enzymes, reactions with transition metals (ie, copper [Cu], iron [Fe]) released during high-oxidative events (ie, injury, drug therapy, during the synthesis of fatty acid metabolites [eg, prostaglandins, leukotrienes]), and the immune system as a deliberate function of innate immune cells [10]. Based on the diversity of radical producers, it is logical that numerous body systems, including cardiopulmonary, endocrine, hematologic, integument, neurologic, and GI systems, are affected by oxidative stress.

The relation of nutrition, disease, and oxidative status is complex. Again, the aspect of molecular immunology surfaces as a technology that is being used to identify mechanisms involved in these relations. Fig. 4 illustrates one example of the complexity of nutrient manipulation focused on immunity (inflammation) and cell growth. In this case, ω-fatty acids are the potential influence on the cell signal cascade and nuclear transcription through inflammatory and tumor cell mediators.

MALNUTRITION, NUTRIENTS, AND IMMUNITY

Malnutrition, associated with a single nutrient or multiple nutrient inadequacies, is consistently associated with metabolic and clinical alterations of immunity. The association of malnutrition with reduced resistance to infection has been observed for centuries. Early work with children in developing countries suggested that the degree of immunocompromise depended on the degree of protein-energy malnutrition, presence of infection, and age at the onset of malnutrition [11]. In industrialized societies, PCM has been described more frequently in the elderly and in hospitalized patients [1]. Malnutrition should not only be considered to be of protein-calorie origin, however, because vitamin and mineral deprivation can also adversely influence the aspects of immunity. Immunocompromise and malnutrition in hospitalized patients contribute to the development of infection, sepsis, organ failure, poor wound healing, and a general increase in morbidity and mortality. Acutely ill patients with sepsis or a sepsis syndrome may exhibit immunosuppression without prior starvation [12].

Marasmus or semistarvation malnutrition is a syndrome that develops gradually over months to years with insufficient energy intake. The body responds by decreasing basal energy expenditure through a decrease in thyroid and sympathetic nervous system activity. Additionally, there is a shift of fuel sources in

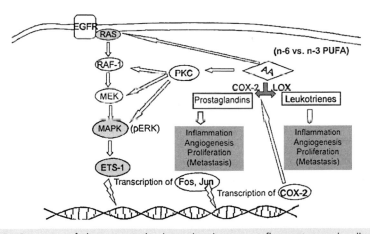

Fig. 4. Overview of the proposed relationship between inflammation and cell growth. Omega-6 and omega-3 fatty acids may influence the cell signaling cascade and nuclear transcription. COX-2, cyclooxygenase-2; EGFR, epidermal growth factor receptor; LOX, lipoxygenase; MAPK, mitogen-activated protein kinase; PKC, protein kinase C; PUFA, polyunsaturated fatty acid; RAS, p21 ras; RAF-1, p74 raf-1; MEK, MAPK (Erk) kinase. (*Adapted with modification from* Cowing BE, Saker KE. Polyunsaturated fatty acids and epidermal growth factor receptor/mitogen-activated protein kinase signaling in mammary cancer. J Nutr 2001;131: 1127; with permission.)

response to the depletion rate of stored nutrients. As glucose and glycogen reserves are depleted, protein and fat are sequestered for energy. To sustain primary protein needs for as long as possible, fat becomes the predominant fuel source. This type of malnutrition can be observed in patients with chronic disease processes that adversely affect energy intake, such as cachexia (cardiac or cancer) or malassimilation disorders [13].

In contrast, hypoalbuminemic malnutrition is a manifestation of the body's response to infection or inflammation with or without nutrient deprivation [14]. The association of malnutrition with metabolic and clinical alterations of immunity is more clearly evident in this situation. Hypoalbuminemic malnutrition is modulated by hormones and cytokines (ie, IL-1, tumor necrosis factor-α [TNFα]) secreted during the acute response to major stressors, such as sepsis, head injury, burns, or trauma [14]. It occurs quickly to deplete visceral protein (albumin) stores, and the multiplicity of sequelae to these events adversely affects metabolism and immune function.

The effects of PCM, regardless of the category, can be quite complex. Humoral immunity can be affected by PCM as a decline in the production of immunoglobulins, secretory antibodies, and complement. Cell-mediated immunity is commonly affected in hypoalbuminemic or severely marasmic patients. The thymus and lymphoid tissues atrophy, peripheral T lymphocytes decrease in number, alterations in cell-mediated delayed cutaneous hypersensitivity and graft-versus-host reactions are apparent, there is an impaired response of lymphocytes to mitogens, and patients exhibit a poor response to contact sensitization or inflammatory reactions as well as a depressed response to vaccines [15]. Neutropenia may occur to varying degrees in patients with PCM. Although neutrophils seem to be morphologically normal, cell function is decreased, specifically the capacity of neutrophils to kill phagocytosed bacteria or molds and to secrete chemokines [16]. Complement components of innate (nonspecific) immunity are depressed. Interferon production, opsonization, plasma lysosome production, and acute-phase reactants (ie, C-reactive protein) are adversely affected. Likewise, alterations in the anatomic barriers to infection included in the nonspecific immune system, such as atrophy of the skin and GI mucosa, may increase the risk of infection [13].

Whether correction of malnutrition improves patient outcome in all cases has yet to be proven, although, intuitively, it is assumed to be associated with a beneficial effect. Several studies [17,18] that clearly demonstrate the acute impact of nutrient deprivation on immune function and the reversal of innate and cell-mediated immune system compromise by appropriate nutrition support are summarized in Table 2. Current research in nutrition support is beginning to focus on exerting organ-specific effects by modulating metabolic processes rather than by simply improving nutrition. The effect of specific nutrients on the immune system is showing great promise in this regard. Many nutrients have a role in immune function. For some, mechanisms of immunomodulation have been clearly delineated, whereas much is yet to be learned in others.

Table 2
Differences in the monocyte phagocytic activity and CD4+/CD8+ lymphocyte expression in response to nutrient deprivation and refeeding in adult cats[a]

Item	Day[b]			
	4	7	11	14
Phagocytic activity[c]	−4.1*	−4.2*	−5.8**	−4.7**
CD4+[d]	−7.0	−9.0	−10.0	+5.0**
CD8+[d]	+15.0*	+9.0	+5.0	+25.0*
Lymphocyte proliferation[e]	−0.04	−0.09	−0.02*	−0.01*

Abbreviations: Con-A, cononavalin-A; DER, daily energy requirement; FITC, fluorescein isothiocyanate.

[a]N = 23 cats.

[b]Cats underwent nutrient deprivation (excluding water) for days 1 through 7 and were then refed to meet DER for days 8 through 14.

[c]Values represent the change from baseline (day 0) in percentage of cells that phagocytosed fluorescent polystyrene beads. Fluorescence detected by flow cytometry.

[d]Values represent the change from baseline in expression of CD4/CD8 on lymphocyte cell membranes after stimulation with con-A and staining with FITC and specific monoclonal antibody. Fluorescence detected by flow cytometry.

[e]Values represent change from baseline in proliferative capacity of 3.0×10^9 cells/mL stimulated with con-A. Proliferation determined by Alamar blue staining.

*Values differ from Day 0 ($P<.01$).

**Values differ from Day 7 ($P<.01$).

KEY NUTRIENTS AS MODULATORS OF IMMUNE FUNCTION

The list of key nutrients that may influence immunity seems to expand almost daily. Several decades ago, the list was short. Protein was the key nutrient, and micronutrient nutrition was a radical concept. Currently, a list of key nutrients includes specific amino acids, fatty acids, vitamins, microminerals, and nucleic acids in addition to the less well-defined micronutrients, such as flavonoids.

PROTEIN AND AMINO ACIDS

Along with total dietary protein content, form of protein delivery as an amino acid or an intact molecule and the individual amino acid concentration in the diet have been shown to influence the immune response. Early human studies evaluated increasing the percentage of protein in diets of children with extensive burn injuries. An increase from 15% to 23% resulted in a twofold increase in survival [19]. The higher dietary protein likewise resulted in significantly higher levels of serum total protein, transferrin (an acute-phase protein), complement C_3, and IgG in these patients. Investigators found no significant enhancement in serum protein levels, nitrogen balance, and complement C_3 in animals fed free amino acids compared with an intact whey protein source [20]. Conversely, there have been numerous reports of immune enhancement resulting from single amino acid enrichment to patient diets, particularly with arginine or GLN.

Arginine

Arginine is an essential amino acid in the cat for growth and maintenance of the urea cycle. It falls into the "semiessential" or "conditionally essential" category under a variety of stress situations, including burns, trauma, sepsis, and rapid growth in other species [21]. Arginine has also been shown to play a necessary role in collagen synthesis for wound healing and is required for nucleotide synthesis. Multiple secretagogue activities have been associated with arginine because it enhances secretion of prolactin, growth hormone, and insulin-like growth factor-1 (IGF-1) [22]. Prolactin induces maturation of dendritic cells by increasing the expression of antigen-presenting MHC class II and costimulatory molecules and stimulates release of T helper (Th) 1 cytokines by T lymphocytes. Growth hormone and IGF-1 can potentiate cytokine responses of T cells, increase progenitor cells in the bone marrow, and increase lymphocyte number [23].

Arginine also has documented immunoregulatory function in the stressed animal. Overall, it augments cellular immunity, and the specific effects can be summarized as increased thymic lymphocyte blastogenesis, responsiveness to mitogens, IL-2 production and IL-2 receptors, natural killer (NK) cells, and macrophage cytotoxicity to tumor cells and bacteria [24]. Arginine also seems to affect induction and development of malignant tumors through its effects on the immune system. These actions seem to be linked to arginine-derived nitric oxide (NO) and, depending on the surrounding microenvironment, the net biologic effect of arginine-derived NO can inhibit or promote tumor growth [25]. Bower [1] summarized numerous studies evaluating the role of arginine in animal tumor models and clinical studies. Arginine was reported to decrease the incidence of tumors after exposure to carcinogens, increase the latency period, shorten the interval required for tumor regression, and increase host survival in animals with malignant lesions [26]. It is thought that retardation of tumor growth and metastatic spread may be caused by the arginine-enhanced phagocytic function of macrophages, increased T-cell blastogenesis, and increased IL-2 production [1]. Adults with a GI malignancy demonstrated a quicker and more advantageous lymphocyte proliferative response to arginine (25 g) versus glycine (43 g) in the postoperative period [27]. These and numerous other studies are suggesting that the antitumorigenic effects of arginine can be via the specific and nonspecific immune systems.

Arginine is an important substrate for the synthesis of NO. The inducible form of nitric oxide (iNOS) is of most relevance to the immune system. iNOS expression, and hence NO production, is induced in monocytes and macrophages in response to stimuli, particularly that of interferon-γ (IFNγ) and lipopolysaccharide (LPS). NO is a regulator of various immune functions, and its inhibition increases host susceptibility to infections, making it essential for host defense [23]. Alternatively, arginine metabolism can involve the enzyme arginase. Arginase is increased in LPS- and cytokine-stimulated macrophages and converts arginine to ornithine. The ornithine produced is involved in the synthesis of polyamines, which are required for maintenance of cell viability. Polyamines act to facilitate DNA, RNA, and protein synthesis; therefore, inhibition of polyamine synthesis leads to a reduction in cell viability and cell differentiation [23]. A profound effect of dietary arginine supplementation was reported some years ago through a series of animal studies. Injured rats exhibited a reduction in trauma-induced thymic involution, increased T-cell response, sustained body weight, improved wound healing, and prolonged survival [26]. Babineau [21] summarized several studies that highlighted the influence of arginine on immune function. One such study demonstrated that arginine-supplemented diets enhanced cytotoxic T-lymphocyte development and increased NK cell activity and IL-2 receptor expression kinetics on activated T cells. In another study, 2% arginine supplementation resulted in increased survival and an improved delayed hypersensitivity response in animal burn patients [21]. A study involving stressed human subjects indicates that dietary arginine enhanced immune function through an increased peripheral blood lymphocyte and blastogenic response to mitogens, concanavalin A, and phytohemagglutinin [21].

Numerous human clinical studies have used commercially available immune-enhancing diets, which are supplemented with a combination of arginine, omega-3 fatty acids, and nucleotides. Although immune-enhancing effects are clearly demonstrated, because of the complexity of the formula, an arginine-specific effect is often not clearly interpretable [23]. Bansal and coworkers [28] investigated the interactions between fatty acids and arginine metabolism and what implications this may have on immune-enhancing diets. They reported that prostaglandin E_2 (PGE_2) from ω-6 fatty acids upregulates expression of arginase 1, which, subsequently, leads to arginine depletion. Conversely, ω-3 fatty acids protected against arginine depletion by attenuating the upregulation of arginase 1. The duality of arginine metabolism has led to some controversy regarding the immunologic value of increased dietary levels of arginine across all critical illness scenarios [29]. Currently, however, the pendulum swings toward supplementation improving outcomes in patients with sepsis, wounds, ischemia-reperfusion, and thermal injury [29,30].

Glutamine

GLN has traditionally been considered to be a nonessential amino acid in health, only taking on a "conditionally essential" status in states of illness or injury. In catabolic states, amino acids, predominantly alanine and GLN, are released from muscle tissue to provide a fuel source for enterocytes of the small bowel and for rapidly dividing leukocytes and macrophages in the immune system [31]. Particularly during stress, GLN is the preferential fuel source for cells of the gut and can be rapidly depleted despite the significant release from muscle tissue. Plasma GLN levels have been shown to decrease by 58% after critical illness or injury and to remain decreased for up to 3 weeks with increased mortality in seriously ill patients [31]. A GLN deficiency-related impairment of lymphocyte and neutrophil function as well as glutathione (GSH) depletion is a likely mechanism for the increased mortality. Several specific immunomodulatory actions of GLN in vitro and in vivo have been nicely summarized and reported by Calder and Yagoob [23]. Increasing the availability of GLN in culture has been shown to enhance T-lymphocyte proliferation and IL-2 and IFNγ production by lymphocytes, B-lymphocyte differentiation into antibody-producing cells, phagocytosis, and antigen-presenting activities of macrophages and neutrophils. Animal studies have reported that GLN enrichment of the diet increases T-lymphocyte proliferation of splenic CD4+ cells and cytokine production (eg, TNFα, IL-1, IL-2, IL-6, IFNγ) in injury- or infection-stressed situations. A study of critically ill patients supplemented with enteral GLN reported a significant decrease in the incidence of sepsis, pneumonia, and bacteremia. The mechanism was thought to be associated with enhanced expression of antigen-presenting receptors on the monocyte cell surface [32]. This, of course, is an important aspect of innate immunity, in which phagocytic cells engulf and process (kill or disassemble) invading pathogens and subsequently jump-start other branches of the immune system for an optimal immune response. Preservation of the gut mucosal barrier to minimize intestinal permeability was another proposed mechanism of GLN supplementation in this study. Fig. 5 summarizes potential pathways for GLN benefits in the critically ill patient.

Interestingly, supplementation of GLN has been reported to demonstrate significant benefit and no added benefit to immunocompetence based on the route of delivery and study design. Hall and coworkers [33] reported that low-dose enteral GLN therapy to critically ill patients resulted in no improvement in the incidence of sepsis, body condition, and mortality compared with unsupplemented controls. There are numerous studies reporting benefit and lack of benefit from parenteral GLN in critically ill patients. Cellular mucosal and peripheral immune cell functions were evaluated in dogs receiving a 2% GLN-fortified parenteral admixture (PA) before and after intestinal resection and anastomosis surgery. PA-GLN resulted in a significantly increased helper and decreased suppressor T-cell population, increased IgM, a mild increase in IgA, significantly less diarrhea days, and a lower hospital cost compared with those parameters in patients receiving a calorie- and GLN-free solution before and after surgery [34]. Again, dosage, timing, and response indices varied and likely influenced the outcome in these studies. In summary, most trials associated with GI disease indicated that larger GLN doses were more beneficial than lower doses of GLN [31]. There is limited availability of studies in critically ill or diseased companion animals supplemented with GLN; therefore, summarizing human studies may support or refute the idea of GLN as a useful immunomodulator in the feeding management of sick pets. The results of a meta-analysis [35], including 14 randomized trials involving 751 patients, of GLN administration in critically ill patients versus standard care indicates a shorter hospital stay, lower rate of infectious complications (risk ratio [RR] = 0.81), and lower mortality rate (RR = 0.78). Subgroup analysis revealed a treatment benefit of high-dose GLN (>0.20 g/kg of body weight [BW] per day) over low-dose GLN (<0.20 g/kg of BW per day) with regard to mortality. Table 3 summarizes only the enteral GLN studies evaluated in the meta-analysis.

GLN is also a nitrogen donor for the synthesis of purines and pyrimidines, a substrate for protein synthesis, and a precursor to glutamate, which is

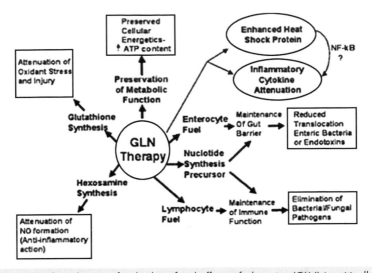

Fig. 5. Potential mechanisms for the beneficial effects of glutamine (GLN) in critically ill patients. ATP, adenosine triphosphate; NF-κB, nuclear factor-κB; NO, nitric oxide. (*Adapted from* Wischmeyer PE. Clinical application of L-glutamine: past, present, and future. Nutr Clin Pract 2003;18(5):378; with permission from the American Society for Parenteral and Enteral Nutrition [ASPEN].)

incorporated into the antioxidant GSH. GSH depletion was associated with diminished IFNγ production. A rise in lymphocyte GSH content was accompanied by an increase in mitogen-induced lymphocyte proliferation and IL-2 production [23]. These studies suggest that GLN promotes a range of cell-mediated and innate immune responses.

Taurine

Taurine is another sulfur amino acid that seems to be involved in immune function, and several studies highlighting this relation are summarized by Calder and Yaqoob [23]. Taurine is derived from the metabolism of methionine and cysteine; thus, it is not considered to be a component of proteins. It is present in high concentrations in cells of the immune system, however, and accounts for 50% of the free amino acid pool within lymphocytes. Although the role of taurine within lymphocytes is not well defined, it is reported that cats fed taurine-deficient diets exhibit atrophy of the lymph nodes and spleen, a decrease in circulating lymphocytes, and impaired oxidative burst by phagocytes. Administration of taurine prevented and reversed adverse T-cell changes in mice of various ages. Taurine chloramine, a complex of taurine with hypochlorous acid (HOCl), protects the host from toxic damage of HOCl derived from oxidative processes and has also been shown to be bacteriocidal in its own right. Because taurine chloramine decreases NO, superoxide, PGE$_2$, TNFα, and IL-6 production by leukocytes, it has been proposed that taurine may offer a therapeutic approach to acute inflammatory events.

Table 3
Randomized trials of enteral glutamine in critically ill human patients

Study	Patient population (no.)	Dosage L-glutamine (g/kg of BW per day)	Mortality (%)		Infectious complications (%)	
			Expt.	Control	Expt.	Control
Houdijk et al, 1998	CI (78)	>25	4/41 (9.8)	3/39 (7.7)	20/35 (57.1)	26/37 (70.2)
Jones et al, 1999	Mixed (165)	−0.16	10/26 (38.5)	9/24 (37.5)	—	—
Brantley and Pierce, 2000	CI (70)	0.50	−0/31 (0.0)	0/41 (0.0)	—	—

Abbreviations: BW, body weight; CI, critically ill; Expt, experiment; Mixed, ICU/hospital; —, not available.

LIPIDS

Lipid metabolism and use can not only yield a useful energy source but can influence metabolic and immunologic parameters during health and illness. Stored body fat is the major energy reserve for nonstressed starvation-adapted patients; however, under circumstances of stress, the protein-sparing effect of fat oxidation is lost. Administration of relatively high levels of lipid in critically ill patients provides a concentrated energy/calorie source and helps to avoid the complications associated with overfeeding CHO. Conversely, excessive fat dosing can itself lead to complications related to cardiopulmonary dysfunction, platelet dysfunction, and immune function compromise. Decreased clearance of bacteria from phagocytosis of lipid globules, subsequently increasing the risk of bacteremia and sepsis, has been reported in human and animal patients receiving excessive lipid in the form of long-chain triglycerides (LCTs) [36]. Replacement of the same fraction of the intravenous (parenteral)-delivered LCTs with medium-chain triglycerides (MCTs) seemed to protect septic patients from these adverse immune system sequelae [36]. This suggests that lipid content and form can influence immune function and that assessment of the patient's immunologic status is paramount when determining lipid content in nutritional support protocols. Evaluation of specific immune cell functions as indicators of immunologic status in patients is realistically more suited for a research setting. Having said this, evaluation of bleeding time could be performed in a clinical setting and would give some measure of platelet function. With its reported relationship to omega-3 FA lipid content (LCT), it could be utilized as a means to assess adequate lipid content nutritional support protocols. A full spectrum, 'quick and dirty' type of immunologic panel for use in daily practice is not currently available.

Although lipids are an essential component of the body, it seems that the immunomodulation of the specific and nonspecific immune systems is profoundly influenced through action of the essential fatty acids (EFAs), omega-6 and omega-3 families. Immune cells, including monocytes, macrophages, lymphocytes, and granulocytes, are able to synthesize non-EFAs but must rely on circulating blood lipids as the source of EFAs. Therefore, the lipid composition of immune cells reflects the fatty acid composition of lipids in the diet [1]. There are numerous reviews outlining the metabolism of the essential polyunsaturated fatty acids (PUFAs) linoleic acid (n6) and linolenic acid (n3). Briefly, linoleic acid is converted to AA, which serves as a precursor to prostanoids (particularly PGE_2), thromboxanes of the 2 series, and leukotrienes of the 4 series. These compounds are largely proinflammatory and have been implicated as mediators in the vascular component of septic shock [21]. Conversely, provision of n3 fatty acids, principally from fish oil, leads to production of eicosapentaenoic acid (EPA) and docosahexaenoic acid (DHA). These compete with AA for cyclooxygenase (COX) and lipoxygenase enzymes, ultimately to yield the 3 series of prostanoids and 5 series leukotrienes, which are reported not only to be less inflammatory and vasoactive but to possess anti-inflammatory action [37]. This indicates that the type of fatty acid in the diet is another avenue to influence immune function.

Omega-6 Fatty Acids

Vegetable oils, including corn, soy, canola and safflower oils, are a primary source of ω-6 fatty acids in the diets of companion animal. Prostanoids derived from metabolism of n6 PUFAs seem to have a dose effect. Extremely low concentrations induce lymphocytes to differentiate into T cells; however, overproduction of PGE_2 depresses measurements of T-cell function, including response to mitogens, clonal proliferation, production of lymphokines, migration and generation of cytotoxic T cells, and killing activity of phagocytes [1]. The leukotrienes are short turn-around activators of leukocytes. They can stimulate leukocytes to aggregate and adhere to endothelial cells. They also influence NK cell activity. The n6 fatty acids, with certainty, play a significant role in immunosuppression, tumorigenesis, and enhancing inflammation (Fig. 6) [38].

Omega-3 Fatty Acids

α-Linolenic acid (18:3ω3) is an essential nutrient for companion animals, thereby necessitating its inclusion in the diet to promote normal growth and development. Dietary omega-3 fatty acids are most commonly derived from marine fish oil, although several agricultural sources for n3 oils also exist. In fish oil–derived n3 fatty acids, EPA is the most active component. Although DHA is also derived from α-linolenic acid and possesses anti-inflammatory as well as other properties, EPA is the form of n3 fatty acid that has been researched most extensively. EPA and DHA attenuate the inflammatory response, stabilize the nuclear factor-κB (NF-κB) complexes, decrease platelet adhesiveness, enhance lymphocyte and neutrophil function, and aid in membrane stability and microvascular perfusion, whereas high levels of AA have the inverse effect [39,40]. Clinically, n3 fatty acids have reportedly shown

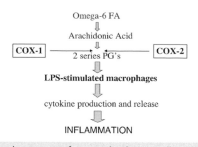

Fig. 6. Overview of the role omega-6 fatty acids play in cell-mediated cytokine production and inflammation. FA, fatty acids; PG, prostaglandin; LPS, lipopolysaccharide; COX-1, cyclooxygenase-1; COX-2, cyclooxygenase 2.

benefit in a variety of disease states, including arthritis, sepsis, cardiac abnormalities, and cancers. The primary mechanism of action underlying the value of n3 fatty acids seems to be, directly and indirectly, their anti-inflammatory focus. Through cell signal cascades, n3 fatty acids influence COX-2 expression and ultimately exhibit COX-2 inhibitor-like action to inhibit PGE_2 production and lessen the inflammatory response. The n3 fatty acids have also been demonstrated to decrease macrophage NF-κB nuclear translocation and subsequently inhibit production of proinflammatory cytokines via NF-κB [40]. It has also been reported that n3 fatty acids alter the proteins and specific nuclear transcription factors in the mitogen-activated protein kinase (MAPK) pathways, including activator protein-1 (AP-1). These pathways ultimately activate or inhibit cell proliferation versus apoptosis (cell death) [40,41]. Numerous commercial (therapeutic and nontherapeutic) diets have focused on the n6:n3 fatty acid ratio in an attempt to maximize immunomodulating properties of the n3 fatty acid family. Currently, there is a range of approximately 12:1 to 1:1 depending on the marketing focus. An overall "optimal" ratio has yet to be established, keeping in mind that the clinical value of dietary n6:n3 may well be disease specific. A second approach is to enhance diets with n3 fatty acids specifically, and thereby focus on the total amount of n3 FA rather than the ratio.

CARBOHYDRATES

Polysaccharides possess immunomodulatory properties as noted by the incorporation of LPS as a stimulating agent in various models of immunity. LPS-associated polysaccharides are not the common CHO source in diets; rather, they are the soluble CHO component of the antigen (eg, CHO, lipid, protein) associated with endotoxins. These endotoxins are localized on the outer surface of gram-negative bacteria and elicit specific antibody responses. Although the three components of endotoxin should potentially elicit antigenic diversity, evidence supports a primary immunodominant role for the specific polysaccharide component of LPS [42]. In the advent of bacterial translocation through compromised GI mucosa, the polysaccharide component of LPS-associated bacterial endotoxins could indeed influence immunomodulation of the GALT. On a different note, Melis and coworkers [43] reported that intake of a CHO-rich beverage before surgery can prevent surgery-induced immunodepression. This is a potential avenue to reduce the risk of infectious complications and maintain barrier and GALT functions in stressed and potentially malnourished patients.

Dietary CHO can be viewed from the perspective of glycemic control, particularly in stressed, critically ill, diabetic, or obese patients. Associated risk factors for increasing the incidence of infection include improving preoperative nutrition, choosing the optimal route of nutrient delivery and type of nutritional supplementation, and tight glycemic control in patients through altering CHO intake. A landmark human study of 1548 patients requiring mechanical ventilation [44] showed that euglycemic patients had fewer episodes of acute renal failure, fewer transfusions, and less polyneuropathy. Compared with a hyperglycemic patient group, infectious complications were 46% lower and the mortality rate was decreased by 42%. Studies have repeatedly indicated the adverse effect of modest hyperglycemia on neutrophil function, including decreased chemotaxis, phagocytosis, oxidative burst, and bacteriocidal capacity [45]. Additionally, modest hyperglycemia has been shown to promote the proinflammatory state through increasing levels of the inflammatory mediator $TNF\alpha$ and activating $NF\text{-}\kappa B$, which promotes production of TNF [46]. The article in this issue covering critical illness provides more details on dietary CHO control, especially during parenteral feeding.

MINERALS AND VITAMINS

These nutrients, although required in small concentrations in the diet, can be considered to be the metabolic glue that is behind nearly all anabolic and catabolic processes in the mammalian system. Electrolytes play key roles in maintaining cell structure, and thus flow of cell regulators. Trace minerals and vitamins alike facilitate complex metabolic reactions and are key components of antioxidant activities, which currently are receiving attention in the scientific arena as modulators of the immunologic components of health and disease.

Copper, Zinc, and Iron

Cu has a profound effect on many aspects of the immune system. Animal models of Cu deficiency have been concisely reported by Lukasewycz and Prohaska [47] and indicate that Cu is important for antibody generation (IgG), for cell-mediated immunity, and for the generation of the inflammatory response. Laboratory animals on a low-Cu diet have demonstrated an increased susceptibility to bacterial infections. Domestic animals with insufficient Cu intake show decreased bactericidal activity, impaired macrophage phagocytosis and MHC class II expression [48], and a higher susceptibility to infection [47]. Mice receiving a Cu-deficient diet showed a decreased reactivity to T- and B-cell mitogens, a low proliferative and delayed type hypersensitivity (DTH) response to stimulation, a redistribution of lymphocyte subsets, a decrease in

NK cell activity [47], and a reduced ability of T cells to produce sufficient quantities of IL-2 to allow cells to progress to the S phase [49]. Many of these aspects of altered immunocompetency have reportedly been reversed by the addition of adequate Cu. Ceruloplasmin, an acute-phase protein, and superoxide dismutase (SOD), an endogenous antioxidant that scavenges damaging ROS in immune cells, are Cu-dependent enzymes whose activity and concentrations reflects dietary Cu intake [47]. These enzyme functions help to define Cu as an integral component of phagocytic cell function.

Dietary Cu deficiency is uncommon in small animal nutrition when feeding most commercially formulated rations. Research strongly suggests that many nutrients, including Cu, may be required in excess of current dietary recommendations during critical illness to compensate for losses and increased use during acute or chronic disease challenge.

The discovery of nutritional zinc (Zn) deficiency in the pathogenesis of disease provided the focus for studies to elucidate the mechanism of Zn-induced changes in immunity. Zn is an important cofactor for numerous enzymes involved in cell metabolism, but deficiency of this mineral can also result in a profound immunodeficiency state. Several common hallmarks of Zn deficiency are lymphopenia and thymic atrophy. Along with atrophy, a decrease in thymic hormone activity is also observed. Deficiency of Zn results in depressed DTH reactions, decreased CD4 (Th) and increased CD8 (T-suppressor) cell populations, a reduced proliferative response to mitogens and NK cell activity, and decreased chemotaxis of monocytes and neutrophils [50]. Lymphopoiesis can likewise be influenced by Zn deficiency. Fraker and King [51] reported that a 30-day period of suboptimal Zn intake in adult mice caused a 40% to 90% depletion of marrow cells in the B-cell compartment. Zn is also a component of the antioxidant enzyme, SOD, which scavenges damaging ROS in immune cells, defining Zn as an integral component of phagocytic cell function and viability [52].

Fe is probably one of the most important trace elements in the body. It plays an important role in the transport of oxygen and in the oxidation-reduction pathways of many systems. Fe is intimately associated with malnutrition as a result of poor intake, poor absorption, or excessive losses. A negative Fe balance can initially lead to decreased tissue stores, a decreased blood hemoglobin concentration, and, finally, the appearance of microcytic hypochromic anemia. Lymphoid cells require Fe for cell division, electron transport, and oxidation-reduction reactions. Fe bound to transferrin is the mode of transport into immune cells. It has been reported that abnormalities in cellular morphology and function of red and white blood cells because of a negative Fe status are associated with decreased DTH reactions, reduced T-cell mitogen response, reduced lymphokine production by T cells, reduced antibody production and phagocytic activity, and enhanced susceptibility to infection [15,53].

Selenium and Vitamin E
Together selenium (Se) and vitamin E share a unique relation through interactions involving the antioxidant enzyme, glutathione-peroxidase (GSH-Px).

These interactions directly and indirectly influence immunity through their combined antioxidant functions. An in-depth discussion of antioxidants in health and disease is presented in another article in this issue. Aside from the antioxidant capacity of Se-dependent GSH-Px, this enzyme has been shown to alter immunity through its impact on lymphocyte differentiation; signal transduction; and regulation of proinflammatory cytokines, such as leukotrienes, thromboxanes, and prostaglandins [10,54]. There are five different forms of GSH-Px, which exhibit their protective functions in unison but at different sites in the body.

Based on recently reported studies, the form of dietary Se should perhaps be considered. The commonly used inorganic sodium selenite is actually capable of promoting O_2^- · formation, and ultimately enhancing oxidative stress [54]. Selenomethionine (Se-Met), an organic Se compound, is nontoxic and noncatalytic and does not produce the superoxide free radical [55]. Lymphocytes treated with Se-Met inhibited peroxyl radical formation in a dose-dependent manner [56]. Seo and coworkers [57] showed that Se-Met induced repair of damaged DNA and protected normal fibroblasts from oxidative damage at easily attainable in vivo diet supplementation levels. Synergistic effects of Se-Met with other antioxidants (ie, ascorbic acid, GSH, mannitol) were not appreciated in enhanced immune cell protection [58,59]. Waters and colleagues [60] reported that Se-Met or Se-enriched yeast lowered the DNA damage in prostate cells and peripheral blood lymphocytes of dogs; however, interestingly, the total activity of plasma glutathione peroxidase was not associated with DNA alterations.

Along with its well-defined role as an antioxidant, it has been reported that vitamin E may indirectly enhance immune factors. This effect is thought to be via inhibition of macrophage secretion of PGE_2, which suppresses IL-1 production, mitogen- and antigen-induced lymphocyte blastogenesis, antibody production, and cytotoxic T-cell activity [61]. A limited number of companion animal studies have evaluated the relation between dietary vitamin E concentrations and immunity. The studies reported by Meydani and coworkers [62] suggested that higher (280-IU/kg diet) dietary vitamin E helped to maintain lymphocyte proliferative activity as compared with lower (27-IU/kg diet) levels in Beagles. Diets supplying vitamin E at a rate of 250 to 500 IU/kg of diet seemed to provide immunologic benefit to older healthy cats [61].

Based on recent reports, perhaps the form of vitamin E supplied in the diet should be a consideration. γ-Tocopherol is the major form of vitamin E in many plants, but α-tocopherol is the predominant form of vitamin E in tissues and the form primarily used in supplements. Recent studies suggest that γ-tocopherol has unique physiologic features that may justify its importance in health and disease. The γ-form seems to be more effective in trapping lipophilic electrophiles compared with α-tocopherol. It is reported to be well absorbed and stored in appreciable concentrations in tissues. Urine is the major route of γ-tocopherol metabolite excretion, and this water-soluble metabolite seems to exhibit natriuretic activity [63]. Unlike the α-form, γ-tocopherol and its major metabolite (γ-carboxyethyl-hydroxychromans [CEHC]) inhibit COX activity and subsequently influence anti-inflammatory properties. Jiang and coworkers [64] reported that γ-tocopherol and γ-CEHC inhibit PGE_2 synthesis in LPS-stimulated macrophages and in Il-1β–activated epithelial cells at significantly lower concentrations than α-tocopherol. The COX-2 inhibitory effects of the γ-form versus the α-form of vitamin E indicate a nonantioxidant property of γ-tocopherol that can be important in the prevention and management of disease, such as autoimmune disease, cancer, and type-1 diabetes. Based on reported properties of α- and γ-tocopherol as well as on the understanding that large doses of α-tocopherol deplete plasma and tissue γ-tocopherol, possible immunomodulatory benefits of γ-tocopherol, the dietary tocopherol form, should be given consideration in nutritional support programs.

Vitamin C

This vitamin was mentioned previously for its role in recycling and reactivating vitamin E. It has more direct implications in immunity as well. Decreased vitamin C (ascorbic acid) is known to be associated with depressed cell-mediated immunity, poor bactericidal activity, and impaired macrophage mobilization. Supplementation with vitamin C enhances T- and B-cell proliferation and bacterial phagocytosis by macrophages [65].

Vitamin A

There are numerous well-documented vitamin A deficiency symptoms, including immune function abnormalities. Deficiency of this vitamin impairs secretory IgA production, decreases mucus production (a component of the innate immune system), and leads to keratinization of secretory epithelia. When vitamin A is bound to RBP and chylomicron remnants, it modulates normal B-cell activation, cytokine production, antibody production, and cell differentiation. β-Carotene, a precursor to vitamin A, has been shown to enhance T-cell and B-cell generation in animals [65].

B-Vitamins

The B-vitamins are generally considered as a "complex," (Table 4) except in specific disease-associated deficiencies, such as small intestinal bacterial overgrowth (SIBO). They all are equally necessary to drive intermediary metabolism in the body; however, with regard to having a specific impact on immune function, there is one B-vitamin in the complex that should be mentioned, pyridoxine (B_6). Deficiency of this B-vitamin is associated with impaired cell-mediated and humoral immune responses. Human beings with poor B_6 intake have been reported to exhibit a decrease in circulating lymphocytes, reduced IgD levels, and a decreased percentage of Th cells [65]. In the human literature, it is suggested that B_6 may be needed in excess of the recommended daily allowances to maintain adequate immune function in compromised patients.

OTHERS
Nucleotides
Nucleotides, which are the precursors of DNA and RNA, can be considered to be the building blocks of life. The supply of nucleotides needed for biochemical

Table 4
Summary of immunomodulatory capabilities of minerals and vitamins

Nutrient		Immunomodulation
Minerals	Iron	Necessary for optimum neutrophil and lymphocyte function; free iron is necessary for bacterial growth
	Copper	Deficiency associated with increased rate of infections, depressed RES and microbicidal activity of granulocytes, impaired antibody response, and depressed thymic hormone; component of the antioxidant enzyme SOD, scavenges immune cell-damaging ROS
	Zinc	Deficiency associated with susceptibility to infection, abnormal cell-mediated immunity, depressed circulating thymic hormones, and altered complement and phagocytic function; component of the antioxidant enzyme SOD, scavenges immune cell-damaging ROS
	Selenium	Deficiency reduces antibody responses; component of the antioxidant enzyme GSH-PX, scavenges immune cell-damaging ROS
	Iodine	Decreased microbicidal activity of neutrophils in hypothyroid patients, and a reversal seen with treatment
	Magnesium	Deficiency causes thymic hyperplasia, impaired humoral and cell-mediated immunologic responsiveness, depressed immunoglobulins (IgG1, IgG2, IgA)
	Manganese	Required for normal antibody synthesis/secretion; excess inhibits antibody formation and chemotaxis and increases susceptibility to pneumococcal infection
	Sodium	Brush border cells in the gastrointestinal tract are dependent on sodium for transport of glutamine, which is pivitol in maintaining an intact gut barrier
Vitamins	A	Deficiency reduces lymphocyte response to mitogens and antigens; β-carotene and retinoids stimulate immune responses
	B complex (B6)	Deficiency associated with decreased antibody response and impaired cellular immunity
	C	Extreme deficiency impairs phagocyte function and cellular immunity
	D	Deficiency causes anergy in the delayed hypersensitivity skin test
	E	Deficiency decreases antibody response to T-cell–dependent antigens; effect is compounded by a Se deficiency; supplementation has been shown to enhance immune responses

Abbreviations: GSH-PX, glutathione peroxidase; RES, reticuloendothelial system; ROS, reactive oxygen species; Se, Selenium; SOD, superoxide dismutase.

processes is mainly supplied through de novo synthesis of purines and pyrimidines. Dietary intake is a secondary source during health but can become of major importance during illness. Animal studies have indicated that a dietary requirement of preformed purine or pyrimidine bases may be required for normal development. Babineau [21] has summarized numerous studies of Van

Buren, Kulkarni, and others in investigating the role of nucleotides in immune function. Uracil seems to be the most important nucleic acid influencing the immune response. Delayed cutaneous hypersensitivity, mitogen-stimulated lymphocyte proliferation, graft rejection, and graft-versus-host disease have all been reported as being suppressed by a diet that lacks nucleotides. Van Buren and coworkers demonstrated that dietary nucleotides were able to reverse malnutrition- and starvation-induced immunosuppression in rats. They also showed that helper/inducer T lymphocytes require exogenous nucleotides to respond normally after immune stimulation. Another study demonstrated that dietary nucleotide restriction negatively influenced the phagocytic cell response to a bacterial sepsis challenge in mice. These studies specifically emphasize the role of nucleotides in lymphocyte and macrophage function and metabolism, although dietary sources are equally as important to support the optimal growth and function of other metabolically active cells, such as intestinal cells.

GUIDELINES WITH A DISCLAIMER

Nutrient guidelines are available for feeding the healthy animal during various life stages and phases of production and/or reproduction. To date, a comprehensive set of recommendations for nutrient support of the immune system does not exist for small or large animals. It may be possible to extrapolate from human or animal studies, but overfeeding a specific nutrient can just as easily diminish one or more aspects of immune function as enhance it. In many circumstances of immune function challenge or malnutrition, increasing a specific nutrient over maintenance recommendations is beneficial to the immune response. The problem lies in exactly how much to enhance. At present, a wiser and safer approach may be to prevent deficiency of identified immunomodulating nutrients in your nutritional support plan. That said, some general guidelines for specific nutrients have been summarized for consideration based on extrapolation from the current literature. The reader should consider these guidelines to be generic, however, because the optimal dose remains controversial. Nutrition support plans need to be individualized based on a thorough and continual assessment of each patient.

Suggestions for clinical use of GLN in the human literature include two categories: (1) critically ill patients can be supplemented with GLN at a rate of 30 to 50 g in addition to the standard enteral diet, with a goal to achieve GLN at a rate of 0.35 to 0.65 g/kg of BW per day, and (2) pre- or postsurgical patients can be supplemented with GLN at a rate of 25 to 50 g in addition to the standard enteral diet, with a goal to supply GLN at a rate of 0.30 to 0.65 g/kg of BW per day. The dose of a powder formula for the small animal patient is reported to be 10 mg/kg/d. A suggested dose of GLN supplementation to PAs for immunomodulation is 2% of the total daily PA as L-GLN. The suggested goal for dietary arginine intake of small animal patients with cancer would be approximately 500 to 600 g per 100 kcal/d. Although values are not available for managing patients with severe sepsis or inflammation, studies suggest a 1.5- to 2.5-fold increase in dietary intake over the standard enteral diet.

Current recommended oral doses for vitamin E in the α-tocopherol isomeric form are in a range of 400 to 500 IU/d for inflammatory disease. This is a dose 2 to 10 times greater than the daily requirement for dogs. Earlier studies suggested that a diet supplying vitamin E at a rate of approximately 250 to 500 IU/kg of diet may help to maintain lymphocyte proliferative activity in healthy cats and dogs. The suggested dose of γ-tocopherol, based on scientific literature, is 50 mg/kg. There are no specific recommendations reported regarding the choice of isomeric form (α or γ) for immunomodulation during critical illness or disease states in small animals.

Reported levels of total n3 fatty acids in commercial diets range between 0.20% and 7.3% dry matter basis (DMB). An initial total dose of n3 fatty acids at 50 to 250 mg/kg of BW per day seems to be effective in a large number of studies for its anti-inflammatory effect. Studies suggest a dietary n3 fatty acid concentration of 7.3% DMB (1348 mg per 100 kcal) as most beneficial for overall management of the canine cancer patient. A dietary n6:n3 fatty acid ratio of 1:1 or less is reported to reduce tumor marker expression significantly and to inhibit tumor growth in feline models.

SUMMARY

The complexity of the immune system allows for a multitude of potential avenues for nutrient modulation, but this also increases the challenge of producing a predictable in vivo response. Numerous studies have attempted to evaluate the clinical usefulness of specific nutrient supplementation as well as the benefit(s) of nutrient-enriched diets in modulating immunity. Because the immune response is a cascade of biologic events, development of nutritional support paradigms cannot and should not be made in a vacuum or with the expectation of a singular response. It is absolutely imperative that the clinician/nutritionist understand the differences in metabolic and physiologic responses to disease states (ie, shock, trauma, organ-specific dysfunction) so as to maximize immunocompetence through specialized feeding practices

More is not always better, especially when it come to immune enhancement. Timing, dosage, and duration criteria of nutritional immunomodulation need to be identified for specific disease states rather than making blanket recommendations. This takes further evaluation of nutrients, diets, and disease scenarios. Much of the human nutrition research takes this stepwise approach, and although progress is sometimes slow, nutrition support recommendations for disease states and health seem to be mechanism based. This level of understanding is invaluable, especially when considering the possible benefit of nutrient combinations for immunomodulation.

References
[1] Bower RH. Nutrition and immune function. Nutr Clin Pract 1990;5:189–95.
[2] Abbas AK, Lichtman AH, Pober JS. Cells and tissues of the immune system. In: Abbas AK, Lichtman AH, Pober JS, editors. Cellular and molecular immunology. Philadelphia: WB Saunders; 1991. p. 13–34.

[3] Shikora SA. Special nutrients for gut feeding. In: Shikora SA, Blackburn GL, editors. Nutrition support. Theory and therapeutics. New York: Chapman & Hall; 1997. p. 285–301.

[4] Rombeau JL. Enteral nutrition and critical illness. In: Borlase BC, Bell SJ, Blackburn GL, et al, editors. Enteral nutrition. New York: Chapman & Hall; 1994. p. 25–36.

[5] McCowen KC, Bistrain BR. Immunonutrition: problematic or problem solving? Am J Clin Nutr 2003;77:764–70.

[6] Smith RJ. Molecular biology in nutrition. Nutr Clin Pract 1992;7:5–15.

[7] Hammarqvist F, Wernerman J, Ali R, et al. Addition of glutamine to total parenteral nutrition after elective abdominal surgery spares free glutamine in muscle, counteracts the fall in muscle protein synthesis, and improves nitrogen balance. Ann Surg 1998;209:455–61.

[8] Jabba A, Chang W, Dryden GW, et al. Gut immunology and the differential response to feeding and starvation. Nutr Clin Pract 2003;18(6):461–82.

[9] Halliwell B. Antioxidants and human disease: a general introduction. Nutr Rev 1997; 55(1 Suppl):S44–52.

[10] Surai PF. Selenium-vitamin E interactions: does 1 + 1 equal more than 2? In: Lyons TP, Jacques KA, editors. Nutritional biotechnology in the feed and food industries. Proceedings of Alltech's 19th Annual Symposium. Nottingham (UK): Nottingham University Press; 2003. p. 59–76.

[11] Chandra RK. Nutrition, immunity and infection: present knowledge and future directions. Lancet 1983;1:688–91.

[12] Cerra FB, Holman RT, Bankley PE, et al. Nutritional pharmacology: its role in the hypermetabolism–organ failure syndrome. Crit Care Med 1990;18:S154–8.

[13] Still C, Apovian C, Jensen GL. Malnutrition and related complications. In: Shikora SA, Blackburn GL, editors. Nutrition support. Theory and therapeutics. New York: Chapman & Hall; 1997. p. 21–9.

[14] McMahon M, Bistrain BR. The physiology of nutritional assessment and therapy in protein calorie malnutrition. Dis Mon 1990;36:373–417.

[15] Shronts EP. Basic concepts of immunology and its application to clinical nutrition. Nutr Clin Pract 1993;8:177–83.

[16] Bistrain BR, Blackburn L, Scrimshaw NS, et al. Cellular immunity in semi-starved states in hospitalized patients. Am J Clin Nutr 1975;28:1148–55.

[17] Freitag KA, Saker KE, Thomas E, et al. Acute starvation and subsequent refeeding affect lymphocyte subsets and proliferation in cats. J Nutr 2000;130:2444–9.

[18] Simon JC, Saker K, Thomas E. Sensitivity of specific immune function tests to acute nutrient deprivation as indicators of nutritional status in a feline model. Nutr Res 2000; 20(1):79–89.

[19] Alexander JW, MacMillan BG, Stinnet JC, et al. Beneficial effects of aggressive protein feeding in severely burned children. Ann Surg 1980;192:505–7.

[20] Trocki O, Mochizuki H, Dominiono L, et al. Intact protein versus free amino acids in the nutritional support of thermally injured animals. JPEN J Parenter Enteral Nutr 1986;10: 139–45.

[21] Babineau TJ. Specific nutrients for the gastrointestinal tract: glutamine, arginine, nucleotides, and structured lipids. In: Borlase BC, Bell SJ, Blackburn GL, et al, editors. Enteral nutrition. New York: Chapman & Hall; 1994. p. 47–59.

[22] Barbul A. Arginine and immune function. Nutrition 1990;6:53–62.

[23] Calder PC, Yagoob P. Amino acids and immune function. In: Cynober LA, editor. Metabolic and therapeutic aspects if amino acids in clinical nutrition, Boca Raton (FL): CRC Press; 2004. p. 305–20.

[24] Luiking YC, Poeze M, Ramsay G, et al. The role of arginine in infection and sepsis. JPEN J Parenter Enteral Nutr 2005;29(1 Suppl):S70–4.

[25] Lind DS. Arginine and cancer. J Nutr 2004;134(Suppl):2837S–41S.

[26] Stechmiller JK, Childress B, Porter T. Arginine immunonutrition in critically ill patients: a clinical dilemma. Am J Crit Care 2004;13:17–23.

[27] Daly JM, Reynolds JV, Thom A, et al. Immune and metabolic effects of arginine in the surgical patient. Ann Surg 1998;208:512–23.

[28] Bansal V, Syres KM, Makarenkova V, et al. Interactions between fatty acids and arginine metabolism: implications for the design of immune-enhancing diets. JPEN J Parenter Enteral Nutr 2005;29(1 Suppl):S75–80.

[29] Ochoa JB, Makarenkova V, Bansal V. A rational use of immune enhancing diets; when should we use dietary arginine supplementation? NCP Bull 2004;19:216–25.

[30] Zaloga GP, Siddiqui R, Terry C, et al. Arginine: mediator or modulator of sepsis? NCP Bull 2004;19:201–15.

[31] Wischmeyer PE. Clinical application of L-glutamine: past, present, and future. Nutr Clin Pract 2003;18(5):377–85.

[32] Wischmeyer PE, Liedel JL, Lunch J, et al. Glutamine reduces gram negative bacteremia in severely burned patients. Crit Care Med 2001;29:2075–80.

[33] Hall JC, Dobb G, Hall J, et al. A clinical trial evaluating enteral glutamine in critically ill patients [abstract]. Am J Clin Nutr 2002;75(2):415S.

[34] Reitz S, Saker KE, Lanz O, et al. Evaluation of a short-term perioperative glutamine-supplemented parenteral nutrition on mucosal and peripheral immunity in dogs. Presented at the First Annual AAVN Clinical Nutrition and Research Symposium. Boston, July 14, 2001.

[35] Novak F, Heyland DK, Avenell A, et al. Glutamine supplementation in serious illness: a systematic review of the evidence. Crit Care Med 2002;30:2022–9.

[36] Ogawa AM. Macronutrient requirements. In: Shikora SA, Blackburn GL, editors. Nutrition support. Theory and therapeutics. New York: Chapman & Hall, 1997. p. 54–65.

[37] Serhan CN. Novel eicosanoid and docosanoid mediators: resolvins, docosatrienes, and neuroprotectins. Curr Opin Clin Nutr Metab Care 2005;8:115–21.

[38] Wan JM-F, Teo TC, Babayan VK, et al. Invited comment: lipids and the development of immune dysfunction and infection. JPEN J Parenter Enteral Nutr 1988;12(Suppl):43s–52s.

[39] Martindale R, Miles I. Is immunonutrition ready for prime time? Two points of view. Nutr Clin Pract 2003;18(6):489–96.

[40] Babcock TA, Dekoj T, Espat NJ. Experimental studies defining ω-3 fatty acid anti-inflammatory mechanisms and abrogation of tumor-related syndromes. Nutr Clin Pract 2005;20(1): 62–74.

[41] Cowing BE, Saker KE. Polyunsaturated fatty acids and epidermal growth factor receptor/mitogen-activated protein kinase signaling in mammary cancer. J Nutr 2001;131:1125–8.

[42] Morrison DC, Ryan JL. Bacterial endotoxins and host immune response. In: Dixon FJ, Kunkel HG, editors. Advances in immunology. New York: Academic Press; 1980. p. 293–450.

[43] Melis GC, van Leeuwen PAM, Von Blomberg-van der Flier BME, et al. A carbohydrate-rich beverage prior to surgery prevents surgery-induced immunodepression: A randomized, controlled, clinical trial. JPEN J Parenter Enteral Nutr 2006;30:21–6.

[44] Van den Berghe G, Wouters P, Weekers F, et al. Intensive insulin therapy in the critically ill patients. N Engl J Med 2001;345:1359–67.

[45] Martindale RG, Cresci G. Preventing infectious complications with nutrition intervention. JPEN J Parenter Enteral Nutr 2005;29(1 Suppl):S53–6.

[46] McCowen KC, Bistrain BR. Hyperglycemia and nutrition support: theory and practice. Nutr Clin Pract 2004;19(3):235–44.

[47] Lukasewycz OA, Prohaska JR. The immune response in copper deficiency. In: Bendich A, Chandra RK, editors. Micronutrients and immune functions. Cytokines and metabolism. New York: The New York Academy of Sciences; 1990. p. 147–59.

[48] Saker KE, Allen VG, Kalnitsky J, et al. Monocyte immune cell response and copper status in beef steers grazed on endophyte-infected tall fescue. J Anim Sci 1998;76: 2694–700.

[49] Failla ML. Nutritional and biochemical considerations of the immunosuppressive influence of copper deficiency. Presented at the International Conference Series on Nutrition and

Health Promotion. Conference of Nutrition and Immunity. Atlanta (GA); May 5–7, 1997. p. 15.

[50] Chandra RK. Micronutrients and immune function. An overview. In: Bendich A, Chandra RK, editors. Micronutrients and immune functions. Cytokines and metabolism. New York: The New York Academy of Sciences; 1990. p. 9–16.

[51] Fraker PJ, King LA. Lymphopoiesis, myelopoiesis, and hematopoiesis in the zinc deficient rodent. Presented at the International Conference Series and Health Promotion. Conference of Nutrition and Immunity. Atlanta (GA); May 5–7, 1997. p. 17.

[52] Bendich A. Antioxidant micronutrients and immune responses. In: Bendich A, Chandra RK, editors. Micronutrients and immune functions. Cytokines and metabolism. New York: The New York Academy of Sciences; 1990. p. 168–80.

[53] Sherman AR. Influences of iron on immunity and disease resistance. In: Bendich A, Chandra RK, editors. Micronutrients and immune functions. Cytokines and metabolism. New York: The New York Academy of Sciences; 1990. p. 140–6.

[54] Surai PF. Antioxidant protection in the intestine: a good beginning is half the battle. In: Lyons TP, Jacques KA, editors. Nutritional biotechnology in the feed and food industries. Proceedings of Alltech's 18th Annual Symposium. Nottingham (UK): Nottingham University Press; 2002. p. 301–21.

[55] Stewart MS, Spallholz JE, Neldner KH, et al. Selenium compounds have disparate abilities to impose stress and induce apoptosis. Free Radic Biol Med 1999;26:42–8.

[56] Sun E, Xu H, Wen D, et al. Inhibition of lipid peroxidation. Biol Trace Elem Res 1997;59: 87–92.

[57] Seo YR, Sweeney C, Smith ML. Selenomethionine induction of DNA repair response in human fibroblasts. Oncogene 2001;21:3663–9.

[58] Roussyn I, Briviba K, Masumoto H, et al. Selenium-containing compounds protect DNA from single-strand breaks caused by peroxynitrite. Arch Biochem Biophys 1996;330:216–8.

[59] Shen CL, Song W, Pence BC. Interactions of selenium compounds with other antioxidants in DNA damage and apoptosis in human normal keratinocytes. Cancer Epidemiol Biomarkers Prev 2001;10:385–90.

[60] Waters DJ, Shen S, Cooley DM, et al. Effects of dietary selenium supplementation on DNA damage and apoptosis in canine prostate. J Natl Cancer Inst 2003;95:237–41.

[61] Hayek MG, Massimino SP, Burr JR, et al. Dietary vitamin E improves immune function in cats. In: Reinhart GA, Carey DP, editors. Recent advances in canine and feline nutrition. Proceedings of the Iams 2000 Nutrition Symposium. Wilmington (OH): Orange Frazer Press; 2000. p. 555–63.

[62] Meydani SN, Hayek MG, Wu D, et al. Vitamin E and immune response in aged dogs. In: Reinhart GA, Carey DP, editors. Recent advances in canine and feline nutrition. Proceedings of the Iams 1998 Nutrition Symposium. Wilmington (OH): Orange Frazer Press; 2000. p. 295–303.

[63] Jiang Q, Christen S, Shigenaga MK, et al. γ-Tocopherol, the major form of vitamin E in the US diet, deserves more attention. Am J Clin Nutr 2001;74:714–22.

[64] Jiang Q, Ames BN. Gamma-tocopherol, but not alpha-tocopherol, decreases proinflammatory eicosanoids and inflammation damage in rats. FASEB J 2003;17(8):816–22.

[65] Baumgartner TG, Henderson G, Baumgartner SL. Micronutrients in clinical nutrition. In: Shikora SA, Blackburn GL, editors. Nutrition support. Theory and therapeutics. New York: Chapman & Hall; 1997. p. 66–90.

Vet Clin Small Anim 36 (2006) 1225–1241

VETERINARY CLINICS
SMALL ANIMAL PRACTICE

ELSEVIER
SAUNDERS

Nutrition in Critical Illness

Daniel L. Chan, DVM, MRCVS[a],*,
Lisa M. Freeman, DVM, PhD[b]

[a]Department of Veterinary Clinical Sciences, The Royal Veterinary College, University of
London, Hawkshead Lane Medicine, North Mymms, Hertfordshire AL97TA, United Kingdom
[b]Department of Clinical Sciences, Cummings School of Veterinary Medicine, Tufts University,
200 Westboro Road, North Grafton, MA 01536, USA

G reat advances have been made recently in the field of critical care nutrition. Although nutrition was once regarded as a supportive measure of low priority, it is increasingly being recognized as an important therapeutic intervention in the care of critically ill patients.

In human ICUs, nutrition not only provides supportive therapy but is also becoming a means to modulate even severe diseases. Although the developing applications are still years away from being standards in veterinary medicine, this trend highlights the possibilities of critical care nutrition in veterinary medicine. The current focus of veterinary critical care nutrition, and the major focus of this article, is on carefully selecting the patients most likely to benefit from nutritional support, deciding when to intervene, and optimizing nutritional support to individual patients.

RATIONALE FOR NUTRITIONAL SUPPORT IN CRITICAL ILLNESS

Critical illness induces unique metabolic changes in animals that put them at high risk for malnutrition and its deleterious effects. An important distinction in the body's response to inadequate nutritional intake occurs in disease (stressed starvation) compared with a healthy state (simple starvation). During acute fasting in the healthy state, use of glycogen stores is the primary source of energy. However, glycogen stores are quickly depleted, especially in strict carnivores such as the cat, and lead to the initial mobilization of amino acids from muscle stores. Within days, a metabolic shift occurs toward the preferential use of stored fat deposits, sparing catabolic effects on lean muscle tissue. In diseased states, the inflammatory response triggers alterations in cytokines and hormone concentrations and shifts metabolism toward a catabolic state. With a lack of food intake, the predominant energy source is derived from accelerated proteolysis, which in itself is an energy-consuming process. Thus, these animals may preserve fat deposits in the face of lean muscle tissue loss.

*Corresponding author. E-mail address: dchan@rvc.ac.uk (D.L. Chan).

0195-5616/06/$ – see front matter
doi:10.1016/j.cvsm.2006.08.009

These shifts in metabolism commonly result in significant negative nitrogen and energy balance. The consequences of continued lean body mass losses include negative effects on wound healing, immune function, strength (both skeletal and respiratory), and ultimately overall prognosis. Although the relationship between malnutrition and clinical outcome has not been proven definitively in companion animals, people experiencing malnutrition and critical illness have been documented to have poorer outcomes [1,2]. The immediate goal of providing nutritional support to hospitalized patients is not to achieve weight gain, per se, which mostly likely reflects shift in water balance, but rather to minimize further loss of lean body mass. Reversal of malnutrition hinges on resolution of the primary underlying disease. Nutritional support has the goal of restoring nutrient deficiencies, providing key substrate for healing and repair, and minimizing the development of malnutrition.

PATIENT SELECTION

As with any intervention in critically ill animals, nutritional support has some risk for complications and the potential to benefit. The risk for complications most likely increases with disease severity and the clinician must consider many factors in deciding to institute nutritional support. Of utmost importance, patients must be cardiovascularly stable before any nutritional support is initiated. In states of shock, perfusion of the gastrointestinal tract is often reduced in favor of maintaining adequate perfusion of heart, brain, and lungs. With reduced perfusion, processes such as gastrointestinal motility, digestion, and nutrient assimilation are altered, and feeding under these circumstances will probably result in more complications. An important goal of nutritional support for critically ill patients is to minimize risk for complications. Other factors that should be addressed before nutritional intervention include dehydration, electrolytes imbalances, and abnormalities in acid–base status.

In animals that have been stabilized, the appropriate time to start nutritional support should also be decided carefully. The number of days an animal has not consumed adequate calories before hospitalization must be determined from the history and added to the number of days during hospitalization that the animal has not consumed any significant amounts of food. Documentation of total days without adequate nutrition should be listed in the patient's daily progress notes to ensure that nutritional support remains an important therapeutic goal. The previous notion that nutritional support is unnecessary until 10 days of inadequate nutritional support have elapsed is certainly outdated and unjustified. Although commencing nutritional support within 3 days of hospitalization, even before diagnosing the underlying disease, is a more appropriate goal in most cases, other factors should be considered.

NUTRITIONAL ASSESSMENT

Because objective measures of nutritional status (eg, anthropometry, bioelectrical impedance, dual energy x-ray absorptiometry, serum indicators of malnutrition) have limited availability in clinical veterinary medicine, subjective assessment of malnutrition is important in identifying patients needing nutritional support. Proposed indicators of malnutrition include unintentional weight loss (typically greater than 10%), poor haircoat quality, muscle wasting, signs of inadequate wound healing, hypoalbuminemia, lymphopenia, and coagulopathy. These abnormalities are not specific to malnutrition and often occur late in the disease process. Evaluating overall body condition is emphasized rather than simply noting body weight. Fluid shifts may significantly impact body weight, whereas body condition scores (BCSs) are not influenced by these changes. BCSs, discussed elsewhere in this issue, have been shown to be reproducible, reliable, and clinically useful measures in nutritional assessment [3]. However, body condition scoring schemes were designed and validated to assess body fat and do not incorporate loss of lean body tissue. A muscle condition score has been proposed to enhance nutritional assessment, but further studies are needed to show its clinical usefulness [4].

Because of the limitations in assessing nutritional status, early risk factors must be identified that may predispose patients to malnutrition, such as anorexia lasting more than 5 days, serious underlying disease (eg, severe trauma, sepsis, peritonitis, acute pancreatitis, major gastrointestinal surgery), and large protein losses (eg, protracted vomiting, diarrhea, protein-losing nephropathics, draining wounds, burns). Nutritional assessment also identifies factors that can impact the nutritional plan, such as specific electrolyte abnormalities, hyperglycemia, hypertriglyceridemia, hyperammonemia, or comorbid illnesses, such as renal, cardiac, or hepatic disease. In the presence of these abnormalities, the nutritional plan should be adjusted accordingly to limit acute exacerbations of any pre-existing condition.

Finally, because many techniques required for nutritional support necessitate anesthesia, (eg, placement of most feedings tubes, intravenous catheters for parenteral nutrition), patients must be properly evaluated and stabilized before undergoing anesthesia, regardless of the urgency to implement nutritional support. When patients are deemed too unstable to undergo general anesthesia, temporary measures of nutritional support that do not require anesthesia (eg, nasoesophageal tube placement, placement of peripheral catheters for partial parenteral nutrition) should be considered. Once patients are deemed stable enough to undergo general anesthesia, more effective means of nutritional support can be implemented.

NUTRITIONAL PLAN

Successful nutritional management of critically ill patients relies on the proper diagnosis and treatment of the underlying disease, although nutritional support should not be delayed until a diagnosis is made. Nutrition should be provided as soon as it is feasible. After the need for support is established, the appropriate route of nutritional support should be determined. Providing nutrition through a functional digestive system is the preferred route of feeding, and the patient's tolerance to enteral feeding routes should be evaluated carefully.

Even if patients can only tolerate small amounts of enteral nutrition, this route of feeding should be pursued and supplemented with parenteral nutrition (PN) as necessary to meet nutritional needs. However, if an animal shows complete intolerance to enteral feeding, some form of PN should be provided. Based on the nutritional and medical assessment, the anticipated duration of nutritional support, and the route of delivery (ie, enteral or parenteral), a nutritional plan is formulated to meet nutritional needs and support healing or recovery from the disease process. The nutritional plan should be instituted gradually with the goal of reaching target level of nutrient delivery in 48 to 72 hours. The nutritional plan is adjusted based on reassessment and the changing medical status.

CALCULATING NUTRITIONAL REQUIREMENTS

Ideally, nutritional support should provide ample substrates for gluconeogenesis, protein synthesis, and energy necessary to maintain homeostasis without causing complications. Sufficient calories should be provided to sustain critical physiologic processes, such as immune function, wound repair, and cell division and growth. Total energy expenditure must be measured to precisely determine caloric needs. Although a few studies have used indirect calorimetry to estimate energy expenditure in select populations of veterinary patients, the use of mathematical formulas remains the only practical means of estimating the patient's daily caloric requirement.

Results of indirect calorimetry studies in dogs support the recent trend of formulating nutritional support to meet resting energy requirements (RER) rather than more generous illness energy requirements [5,6]. Until recently, many clinicians multiplied the RER by an illness factor between 1.1 and 2.0 to account for a presumed increase in metabolism associated with different diseases and injuries. More conservative energy estimates (ie, starting with the animal's RER) are currently recommended to avoid overfeeding and its associated complications [7,8]. A recent study showed an association between the use of illness factors and the development of hyperglycemia in cats administered total parenteral nutrition (TPN) [9], whereas another found a negative association between the development of hyperglycemia and poor outcome [10]. Furthermore, overfeeding energy can result in gastrointestinal complications, hepatic dysfunction, and increased carbon dioxide production [11].

Although several formulas have been proposed to calculate the RER, a widely used allometric formula can be applied to both dogs and cats of all weights. This formula, most commonly used by the authors, is:

$$RER = 70 \times (\text{current body weight in kg})^{0.75}$$

Alternatively, for animals weighing between 3 and 25 kg, the following may be used:

$$RER = (30 \times \text{current body weight in kg}) + 70$$

Other veterinary nutritionists recommend using the animal's ideal body weight in these equations, which differs from the authors' recommendations, particularly in critically ill animals for which the authors believe using ideal body weight is inappropriate. To avoid overfeeding underweight animals, the authors recommend using the animal's current weight for the RER calculation. Animals that are overweight should be fed the appropriate number of calories to avoid weight loss, because seriously ill or injured animals lose more lean body mass than fat. Nutritional requirements in significantly overweight animals (ie, >25% above ideal body weight) can be calculated in several ways. One is to use the animal's current body weight for the RER calculation and adjust to maintain weight. Another option assumes that 25% of excess weight is lean tissue and the remaining 75% is metabolically inactive fat (ie, if a dog's ideal weight is 20 kg and he weighs 30 kg, he has 10 kg of excess weight, 2.5 kg of which is lean tissue and 7.5 kg of which is fat). Therefore, the ideal weight plus 25% of the excess weight (to account for the extra lean body mass) can be used to calculate RER. Using the 30-kg dog whose ideal weight is 20 kg, the adjusted body weight to use to calculate RER would be 20 kg + (25% × 10 kg) or 20 kg + 2.5 kg = 22.5 kg. Thus, the RER for this overweight dog would be 723 kcal/d.

Although nitrogen balance is often used to determine the protein requirements of critically ill people, this is not commonly measured in critically ill animals. One method of estimating the extent of amino acid catabolism is to measure 24-hour urinary urea nitrogen content. Although measuring urinary urea nitrogen in critically ill dogs has been shown to be a feasible tool in assessing nitrogen balance, further studies are warranted to better characterize the protein requirements of critically ill animals [12]. Experts currently recommend that hospitalized dogs be supported with 4 to 6 g of protein per 100 kcal (15%–25% of total energy requirements), whereas cats are usually supported with 6 or more grams of protein per 100 kcal (25%–35% of total energy requirements) [8]. Protein requirements are usually estimated based on clinical judgment and the recognition that protein requirements are markedly increased during certain diseases (eg, peritonitis, draining wounds). Further studies are clearly needed to better characterize the protein requirements of critically ill animals.

PARENTERAL NUTRITIONAL SUPPORT

PN can be delivered through a central vein (total parenteral nutrition) or a peripheral vein (peripheral or partial parenteral nutrition). TPN, as defined in this article, is the provision of all of the animal's calorie and protein requirements. Partial parenteral nutrition (PPN) only supplies part of the animal's energy, protein, and other nutrient requirements [7], which can be administered through either a peripheral or central vein.

Because TPN supplies all calorie and protein requirements, it is often the preferred modality for an animal requiring PN. The disadvantages are that it requires a jugular venous catheter, is slightly more expensive (with solutions costing typically approximately 10%–20% more than a PPN solution for the same sized animal), and may be associated with more metabolic complications. PPN may be an alternative to TPN in selected cases, but clinicians must be aware that it will not provide all of the animal's requirements. Both TPN and PPN are typically a combination of dextrose, an amino acid solution, and a lipid solution. The concentration of some components (eg, dextrose, lipid) varies depending on the disease state and whether TPN or PPN is chosen.

Crystalline amino acid solutions are essential components of PN. The importance of supplying amino acids relates to the maintenance of positive nitrogen balance and repletion of lean body tissue, which may be vital in the recovery of critically ill patients. Supplementation of amino acids may support protein synthesis and spare tissue proteins from being catabolized through gluconeogenesis. The most commonly used amino acid solutions contain most essential amino acids for dogs and cats, except taurine. However, because PN is typically not used beyond 10 days, the lack of taurine does not become a problem in most circumstances. Amino acid solutions are available in different concentrations from 3.5% to 15%, but the most commonly used concentration is 8.5%. Amino acid solutions are also available with and without electrolytes. Animals that have normal serum electrolytes typically receive amino acid solutions with electrolytes, whereas patients who have electrolyte disturbances may benefit from amino acid solutions without electrolytes so that they can be individually corrected.

Lipid emulsions are the calorically dense component of PN and a source of essential fatty acids. Lipid emulsions are isotonic and are available in 10% to 30% solutions. These commercially available lipid emulsions are made primarily of soybean and safflower oil and provide predominantly long-chain polyunsaturated fatty acids, including linoleic, oleic, palmitic, and stearic acids. These solutions are emulsified with egg yolk phospholipids and their tonicity is adjusted with glycerol. The emulsified fat particles are comparable in size to chylomicrons and are removed from the circulation through the action of peripheral lipoprotein lipase.

A common misconception exists regarding the use of lipids in pancreatitis. Although hypertriglyceridemia may be risk factor for pancreatitis, infusions of lipids have not been shown to increase pancreatic secretion or worsen pancreatitis and are therefore considered safe [13], The one exception, however, is in cases where serum triglycerides are elevated, indicating a clear failure of triglyceride clearance. According to the most recent guidelines provided by the American Society for Parenteral and Enteral Nutrition, human patients with serum triglycerides exceeding 400 mg/dL should have the lipid proportion in PN markedly reduced or eliminated altogether [13]. Although specific data on the maximal safe level of lipid administration in veterinary patients are not available, maintaining normal serum triglycerides levels in patients undergoing PN seems prudent. Another concern about using lipids in PN is their purported immunosuppressive effects from impairing the reticuloendothelial system, particularly in PN solutions containing a high percentage of lipid. Despite in vitro evidence supporting the notion that lipid infusions can also suppress neutrophil and lymphocyte function, studies have not correlated lipid use and increased rates of infectious complications.

Electrolytes, vitamins, and trace elements also may be added to the PN formulation. Depending on the hospital and the individual patient, electrolytes can be added individually to the admixture, added as an electrolyte mixture, included as part of the amino acid solution, or left out altogether and managed separately through the animal's other fluids. Amino acids with or without electrolytes can be included, based on clinician preference. Because most animals undergo PN for only a short duration, fat-soluble vitamins usually are not limiting and therefore supplementing human TPN with vitamin preparations is usually not indicated. The exception is obviously malnourished animals in which supplementation may be desirable.

However, because B vitamins are water soluble, they are more likely to become deficient, particularly in anorectic animals and those with high-volume diuresis (eg, renal failure, diabetes). Therefore, supplementing B vitamins in the PN admixture may be appropriate in certain animals. Some authors recommend vitamin K supplements for animals undergoing PN because PN is believed to be low in vitamin K (it is generally administered subcutaneously on day 1 of TPN and then once weekly). Because vitamin K deficiency is unlikely to occur, particularly when a lipid emulsion is used, the authors do not routinely supplement vitamin K unless the animal's underlying disease indicates the need. Trace elements serve as cofactors in various enzyme systems and can become deficient in malnourished animals or those undergoing long-term PN. In people undergoing PN, zinc, copper, manganese, and chromium are routinely included in the PN admixture. These nutrients are sometimes added to PN for malnourished animals, but the authors do not routinely include them. Nonetheless, because zinc and vitamin B status may be important for normal smell, taste, and appetite, supplementing these nutrients could be considered.

Although adding other parenteral medications to the PN admixture is possible, their compatibility must be verified first. Drugs that are known to be compatible and are sometimes added to PN include heparin, insulin, potassium chloride, and metoclopramide. Although the addition of insulin to PN is often required in people undergoing PN, the hyperglycemia seen in veterinary patients undergoing PN does not usually require insulin administration, except in those with diabetes who will require adjustments to their insulin regimen.

PARENTERAL NUTRITION COMPOUNDING

Based on the nutritional assessment and plan, PN can be formulated according to the worksheets found in Appendices 1 and 2. For TPN (see Appendix 1), the first step is calculating the patient's energy needs or RER. Protein requirements (grams of protein required per day) are then determined, taking into consideration factors such as excessive protein losses or severe hepatic or renal disease. Although some nutritionists believe that the energy requirements are supplied by the dextrose and lipid portion of the PN, the authors apply the energy provided by amino acids to the energy calculations, subtracting it from the daily RER to establish the total nonprotein calories required. The nonprotein calories are then usually provided as a 50:50 mixture of lipids and dextrose, although this ratio can be adjusted in cases of persistent hyperglycemia or hypertriglyceridemia (eg, a higher proportion of calories would be provided by lipids in an animal with hyperglycemia). The calories provided by each component (amino acids, lipids, and dextrose) are then divided by their respective caloric densities and the exact amounts of each component are added to the PN bags in an aseptic fashion. The amount of TPN delivered often provides less than the patient's daily fluid requirement. Additional fluids can be either added to the PN bag at compounding or provided as a separate infusion.

Appendix 2 provides a step-by-step protocol for formulating PPN, in which patients of various sizes can receive 70% of their RER and approximately meet their daily maintenance fluid requirement. In very small animals ($\leq$3 kg), the amount of PPN will exceed the maintenance fluid requirement and increase the risk for fluid overload, so adjustments may be necessary. Furthermore, in animals requiring conservative fluid administration (eg, those with congestive heart failure), these calculations for PPN may provide more fluid then would be safe. In this formulation, the proportion of each PN component depends on the weight of the patient, so that a smaller animal (between 3 and 5 kg) receives proportionally more calories from lipids than a large dog (>30 kg), which would receive more calories in the form of carbohydrates. Therefore, the resulting formulation approximates the patient's daily fluid requirement.

Ideally, PN should be compounded aseptically under a laminar flow hood using a semiautomated, closed-system, PN compounder (eg, Automix compounder, Clintec Nutrition, Deerfield, Illinois). If an automated compounder is not available, manual compounding can be performed in a clean, low-traffic area with strict adherence to aseptic technique using a 3-in-1 bag (eg, All-In-One EVA container, Clintec Nutrition, Deerfield, Illinois). Because of these ideal conditions, having a local human hospital, compounding pharmacies, or a human home health care company compound PN solutions is often easier and more cost-effective. Alternatively, commercial ready-to-use preparations of glucose or glycerol and amino acids suitable for (peripheral) intravenous administration are available. Although ready-to-use preparations are convenient, they provide only 30% to 50% of caloric requirements when administered at maintenance fluid rates and therefore should only be used for interim nutritional support or to supplement low-dose enteral feedings.

PARENTERAL NUTRITION ADMINISTRATION

Administering any PN requires a dedicated catheter used solely for PN administration that is placed using aseptic technique. In most cases, additional catheters are required because PN should not be administered through existing catheters that were placed for reasons other than PN. Long catheters composed of silicone, polyurethane, or tetrafluoroethylene are recommended for any type of PN to reduce the risk for thrombophlebitis. Multilumen catheters are often recommended for TPN because they can remain in place for long periods, and separate ports can be used for blood sampling and administering additional fluids and intravenous medications without needing separate catheters at other sites. Although placement of multilumen catheters requires more technical skills than conventional jugular catheters, they can be effective in treating critically ill patients. Because of the high osmolarity of TPN solutions (often 1200 mOsm/L), they must be administered through a central venous (jugular) catheter, whereas PPN solutions can be administered through either a jugular catheter or catheters placed in peripheral veins. High osmolarity is a concern because it may increase the incidence of thrombophlebitis, although this has not been well characterized in veterinary patients.

Because of the various metabolic derangements associated with critical illness, TPN should be instituted gradually over 48 hours. In the authors' respective institutions, TPN is typically initiated at 50% of the RER on the first day and then increased to the targeted amount by the second day. In most cases, PPN can be started without gradual increase. Adjusting the rates of other fluids being administered concurrently is also important. For TPN and PPN, the animal's catheter and infusion lines must always be handled aseptically to reduce the risk for PN-related infections. Even with aseptic technique, injections into the PN catheter infusion port or administration lines should be strictly prohibited because many drugs and solutions are incompatible with PN solutions. Drug incompatibilities can result in precipitates, alter the lipid emulsion, and possibly lead to pulmonary embolism and patient death.

PN should be administered as continuous rate infusions over 24 hours through fluid infusion pumps. Inadvertent delivery of massive amounts of PN can result if administration is not properly regulated. Once a bag of PN is set up for administration, it is not disconnected from the patient even for walks or diagnostic procedures; the drip regulator is decreased to a slow drip and accompanies the patient throughout the hospital. Administering PN through an 1.2-μm in-line filter is also recommended and is attached at setup. This setup process is performed daily with each new bag of PN. Each bag should only hold a day's worth of PN, and the accompanying fluid administration sets and in-line filter are also changed using aseptic technique. PN should discontinue when the animal resumes consuming an adequate amount of calories of at least 50% of RER. TPN should be gradually discontinued over 6 to 12 hours. Abrupt discontinuation can cause hypoglycemia when the concentrated dextrose solution is discontinued in the face of high endogenous insulin secretion by the patient. PPN can be discontinued without weaning.

ENTERAL NUTRITIONAL SUPPORT

Feeding tubes are the standard mode of nutritional support in critically ill animals that have a functional gastrointestinal tract. Nasoesophageal, esophagostomy, gastrostomy, and jejunostomy feeding tubes are the most commonly used. In animals undergoing laparotomy, placing gastrotomy or jejunostomy feeding tubes should particularly be considered. Newer techniques that incorporate an intraluminal jejunal tube through a gastrostomy tube were also developed. The decision to use one tube over another is based on the anticipated duration of nutritional support (eg, days vs. months), the need to circumvent certain segments of the gastrointestinal tract (eg, oropharnyx, esophagitis, pancreatitis), clinician experience, and the patient's ability to withstand anesthesia (very critical animals may only tolerate placement of nasoesophageal feeding tubes). In-depth instructions for placing feeding tubes have been provided in the literature [14–19].

The major advantages of nasoesophageal feeding tubes are that they are simple to place; require minimal, if any, sedation; and require no special equipment. Because this procedure is largely blind, verifying placement of the tube within the esophagus using radiography or an end-tidal carbon dioxide monitor is recommended [20]. Tubes placed within the gastrointestinal tract should yield no carbon dioxide when checked [20]. Disadvantages of nasoesophageal tubes include patient discomfort and the exclusive use of liquid diets because tubes typically measure 3.5 to 5 Fr.

Esophageal feeding tubes are an excellent choice for many critically ill animals and have completely supplanted the need for pharyngostomy tubes. They are also easy to place, require only brief anesthesia, and can accommodate more calorically-dense diets (ie, >1 kcal/mL), making them ideal for patients that have feeding-volume limitations. Tubes ranging from 12 to 19 Fr are commonly used and patient discomfort is usually not an issue. The most common problems associated with this tube are tube obstruction and cellulitis at the stoma site. Intermittent bolus feeding is usually used with these tubes, but low-rate continuous infusions can be used for animals that cannot tolerate bolus feeding.

Surgically placed and percutaneous-guided gastrostomy tubes (PEG) are good options for patients undergoing laparotomy and endoscopy, respectively. These tubes can be used for long-term nutritional support (ie, months) and feeding is usually performed through bolus feeding. Gastrostomy feeding tubes are the largest feeding tubes (16–32 Fr) and can deliver most diets after blenderizing. Placing PEG tubes requires special equipment and considerable experience, but can be effective. Complications associated with these tubes range from mild cellulitis around the stoma site to more serious life-threatening peritonitis. Premature tube dislodgement (before 14 days) should be immediately evaluated for the need for possible surgery.

Animals requiring laparotomy and deemed to require bypass of the stomach or pancreas (eg, significant stomach wall resection, severe pancreatitis, pancreatectomy) should have a jejunostomy feeding tube placed. These tubes are similar in size to nasoesophageal tubes and therefore can only accommodate liquid diets. Feeding through these tubes should also be performed through continuous infusions (eg, 1 mL/kg/h initially and slowly increased) rather than bolus feeding. Complications associated with these feeding tubes include tube occlusion, diarrhea, and dislodgement resulting in peritonitis [21]. Placing jejunal tubes through gastrostomy tubes offers a certain degree of versatility in that the nutrients can be administered to the mid-distal jejunum without the need for a jejunostomy [15,19]. However, this technique has limited experience and possible complications have not been adequately described.

A common misconception is that animals fed through feeding tubes will not eat voluntarily, and therefore feedings are withheld to evaluate the animal's appetite. However, the main purpose of nutritional support is to provide nutrients and calories that the animal needs, and therefore less emphasis should be placed on appetite per se. Anorexia should be corrected once the primary disease is addressed. Weaning animals from tube feedings while they are still hospitalized is discouraged; this is more appropriate after discharge while the animal is recovering in its own environment. Because feeding regimens should have been reduced to three or four times daily by discharge, owners can be instructed to offer oral feeding before each tube feeding so they can monitor for the return of adequate spontaneous feeding. Based on reassessment by the clinician, tube feedings can then be reduced or discontinued depending on progress made.

MONITORING FOR COMPLICATIONS

Because the development of complications in critically ill animals can have serious consequences, it is an important aspect of nutritional support that involves close monitoring. With implementation of enteral nutrition, possible complications include vomiting, diarrhea, fluid overload, electrolyte imbalances, feeding tube malfunction, and infectious complications associated with insertion sites of feeding tubes. Metabolic complications are more common with PN and include the development of hyperglycemia, lipemia, azotemia, hyperammonemia, cholestasis, and electrolyte abnormalities. Rarely, nutritional support can be associated with severe abnormalities that are sometimes referred to as the *refeeding syndrome* [22,23]. Strategies to reduce risk for complications include using aseptic techniques when placing feeding tubes and intravenous catheters, using conservative estimates of energy requirements (ie, RER), and paying careful attention to nutritional assessment. Frequent monitoring and adjusting the nutritional plan if complications arise are important aspects of reassessment. Parameters that should be monitored during nutritional support include body temperature, respiratory rate and effort, signs of fluid overload (eg, chemosis, increased body weight), and serum concentrations of glucose, triglyceride, electrolytes, packed cell volume, total protein, and blood urea nitrogen/creatinine.

PHARMACOLOGIC AGENTS IN NUTRITIONAL SUPPORT

Because critically ill animals are often anorexic, the temptation exists to use appetite stimulants to increase food intake. Unfortunately, appetite stimulants are generally unreliable and seldom result in adequate food intake in critically ill animals. Pharmacologic stimulation of appetite is often short-lived and only delays true nutritional support. The authors do not believe appetite stimulants should be used to manage hospitalized animals when more effective measures of nutritional support, such as placement of feeding tubes, are more appropriate. Appetite stimulants may be considered in recovering animals once they are home in their own environment, because the primary reason for loss of appetite should ideally be reversed by discharge. As with many drugs, appetite stimulants also have negative side effects, such as behavioral changes associated with cyproheptadine and sedation associated with diazepam, and therefore should be used with caution.

Other agents commonly used in critically ill animals that have gastrointestinal dysfunction include antiemetics, H_2 blockers, and prokinetics. Similar to appetite stimulants, these drugs have not been formally evaluated in critically ill animals. A recent prospective study in dogs with parvoenteritis and early enteral nutrition incorporated the use of metoclopramide (an antiemetic and prokinetic agent) in the treatment of all dogs enrolled [24]. Tolerance to enteral feeding was remarkably good considering the usual clinical course of parvoenteritis [24]. A more recent retrospective study of parvoenteritis in dogs proposed that metoclopramide was associated with increased hospitalization and did not show a benefit [25]. Although phenothiazine derivatives, such as prochlorperazine and chlorpromazine, also have antiemetic properties, the risk for hypotension precludes their use in many critically ill animals. A more potent class of antiemetics, the $5HT_3$ antagonists, is increasingly being used despite a lack of formal evaluation in animals. Drugs in this class include ondansetron and dolasetron, which were first used to treat chemotherapy-induced nausea in people and then animals and are now used routinely to treat critically ill animals. Although antiemetics and prokinetic agents probably have a place in veterinary critical care, further studies are needed to define their role and optimal use.

FUTURE DIRECTIONS IN CRITICAL CARE NUTRITION

The current state of veterinary critical care nutrition revolves around proper recognition of animals requiring nutritional support and implementing strategies to best provide nutritional therapies. Important areas needing further evaluation in critically ill animals include the optimal composition and caloric target of nutritional support and strategies to minimize complications and optimize outcome. Recent studies implicating poor clinical outcome in the development of hyperglycemia in critically ill people have led to more vigilant monitoring and stricter control of blood glucose, with obvious implications for nutritional support [26–29]. Evidence of a similar relationship in dogs and cats is mounting, and ongoing studies are focusing on the possible consequences of hyperglycemia for clinical outcome in the veterinary ICU [9,10,30–32]. Until further studies suggest otherwise, efforts to reduce the incidence of hyperglycemia in critically ill animals, especially those undergoing nutritional support, should be strongly pursued.

Other exciting areas of clinical nutrition in critical care include the use of special nutrients that possess immunomodulatory properties, such as glutamine, arginine, n-3 fatty acids, and antioxidants. In specific patient populations, these nutrients, used singly or in combination, have shown promising results [33–35]. However, the response has not been consistent, and ongoing trials continue to evaluate their efficacy [36–38]. Limited information is available on using these nutrients to specifically modulate disease in clinically affected animals. Two studies using enteral glutamine have not shown any benefit [39,40]. A recent study did not show a depletion of glutamine in critically ill dogs that had several illnesses, but showed a marked decrease in arginine compared with healthy controls [41]. Future studies should focus on whether manipulating these nutrients offers any benefit in animals. Further development of veterinary critical care nutrition may transition nutrition from a strictly supportive measure to one designed to modulate disease and outcome.

APPENDIX 1. WORKSHEET FOR CALCULATING A TOTAL PARENTERAL NUTRITION FORMULATION

1. Resting energy requirement (RER):
   $70 \times$ (current body weight in kg)$^{0.75}$ = kcal/d
   or for animals 3–25 kg, can also use:
   $30 \times$ (current body weight in kg) + 70 = kcal/d
   RER = _____kcal/d

2. Protein requirements:

	Canine	Feline
Standard	4–5 g/100 kcal	6 g/100 kcal
Decreased requirements (hepatic/renal failure)[a]	2–3 g/100 kcal	3–4 g/100 kcal
Increased requirements (protein-losing conditions)[a]	6 g/100 kcal	6 g/100 kcal

   (RER ÷ 100) × _____g/100 kcal = _____g protein required/d
   Protein requirement:_____

3. Volumes of nutrient solutions required each day:

   a. 8.5% amino acid solution = 0.085 g protein/mL
   _____g protein/d required ÷ 0.085 g/mL = _____mL of amino acids/d

   b. Nonprotein calories:
   The calories supplied by protein (4 kcal/g) are subtracted from the RER to get total nonprotein calories needed:
   _____g protein required/d × 4 kcal/g = _____kcal provided by protein
   RER − kcals provided by protein = _____nonprotein kcal needed/d

   c. Nonprotein calories are usually provided as a 50:50 mixture of lipid to dextrose. However, if the patient has a pre-existing condition (eg, diabetes, hypertriglyceridemia), this ratio may need to be adjusted
   20% lipid solution = 2 kcal/mL
   To supply 50% of nonprotein kcal:
   _____lipid kcal required ÷ 2 kcal/mL = _____mL of lipid
   50% dextrose solution = 1.7 kcal/mL
   To supply 50% of non-protein kcal:
   _____dextrose kcal required ÷ 1.7 kcal/mL = _____mL dextrose

4. Total daily requirements:
_____mL 8.5% amino acid solution
_____mL 20% lipid solution
_____mL 50% dextrose solution
_____mL total volume of TPN solution[a]

5. Administration rate:
Day 1: _____mL/h
Day 2: _____mL/h
Day 3: _____mL/h

[a]Be sure to adjust the patient's other fluids accordingly!

APPENDIX 2. WORKSHEET FOR CALCULATING A PARTIAL PARENTERAL NUTRITION FORMULATION

1. Resting energy requirement (RER):
$70 \times$ (current body weight in kg)$^{0.75}$ = kcal/d
or for animals 3–25 kg, can also use:
$30 \times$ (current body weight in kg) + 70 = kcal/d
RER = _____kcal/d

2. Partial energy requirement (PER):
Plan to supply 70% of the animal's RER with PPN:
PER = RER $\times$ 0.70 = _____kcal/d

3. Nutrient composition:
(Note: For animals ≤3 kg, the formulation will provide a fluid rate higher than maintenance fluid requirements. Be sure that the animal can tolerate this volume of fluids.)

a. Cats and dogs 3–5 kg:
PER $\times$ 0.20 =_____kcal/d from carbohydrate
PER $\times$ 0.20 =_____kcal/d from protein
PER $\times$ 0.60 =_____kcal/d from lipid

b. Cats and dogs 6–10 kg:
PER $\times$ 0.25 =_____kcal/d from carbohydrate
PER $\times$ 0.25 =_____kcal/d from protein
PER $\times$ 0.50 =_____ kcal/d from lipid

c. Dogs 11–30 kg:
PER $\times$ 0.33 =_____kcal/d from carbohydrate
PER $\times$ 0.33 =_____kcal/d from protein
PER $\times$ 0.33 =_____kcal/d from lipid

d. Dogs >30 kg:
PER $\times$ 0.50 =_____kcal/d from carbohydrate
PER $\times$ 0.25 =_____kcal/d from protein
PER $\times$ 0.25 =_____kcal/d from lipid

4. Volumes of nutrient solutions required each day:

    a. 5% dextrose solution = 0.17 kcal/mL
    _____kcal from carbohydrate ÷ 0.17 kcal/mL =_____mL
      dextrose/d

    b. 8.5% amino acid solution = 0.085 g/mL = 0.34 kcal/mL
    _____kcal from protein ÷ 0.34 kcal/mL = _____mL amino acids/d

    c. 20% lipid solution = 2 kcal/mL
    _____kcal from lipid ÷ 2 kcal/mL = _____mL lipid/d

5. Total daily requirements:
    _____mL 5% dextrose solution
    _____mL 8.5% amino acid solution
    _____mL 20% lipid solution
    _____mL total volume of PPN solution[a]

6. Administration rate:
    This formulation provides approximately a maintenance fluid rate.
    _____mL/hr PPN solution

[a]Be sure to adjust the patient's other fluids accordingly!

References

[1] Barton RG. Nutrition support in critical illness. Nutr Clin Pract 1994;9(4):127–39.
[2] Wray CJ, Mammen JM, Hasselgren P. Catabolic response to stress and potential benefits of nutritional support. Nutrition 2002;18(11–12):960–5.
[3] Mawby DI, Bartges JW, D'Avignin A, et al. Comparison of various methods for estimating body fat in dogs. J Am Anim Hosp Assoc 2004;40(2):109–14.
[4] Buffington T, Holloway C, Abood A. Nutritional assessment. In: Buffington T, Holloway C, Abood S, editors. Manual of veterinary dietetics. St. Louis (MO): WB Saunders; 2004. p. 1–7.
[5] O'Toole E, Miller CW, Wilson BA, et al. Comparison of the standard predictive equation for calculation of resting energy expenditure with indirect calorimetry in hospitalized and healthy dogs. J Am Vet Med Assoc 2004;255(1):58–64.
[6] Walton RS, Wingfield WE, Ogilvie GK. Energy expenditure in 104 postoperative and traumatically injured dogs with indirect calorimetry. J Vet Emerg Crit Care 1998;6(2):71–9.
[7] Freeman LM, Chan DL. Total parenteral nutrition. In: DiBartola SP, editor. Fluid, Electrolyte, and acid-base disorders in small animal practice. 3rd edition. St. Louis (MO): Saunders Elsevier; 2006. p. 584–601.
[8] Chan DL. Nutritional requirements of the critically ill patient. Clin Tech Small Anim Pract 2004;19(1):1–5.
[9] Crabb SE, Chan DL, Freeman LM. Retrospective evaluation of total parenteral nutrition in cats: 40 cases (1991–2003). J Vet Emerg Crit Care 2006;16(S1):S21–6.
[10] Pyle SC, Marks SL, Kass PH. Evaluation of complications and prognostic factors associated with administration of total parenteral nutrition in cats: 75 cases (1994–2001). J Am Vet Med Assoc 2004;255(2):242–50.
[11] Lippert AC. The metabolic response to injury: enteral and parenteral nutritional support. In: Murtaugh RJ, Kaplan PM, editors. Veterinary emergency and critical care medicine. St Louis (MO): Mosby Yearbook; 1992. p. 593–617.

[12] Michel KE, King LG, Ostro E. Measurement of urinary urea nitrogen content as an estimate of the amount of total urinary nitrogen loss in dogs in intensive care units. J Am Vet Med Assoc 1997;210(3):356–9.

[13] ASPEN Board of Directors and the Clinical Guidelines Task Force. Guidelines for the use of parenteral and enteral nutrition in adults and pediatric patients. JPEN J Parenter Enteral Nutr 2002;26(1 Suppl):1SA–6SA.

[14] Abood SK, Buffington CA. Improved nasogastric intubation technique for administration of nutritional support in dogs. J Am Vet Med Assoc 1991;199(5):577–9.

[15] Heuter K. Placement of jejunal feeding tubes for post-gastric feeding. Clin Tech Small Anim Pract 2004;19(1):32–42.

[16] Mazzaferro EM. Esophagostomy tubes: don't underutilize them!. J Vet Emerg Crit Care 2001;11(2):153–6.

[17] Bright RM. Use of percutaneous gastrostomy tubes and low profile feeding devices. In: Bojrab MJ, editor. Current techniques in small animal surgery. 4th edition. Baltimore (MD): Williams & Wilkins; 1998. p. 170–6.

[18] Devitt CM, Seim HB. Use of jejunostomy and enterostomy tubes. In: Bojrab MJ, editor. Current techniques in small animal surgery. 4th edition. Baltimore (MD): Williams & Wilkins; 1998. p. 177–82.

[19] Jennings M, Center SA, Barr SC. Successful treatment of feline pancreatitis using an endoscopically placed gastrojejunostomy tube. J Am Anim Hosp Assoc 2001;37(2):145–52.

[20] Johnson PA, Mann FA, Dodam J, et al. Capnographic documentation of nasoesophageal and nasogastric feeding tube placement in dogs. J Vet Emerg Crit Care 2002;12(4): 227–33.

[21] Swann HM, Sweet DC, Michel K. Complications associated with use of jejunostomy tubes in dogs and cats: 40 cases (1989 – 1994). J Am Vet Med Assoc 1997;210(12):1764–7.

[22] Miller CC, Bartges JW. Refeeding syndrome. In: Bonagura JD, editor. Current veterinary therapy XIII. Philadelphia: WB Saunders; 2000. p. 87–9.

[23] Justin RB, Hoenhaus AE. Hypophosphatemia associated with enteral alimentation in cats. J Vet Intern Med 1995;9(4):228–33.

[24] Mohr AJ, Leisewitz AL, Jacobson LS, et al. Effect of early enteral nutrition on intestinal permeability, intestinal protein loss, and outcome in dogs with severe parvoviral enteritis. J Vet Intern Med 2003;17(6):791–8.

[25] Mantione NL, Otto CM. Characterization of the use of antiemetic agents in dogs with parvoviral enteritis treated at a veterinary teaching hospital:77 cases (1997–2000). J Am Vet Med Assoc 2005;227(11):1787–93.

[26] Van den Berghe G, Wouters PJ, Weekers F, et al. Intensive insulin therapy in critically ill patients. N Engl J Med 2001;345(19):1359–67.

[27] Yu WK, Li WQ, Li JS. Influence of acute hyperglycemia in human sepsis on inflammatory cytokines and couter-regulatory hormone concentrations. World J Gastroenter 2003;9(8):1824–7.

[28] Krinsley JS. Effect of am intensive glucose management protocol on the mortality of critically ill adult patients. Mayo Clin Proc 2004;79(8):992–1000.

[29] Grey NJ, Perdrizer GA. Reduction of nosocomial infections in the surgical intensive care unit by strict glycemic control. Endocr Pract 2004;10(Suppl 2):46–52.

[30] Brady CA, Hughes D, Drobatz KJ. Association of hyponatraemia and hyperglycemia with outcome in dogs with congestive heart failure. J Vet Emerg Crit Care 2004;14(3):177–82.

[31] Chan DL, Freeman LM, Rozanski EA, et al. Prevalence of hyperglycemia in cats presented to the emergency service. (Abstr.) J Vet Emerg Crit Care Med 2002;12(3):1999.

[32] Torre DM, deLaforcade AM, Chan DL. Incidence and significance of hyperglycemia in critically ill dogs. [abstract]. J Vet Emerg Crit Care 2005;15(3 Suppl. 1):S7.

[33] Heyland DK, Novak F, Drover JW, et al. Should immunonutrition become routine in critically ill patients? A systematic review of the evidence. J Am Med Assoc 2001;286(8): 944–53.

[34] Dhaliwal R, Heyland DK. Nutrition and infection in the intensive care unit: what does the evidence show? Curr Opin Crit Care 2005;11(5):461–7.

[35] Novak F, Heyland DK, Avenell A, et al. Glutamine supplementation in serious illness: a systematic review of the evidence. Crit Care Med 2002;30(9):2022–9.

[36] Mendez C, Jurkovich GJ, Garena I, et al. Effects of an immune-enhancing diet in critically injured patients. J Trauma 1997;42(5):933–40.

[37] McClave SA. The effects of immune-enhancing diets (IEDs) on mortality, hospital length of stay, duration of mechanical ventilation, and other parameters. JPEN J Parenter Enteral Nutr 2001;25(2 Suppl):S44–9.

[38] Bertolini G, Iapichino G, Radrizzani D, et al. Early enteral immunonutrition in patients with severe sepsis: results of an interim-analysis of a randomized multicentre clinical trial. Intensive Care Med 2003;29(5):834–40.

[39] Marks SL, Cook AK, Reader R, et al. Effects of glutamine supplementation of an amino acid-based purified diet on intestinal mucosal integrity in cats with methotrexate-induced enteritis. Am J Vet Res 1999;60(6):755–63.

[40] Lana SE, Hansen RA, Kloer L, et al. The effects of oral glutamine supplementation on plasma glutamine concentration and PGE_2 concentration in dogs experiencing radiation-induced mucositis. J Appl Res Vet Med 2003;1(4):259–65.

[41] Chan DL, Rozanski EA, Freeman LM. Relationship between plasma amino acids, C-reactive protein, illness severity and outcome in critically ill dogs. [abstract]. J Vet Intern Med 2006;20(3):755.

Vet Clin Small Anim 36 (2006) 1243–1249

VETERINARY CLINICS
SMALL ANIMAL PRACTICE

Management of Anorexia in Dogs and Cats

Sean J. Delaney, DVM, MS[a,b,*]

[a]Davis Veterinary Medical Consulting, PC, 707 Fourth Street, Suite 307, Davis, CA 95616, USA
[b]Department of Molecular Biosciences, School of Veterinary Medicine, University of California, Davis, Davis, CA, USA

norexia is defined as the lack or loss of appetite for food. In veterinary medicine, it is one of the most common presenting complaints for a myriad of disease processes with greatly varying pathogenesis. Given this variation in cause, one set of guidelines cannot be applicable to all anorexic patients; however, certain standard approaches that do not use assisted feeding may still prove helpful in differing diseases. The following article discusses these approaches and, where appropriate, highlights some disease-specific recommendations. In addition, guidelines for when to turn to assisted feeding are provided.

ANOREXIA VERSUS HYPOREXIA

Before beginning a discussion on the management of anorexia, it might prove useful to introduce the term *hyporexia*, because it may be more descriptive of the condition that many veterinary patients who may benefit from this article are actually experiencing. Hyporexia, although not classically defined, means a reduction in appetite rather than a total loss. It is the experience of this author that canine and feline patients that are completely unwilling to eat anything voluntarily can rarely be made to eat enough to meet their energy requirement despite using the techniques and approaches that follow. These patients typically have an underlying reason for their anorexia that may need other therapeutics and time before they even become hyporexic. In the interim, they need to be supported with assisted feeding (nutrition provided parenterally or by feeding tube) until they become hyporexic, which then may be manageable without assisted feeding. Thus, a more accurate title for this article might be management of hyporexia.

*Davis Veterinary Medical Consulting, PC, 707 Fourth Street, Suite 307, Davis, CA 95616, USA. *E-mail address:* sjdelaney@dvmconsulting.com

0195-5616/06/$ – see front matter
doi:10.1016/j.cvsm.2006.08.001

FEEDING STRATEGIES TO ENHANCE ORAL INTAKE

Before attempting any of the following techniques or approaches to get patients to eat, medical therapy should have been implemented to correct electrolyte abnormalities, rehydrate the patient, reduce uremic toxins, and reduce pain. It should be noted that opiates commonly used in pain management have antimotility effects that can result in anorexia. Therefore, a balanced approach to pain management and anorexia should be used, with pain management favored during the initial care of patients.

Although a common nutritional quote is "...it is always better for a patient to eat some of the 'wrong' diet than none of the 'right' diet," there are many exceptions to this statement. For example, it is not advisable to give an extremely high-protein meal to a uremic patient, a high-fat meal to a pancreatitic patient, a high-salt treat to a patient with pulmonary edema or ascites attributable to congestive heart failure, or a high organ meat meal to a hepatoencephalopathic patient. Thus, caution should be practiced when using an approach or nutritional strategy that may be effective in getting a patient to eat a single meal but may make the patient's condition worse, and may consequently prevent subsequent more appropriate meals from being consumed.

Creating Ambiance and Improving Service

Although the most commonly used strategy to get an anorexic pet to eat is to increase the palatability of the food offered, this is probably not where one should start. A restaurant's success can hinge as much on ambiance and service as its food. A restaurant that rudely served the most delicious food at odd hours, had no place to sit, and insisted on loudly playing bad music is unlikely to have many diners. Unfortunately, this type of dining experience is not uncommon in veterinary practice. Therefore, an attempt should be made to create a place to feed patients wherein stressors are minimized. This may be achievable in the patient's cage or run; however, a special place may often need to be used. Ideally, this area would be quiet and comfortable. Although comfort can mean different things to different pets, it typically means using an area that more similarly mimics the feeding circumstances of the pet at home. Many areas and places in which a pet is typically fed parallel possible locations in most veterinary practices, such as a laundry area, kitchen, office, outside patio, or yard.

Finding a quiet and less foreign feeding area should not be the only strategy pursued. Attempts to normalize feeding times may also be helpful. Many dogs have fixed times for feedings in their home that should be followed. Care should be taken to ensure environmental cues that indicate time are retained as much as possible. Twenty-four–hour lighting should be avoided, and light-dark cycles should be considered, because not only does this provide visual cues as to time for the pets, but some pets, such as cats, can have different consumption patterns during the light or dark cycle [1]. Efforts should also be made not to have food bowls located right next to the area for defecation or urination, because this location does not increase a food's acceptance.

Finally, addressing food service can be quite important. Do not attempt to "poke" or restrain a patient every time the cage or run door is opened. The practice of "poking" or restraining can elicit fear in the patient and is likely to reduce the chance of a patient eating. At the same time, the actual food server may be significant. It has been the experience of this author that the likelihood of patients eating from a server increases in direct proportion to the time that they have spent or spend with the server in a nonstressed situation. Thus, the following order for preferred servers is ideal for feeding success: (1) client, (2) technician (assuming he or she is not the main "poker" or restrainer), and (3) kennel person. Alternately, kennel personnel should be favored over technical staff if the former are the most frequently encountered people who are providing comfort. There is one caveat to client feeding. This author is reluctant to have a client feed a pet if he or she is basing life and death decisions on whether a patient eats or not. This creates a stressful environment for all involved and should be avoided. Thus, the first step in attempting to get an anorexic patient to eat does not involve food but rather involves creating an environment that only enhances the likelihood of a patient eating when offered a highly palatable food.

Increasing Palatability

After appropriate medical therapy, the most common initial strategy to get a patient to eat is to increase the palatability of the meal offered. Several methods that can be used to improve palatability are discussed.

Increasing moisture

Switching from a dry food to a canned or pouched food may be an effective means of increasing palatability. Although the major difference between dry and canned or pouched foods is moisture level ($\sim$10% versus $\sim$75%), it should be noted that canned or pouched foods are also typically higher in fat and protein. Increasing fat and protein may also improve palatability, but care should be taken to ensure that there are no adverse effects from increasing fat or protein, as discussed previously. In addition, the clinician should not assume that the canned or pouched version of a commercial food, including therapeutic formulations, is the same as the dry food. Thus, just because a dry food has been tolerated, the clinician cannot assume that the canned or pouched form is also going to be equally tolerated. An alternative to switching to a canned or pouched food is to simply soak dry kibble. Although most kibble absorbs an equal volume of water, this does not represent a moisture content equivalent to most canned or pouched foods, which would require at least 2.5 parts water to 1 part kibble. Finally, caution should be taken when increasing the moisture of foods fed to cats. Cats raised lifelong on dry food may not find higher moisture foods more palatable but rather less palatable because of a learned texture preference for dry kibble.

Increasing fat

The second most commonly used strategy to improve palatability is to increase dietary fat. This strategy is commonly used in therapeutic foods and increases the energy density so that less food can be consumed to meet a patient's energy requirement. Although this strategy can be quite effective, it should be used cautiously, because fat is not innocuous. Concerns include those for patients with pancreatitis (although the role of dietary fat in pancreatitic cats remains controversial) and slowing of gastric emptying and overall gastrointestinal (GI) transit time in patients at risk of aspirating or with ileus. In general, this author prefers not to increase the dietary fat content of foods offered to patients as an initial strategy and to do so only when there is good evidence that the patient is not experiencing or at risk for pancreatitis and there are no concerns regarding GI motility.

Increasing protein
Increasing dietary protein may be beneficial in some pets, but it can be difficult to determine whether the effect of protein is independent of the frequent concurrent increase in moisture and fat. There is evidence that dogs select foods with a higher dietary protein level [2]. In addition, certain amino acids present in protein may increase a food's palatability. Much like increasing dietary fat, care should be taken when increasing dietary protein in certain disease processes, such as hepatic failure with hepatic encephalopathy and renal failure with acute uremia.

Sweet and salty
Adding a sweet flavor with the use of sugars or syrups as a top dressing can increase the palatability of a food for dogs [2]. Artificial sweeteners should be avoided because they have little to no nutritive value and a common artificial sweetener, xylitol, can cause a hypoglycemic crisis in dogs [3]. This strategy is not effective in cats because they do not have sweet receptors [4], and it should be noted that the use of sucrose (fructose plus glucose) or syrups containing fructose (eg, corn syrup) should not be used in cats because it can cause fructosuria [5]. Although the addition of carbohydrates is generally better tolerated than increasing fat or protein, caution should be exercised in the diabetic patient. One should also be aware of the concept of caloric dilution of nutrients. This occurs when an incomplete and unbalanced food is added to a complete and balanced food in a large enough amount to reduce the amount of essential nutrients a patient consumes to a point that results in a deficiency. This occurs because patients eating or being fed to meet their energy requirement consequently take in less of other nutrients per day. Thus, sugar or syrup added to the patient's food should constitute less than 10% of the total daily calories. It has been the experience of this author that many dogs need to have a small amount of sugar- or syrup-enhanced food placed under their lip to realize that their food has been sweetened.

Adding salt or using a salty food can also be effective in getting some dogs to eat. Cats seem to be insensitive to the addition of salt. Again, caution should be used in adding salt to foods fed to patients with hypertension, edema, ascites, or renal disease. Although included here, this author has not personally found the addition of salt to be an effective strategy and believes that the reported preference some patients have for "salty" foods (eg, potato chips, salted nuts, peanut butter) may, in fact, be a preference for fat or treats in general that is somewhat independent of the food's salt level.

Freshness, aroma, and food temperature
Although much more difficult to quantify, clinical experience indicates that a food's freshness can play a role in increasing a patient's appetite. The effectiveness of fresh canned food or even nonprocessed foods, such as freshly prepared human meats and starches, in getting patients to eat may be related to freshness, which may also be tied to aroma, because more chemicals are released for sensing. In a similar grain, warming food (to no greater than body temperature to prevent burning the patient's mouth) may be quite helpful, possibly because of the additional release of aromas. This may play an even greater role in patients with a diminished sense of smell, such as older patients, because it has been shown that the sense of smell is reduced in elderly human beings [6]. In addition, the sense of smell may be reduced in certain disease states, such as chronic renal failure, based on human data [7]. Therefore, enhancing the aroma or smell of foods may be helpful in getting patients to eat.

This also supports the need to keep food fresh during storage at a clinic or hospital and during feeding. Leaving a meal of canned food with a patient all day should be avoided, because it is likely that the food becomes less palatable with time and dehydration.

Rarity
Many patients may be more likely to eat a food that is rare but not completely foreign. A rare food may be more enticing than a common food; however, it can be helpful to try first to feed the patient's regular food if a learned aversion is not suspected or likely to develop. It has been shown in cats that rarity can lead cats to eat a food more readily. Interestingly, it has also been shown that a seemingly palatable food, such as raw beef (this author does not advocate feeding raw meat), is refused by cats that have not been exposed to it previously [8]. This is further supported by the clinical experience of cats fed dry food exclusively refusing canned or pouched food as discussed previously. Therefore, uncommon or rare food can be offered, but types of food that are completely novel may not be the best choice.

Variety
A common approach to feeding the anorexic patient is the cafeteria-style feeding method, where numerous foods are offered to patients so as to allow them to select a food they are interested in. This can be an effective "shotgun" approach, and there is supportive canine and human data that variety can increase food intake in healthy subjects [2,9]. There are a couple of cautionary points when using this feeding approach, however. First, a careful measure of the amount of each "cafeteria item" should be made to allow for accurate accounting of

food intake. This should prevent positive or negative assumptions from being made regarding the effectiveness of this feeding strategy. Second, this approach should not be used in patients with diseases that commonly have a learned food aversion as a sequela or have limited commercial therapeutic food options. For example, providing a patient with renal failure in the midst of a uremic crisis with all the available commercial therapeutic foods for sampling should be avoided. This minimizes the likelihood of a patient developing a learned aversion to all the foods that the patient may need to be fed in the long term.

Polypharmacy Avoidance

Many commonly used drugs can affect appetite by causing nausea or altering smell or taste. Common pain medications, antibiotics, antifungals, diuretics, anti-inflammatories, immunosuppressives, and chemotherapeutics can reduce appetite. This brief article cannot provide a comprehensive list of all potentially offending medications but can recommend that the potential effects of medications on appetite be reviewed in anorexic patients. Although certain medications may be necessary, dose alterations may be possible or alternative medications or routes of administration may be used that might mitigate some medications' adverse effects on appetite. Redundant drugs or drugs unnecessary for patient short-term management should be stopped to determine if they may be having adverse effects on appetite. In addition, awareness of a drug's potential adverse effect on appetite may be helpful, simply because it may improve the patient's perceived prognosis.

Eliminating Physical Barriers to Eating

Although it may seem intuitive, it is this author's clinical experience that physical barriers to eating are often unrecognized as preventing or reducing food intake. Examples of barriers include Elizabethan collars (E-collars), poor bowl location, and dental or oral pain. It is recommended that E-collars be removed at meals with close observance that the patient eats and does not use this freedom to disturb areas protected by the E-collar. In addition, bowls should be easily accessible, accounting for any limitations in movement the patient may have. This may mean raising bowls for large dogs or moving bowls closer to immobile patients. Finally, poor appetite because of dental or oral pain may be somewhat improved in the short term with higher moisture foods, including slurries and liquid foods.

Appetite-Stimulating Drugs

The commonly used or reported appetite-stimulating drugs diazepam, cyproheptadine, and low-dose propofol [10] are not used by this author because their effects seem to be unpredictable, intermittent, and short lasting. Therefore, this author recommends that the previously discussed techniques or approaches be attempted; if they do not work, assisted feeding may be used.

GUIDELINES FOR WHEN TO INITIATE ASSISTED FEEDING

Despite perfect execution of these approaches in getting an anorexic patient to eat, some patients do not eat and assisted feeding should be initiated. Although there is debate as to when assisted feeding should be begun, assisted feeding is generally indicated in dogs and cats when consumption is less than the resting energy requirement [RER $= 70 \times$ (body weight$_{kg}^{0.75}$)] for greater than 3 to 5 days with no trend toward improving. Three to 5 days is arbitrary and based loosely on when a patient has exhausted carbohydrate reserves, such as glycogen, and altered metabolism to generate glucose primarily from fat and some protein through gluconeogenesis. This time frame should be shortened if the patient's body condition score is low or the patient shows other signs of malnutrition, if the patient is growing, if the disease process is expected to worsen without nutritional support (eg, hepatic lipidosis), or to inhibit voluntary intake for a protracted length of time (eg, severe pancreatitis).

SUMMARY

The management of anorexia should center first on the urgent and emergent medical management of the patient and be followed by feeding of a highly palatable food in a low-stress environment and manner. Diet palatability can potentially be improved by increasing dietary moisture, fat, or protein and, in the dog, by adding sugar or salt as well as by using a variety of fresh pleasantly aromatic and uncommon foods. Caution should be used when increasing or adding nutrients that may be harmful to patients with specific diseases. Concurrent drug therapy that may reduce appetite should be minimized, and physical barriers to eating should be removed. Patients that consume less than their RER for greater than 3 to 5 days with no trend toward improving should receive parenteral or enteral nutrition.

References

[1] Kane E, Leung PMB, Rogers QR, et al. Diurnal feeding and drinking patterns of adult cats as affected by changes in the level of fat in the diet. Appetite 1987;9:89–98.

[2] Torres CL, Hickenbottom SJ, Rogers QR. Palatability affects the percentage of metabolizable energy as protein selected by adult beagles. J Nutr 2003;133:3516–22.

[3] Dunayer EK. Hypoglycemia following canine ingestion of xylitol-containing gum. Vet Hum Toxicol 2004;46(2):87–8.

[4] Li X, Li W, Wang H, et al. Pseudogenization of a sweet-receptor gene accounts for cats' indifference toward sugar. PLoS Genet 2005;1(1):27–35.

[5] Kienzle E. Blood sugar levels and renal sugar excretion after the intake of high carbohydrate diets in cats. J Nutr 1994;124(12 Suppl):2563S–7S.

[6] Duffy VB, Cain WS, Ferris AM. Measurement of sensitivity to olfactory flavor: application in a study of aging and dentures. Chem Senses 1999;24(6):671–7.

[7] Frasnelli JA, Temmel AF, Quint C, et al. Olfactory function in chronic renal failure. Am J Rhinol 2002;16(5):275–9.

[8] Bradshaw JWS, Healey LM, Thorne CJ, et al. Differences in food preferences between individuals and populations of domestic cats Felis sylvestris catus. Appl Anim Behav Sci 2000;68:257–68.

[9] Hetherington MM, Foster R, Newman T, et al. Understanding variety: tasting different foods delays satiation. Phys Behav 2006;87:263–71.

[10] Long JP, Greco SC. The effect of propofol administered intravenously on appetite stimulation in dogs. Contemporary Topics in Laboratory Animal Science 2000;39(6):43–6.

Vet Clin Small Anim 36 (2006) 1251–1268

VETERINARY CLINICS
SMALL ANIMAL PRACTICE

Hydrolyzed Protein Diets for Dogs and Cats

Nicholas J. Cave, BVSc, MVSc, MACVSc

Institute of Veterinary, Animal, and Biomedical Sciences, Massey University,
Private Bag 11-222, Palmerston North, New Zealand

Hydrolyzed proteins have been used as the source of essential and dispensable amino acids in breast-milk replacer formulae for more than 50 years, mainly for the management of infant cow's milk allergy [1–3]. In contrast, diets formulated for dogs and cats that use hydrolysates as the amino acid source have been available for less than a decade, and experience and knowledge in veterinary medicine are still rudimentary.

The primary aim of hydrolyzing proteins for specialized diets is to sufficiently disrupt the protein structure within the diet to remove any existing allergens and allergenic epitopes and thereby prevent immune recognition by patients already sensitized to the intact protein. A secondary aim might be to disrupt the proteins to such an extent that there are no antigens capable of eliciting an immune response and leading to sensitization in a naive individual. An "antigen" is defined as a substance capable of stimulating antibody production. Antigens are usually, although not always, proteins. An "allergen" is an antigen that is capable of eliciting and binding to specific immunoglobulin E (IgE) antibodies and inducing mast cell degranulation after binding to IgE on the cell surface [4]. Ideally, protein hydrolysis prevents mast cell degranulation that would occur in response to the intact protein and enables a patient hypersensitive to the protein to ingest the hydrolysate without clinical signs.

The term *hypoallergenic diet* is, at best, an ambiguous one and has been widely misused. It should be reserved for diets that have at least been demonstrated to possess a substantial reduction in antigenicity and have preferably been shown to be tolerated by the most patients known to be hypersensitive to the intact source protein [5–7]. Any reduction in antigenicity or clinical reactivity at which point a diet could be considered "hypoallergenic" is arbitrary, however, unless it is absolute. Therefore, the use of the term is discouraged, and it is not used further in this review.

E-mail address: n.j.cave@massey.ac.nz

0195-5616/06/$ – see front matter
doi:10.1016/j.cvsm.2006.08.008

FOOD ALLERGENS

Foods contain an enormous variety of proteins, most of which are potentially antigenic, and yet only a few have been shown to be allergenic. It is generally thought that the biochemical properties that make a particular substance an allergen are not species specific and that, in general, significant homology might be preserved in the recognition of allergens. Indeed, that seems to hold true for the allergenic potential of immunoglobulins [8]. Nonetheless, there are species differences in the relative importance of most allergens. For instance, although beef is the most common allergen in dogs and cats, it is not a common cause of allergy among people living in North America, despite its being a significant source of protein in their diets [9–12].

Adverse food reactions in dogs and cats include both non-immunologic (food intolerance) and immunologic (food hypersensitivity) mechanisms. It is probably the case that the majority of true food hypersensitivities are a type-I hypersensitivity that involves mast cell degranulation for the development of clinical signs. Mast cell degranulation requires cross-linking of two or more IgE molecules bound by high-affinity IgE receptors ($F_c \varepsilon R1s$) on the mast cell membrane (Fig. 1A). This requirement for divalency places a minimum size limit on molecules that can stimulate IgE-mediated reactions. Most publications refer to this lower limit as being 10 kd, although smaller peptides could act as haptens [12–14]. Work by van Beresteijn and colleagues [15] and, more recently, by Van Hoeyveld and coworkers [16] suggests that the limit may be much smaller, possibly between 3 and 5 kd. The minimum molecular mass for simple IgE binding seems to be somewhere between 0.97 kDa and 1.4 kDa (see Fig. 1B).

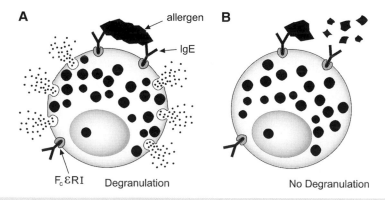

Fig. 1. Requirements for mast cell activation. (A) Mast cells are sensitized by IgE binding to the high affinity IgE receptor, to $F_c \varepsilon RI$. Allergen binding to IgE cross-links the $F_c \varepsilon RI$ molecules and induces the release of preformed and de novo synthesized mediators, such as histamine, prostaglandins, enzymes, and cytokines. (B) If the allergenic protein is sufficiently hydrolyzed, cross-linking does not occur and the mast cell does not degranulate. This is the case even if some of the fragments retain the ability to bind IgE.

In human beings, peptides as small as 4.5 kd have been shown to retain allergenicity [17]. In contrast, proteins of greater than 70 kd are unlikely to be efficiently absorbed intact through the enteric mucosa, and few food allergens are of that size. However, the size of the smallest fragments that retain allergenicity varies greatly between food protein sources.

Although most of the known food allergens are naturally occurring food proteins or glycoproteins, there is evidence that nonprotein molecules can function as allergens. Certain carbohydrates free of proteins, such as pneumococcal polysaccharides and highly cross-linked dextran, have been demonstrated to induce allergic reactions in human beings [12,18]. Carbohydrate determinants have been implicated as protein-binding haptens (eg, inulin) and as parts of antigenic glycoproteins (eg, β-fructofuranosidase) [19–21]. They are also claimed to be responsible for cross-reactivity between plant allergies and are incriminated in false-positive IgE-binding assays, such as those used in serum ELISA allergy tests [11]. The role of true carbohydrate antigens in human allergology is still controversial and poorly defined, however, and nothing is yet known about their existence in canine and feline patients.

In cases in which a dietary carbohydrate is implicated as a source of allergen (eg, corn [maize]), it is more likely that there is a protein allergen within the carbohydrate source than the existence of a true hypersensitivity to the carbohydrate molecules. Maize zeins, which are 20- to 23-kDa prolamine proteins, have been detected in hydrolyzed casein formulae when corn starch is used as the carbohydrate source [22]. Similarly, lipophilic protein allergens have been isolated in refined vegetable oils [23]. Thus, the carbohydrate and lipid sources chosen for incorporation into hydrolyzed protein diets may be important sources of conventional protein allergens because they are not commonly subjected to enzymatic hydrolysis and should be considered when evaluating commercial diets.

It is important to recognize the limitations of our understanding of canine and feline adverse reactions to food. The precise nature of the immunologic responses in most cases has not been defined. Thus, although type 1 IgE-mediated hypersensitivities are thought to be present in some cases, it is likely that other mechanisms exist in a subset of cases. This is especially true for cases in which only gastrointestinal signs are present. The degree of hydrolysis needed to prevent an adverse reaction may be different when non–IgE-mediated immune responses are present.

REDUCING THE ANTIGENICITY OF FOOD PROTEINS

The antigenicity of a protein is determined by its primary structure (ie, its amino acid sequence), its secondary structure (folding of the amino acid chain into helices or sheets), and its tertiary structure (further folding of the helices and sheets). Reducing the antigenicity can be achieved by (1) disrupting the three-dimensional structure of the protein (secondary and tertiary structures), (2) altering the structure of amino acid side chains (eg, conjugation of amino acids with sugars, oxidation of amino acids), or (3) cleaving peptide bonds (hydrolysis).

The specific methods by which antigenicity can be reduced include heat treatment, pH manipulation, enzymatic hydrolysis, and filtration [24]. The effectiveness of heat treatment depends on the inherent lability of the protein to increased temperatures [25]. Among milk proteins, for example, casein is relatively heat stable and can withstand temperatures of 130°C for longer than 1 hour without significant denaturation [26]. In contrast, whey proteins are much more heat labile, denaturing at around 80°C [27].

Accordingly, in human beings, it has been shown that although heat treatment may reduce the number of whey protein antigens, it has little effect on the casein antigens, despite heating at 121°C for 15 minutes [25]. Thus, heat treatment used alone to reduce the allergenicity of a milk product is of no use in those individuals sensitized to the casein component [28].

It can be assumed that there are a significant number of heat-stable allergens, because many of the food allergies identified in domestic animals include reactions to protein components in commercial diets (dry or canned) that are subject to heat treatment during manufacturing. Alternatively, it may be that some proteins increase in allergenicity with heat treatment. The effect of heat treatment is mostly to change the three-dimensional conformation of the protein [29]. Although this may disrupt some allergens, it may equally uncover previously hidden allergenic determinants. Other reactions occurring at high temperatures include the Maillard reactions, which involve the reactions between certain amino acids and reducing sugars to produce compounds called melanoidins, which give a characteristic brown color. Melanoidins can be more or less allergenic than the original protein by acting as haptens or by reducing peptide absorption, respectively [30,31]. These findings may explain some of the observations pertaining to differences between home-prepared elimination diets and commercial diets. It has been demonstrated recently that heat treatment during canning of a purified diet containing casein, starch, sucrose, and corn oil can create new antigens that are more immunogenic than the uncooked diet [32].

Alterations in the pH of the solution can be used to reduce the antigenicity of a protein further in addition to the conformational changes that occur at high temperatures. Most food allergens are usually quite resistant to moderate acid treatments, however, particularly those acid concentrations simulating stomach acid conditions [13]. For example, the peanut allergen "Ara h 2," soy allergen "Gly m 1," and milk β-lactoglobulin are resistant to acid digestion at pH 2.8 in contrast to the nonallergenic peptides [33,34].

Therefore, heat treatment and pH adjustments alone cannot be relied on to reduce the allergenicity of parent compounds significantly, and, as discussed, some reactions may actually increase allergenicity.

Enzymatic Hydrolysis

Cleavage of a protein molecule by enzymatic hydrolysis into small fragments is the most reliable way of reducing antigenicity. If the cleavage occurs within an antigenic peptide sequence, it is immunologically inactive. Additionally, because many antigenic determinants rely to some degree on the three-dimensional structure of the peptide, disruption of the surrounding amino acid sequence may lead to a sufficient change in three-dimensional conformation so that loss of antigenicity occurs.

Hydrolysis of proteins is achieved by using food-grade proteolytic enzymes. The resultant hydrolysate varies in composition according to the composition of the parent compound, the specificity of the proteolytic enzymes chosen, the method by which the hydrolysis is conducted, and any further processing of the resultant product.

The selection of enzymes is important, because the specific site at which the particular enzymes act determines the likelihood of degradation of the particular epitopes responsible for the hypersensitivity reactions. Because the amino acid sequence and three-dimensional structure of the individual epitopes are rarely known, trial and error with in vitro evaluation is usually the method by which a particular hydrolytic enzyme is selected. A variety of proteases have been used from various sources, including mammalian pancreas, porcine stomach, bacteria, fungi, and some fruits [25].

Ultrafiltration

Hydrolysates usually contain residual amino acid sequences that were resistant to the hydrolysis plus traces of the enzymes used in the hydrolysis process. The hydrolysates therefore contain a variety of fragments, which may range from single amino acids to large-molecular-weight polypeptides depending on the degree of hydrolysis. Removal of the larger fragments via physical separation or molecular filtration can have a significant influence on the "quality" of the finished product. Currently, ultrafiltration of the hydrolysate is the most widely used method to remove the large-molecular-weight fragments. The size of the filter and the efficiency of the filtration process determine the success of ultrafiltration. Understandably, ultrafiltration of a protein hydrolysate would add a considerable cost to the final product if used.

EVALUATING AND COMPARING HYDROLYZED PROTEIN DIETS

Ingredients

Initial selection of a commercial hydrolyzed protein diet for a particular patient should probably be based on the protein source. None of the currently available commercial diets are sufficiently hydrolyzed to guarantee the complete absence of all allergens. Therefore, it is prudent to select a diet that does not contain a protein source that the patient is known or suspected to be sensitized to. Secondary consideration should be given to the sources of carbohydrate and lipid as sources of potential protein allergens and (unproven) as sources of carbohydrate or lipid antigens. The hydrolyzed protein diets currently widely available are presented in Table 1.

Table 1
Complete and balanced hydrolyzed protein diets available for dogs

Diet[a]	Protein source	Carbohydrate source	Lipid source
Hill's z/d Ultra Allergen Free	Chicken	Corn starch, cellulose	Soybean oil
Hill's z/d Low Allergen	Chicken, potato	Potato, potato starch, cellulose	Soybean oil
Nestle-Purina HA	Soy	Corn starch, cellulose, vegetable gums (gum arabic and guar gum)	Coconut oil, canola oil, corn oil
Royal Canin Hypoallergenic	Soy, poultry liver	Rice, beet pulp, fructo-oligosaccharides	Poultry fat, soybean oil, borage oil, fish oil

Ingredients taken from manufacturers' product guides (January 2006).
[a]Hill's Pet Nutrition, Inc. Topeka, Kansas, USA; Nestlé Purina PetCare Company, St. Louis, Missouri, USA; Royal Canin, Aimargues, France.

Nutritional Evaluation

The digestibility of a protein hydrolysate is predicted to be superior to that of the intact protein source. In fact, numerous studies have shown that small peptides are even better absorbed from the intestine than free amino acids [35,36]. Thus, extensively hydrolyzed proteins seem to be the ideal source of amino acids for maximal digestibility. The digestibility of the protein fraction of a soy-hydrolysate–based diet is reported by the manufacturer to be 90.7% [37]. By comparison, intact soy protein isolates have been shown to have apparent total tract digestibilities of 84.7% to 89.3% [38]. In addition, the apparent ileal protein digestibility of a chicken-based hydrolysate diet has been found to be 82.4% [39]. Thus, although the digestibility may be higher, it is not dramatically so compared with some forms of the intact protein source.

Despite the higher digestibility and absorption of protein hydrolysates, use of the amino acids seems to be different in extensively hydrolyzed formulae compared with the intact protein. Nitrogen use seems to be reduced when compared with conventional formulae [40]. Reduced growth, decreased serum albumin, and increased serum urea have been observed in newborn human infants fed from birth to 1 month with various hydrolysates when compared with feeding intact protein or breast milk [40,41]. Alterations in calcium and phosphorus absorption and differences in the serum amino acid profiles can occur between infants fed whey-protein and those fed a whey hydrolysate [40,41]. These reduced nutritional aspects of protein hydrolysates are seen with extensively hydrolyzed formulae and not with moderately hydrolyzed formulae, such as those currently available in commercial veterinary diets.

Therefore, although the digestibility and nutritional value of hydrolysates cannot be assumed to be the same as those of the parent protein, it is unlikely that the degree of hydrolysis used by the currently available hydrolyzed protein diets is associated with a detrimental effect on nitrogen balance. In addition, products that have been subjected to suitable feeding trials, such as the protocols recommended by the American Association of Feed Control Officials (AAFCO), have been demonstrated to be suitable for long-term feeding.

Physicochemical and Immunologic Evaluation

Laboratory-based testing provides manufacturers with the opportunity to characterize various molecular and immunologic properties of hydrolysates before their incorporation into complete feeds. The antigenicity and allergenicity of a hydrolysate are partly but not wholly dependent on the molecular weight of the remaining peptides. As stated previously, the smaller the resulting fragments are, the less likely it is that residual epitopes remain. Physicochemical analyses of hydrolysates describe the extent of the hydrolysis and the distribution of the molecular weights of the remaining peptide fragments. This is often the starting point in the selection of a candidate hydrolysate [42]. High-performance size-exclusion chromatography has been commonly used to describe the molecular weight profile of infant formulae and has been applied to the peptide component of one veterinary hydrolysate diet [6]. The molecular weight profile and the accumulative percentage curve of the hydrolysate are presented in Fig. 2, and the molecular weight distribution and peptide concentrations are presented in Table 2. As can be seen from Fig. 2, molecular weight profiles are complex data sets that cannot, and should not, be reduced to simple

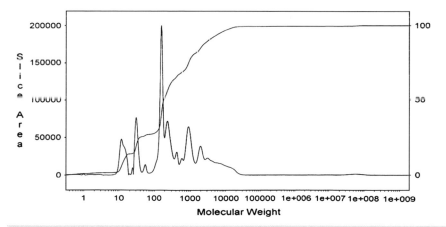

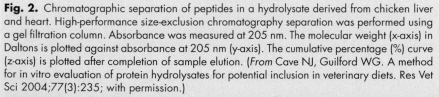

Fig. 2. Chromatographic separation of peptides in a hydrolysate derived from chicken liver and heart. High-performance size-exclusion chromatography separation was performed using a gel filtration column. Absorbance was measured at 205 nm. The molecular weight (x-axis) in Daltons is plotted against absorbance at 205 nm (y-axis). The cumulative percentage (%) curve (z-axis) is plotted after completion of sample elution. (*From* Cave NJ, Guilford WG. A method for in vitro evaluation of protein hydrolysates for potential inclusion in veterinary diets. Res Vet Sci 2004;77(3):235; with permission.)

Table 2
Molecular weight distribution of a chicken-protein hydrolysate

Molecular weight range (kd)	Percentage of total sample (wt/wt)
< 0.5	67.6
0.5–1	10.8
1–3	10.8
3–5	3.7
5–10	4.0
> 10	3.1

From Cave NJ, Guilford WG. A method for in vitro evaluation of protein hydrolysates for potential inclusion in veterinary diets. Res Vet Sci, 2004; 77(3):232.

molecular weight averages. Clearly, the expression of a hydrolysate in terms of its average molecular weight provides limited information on the potential for and significance of intact antigens within the formulation.

It is difficult to determine the limit under which the remaining peptide fragments are small enough to prevent clinical signs in sensitized patients, however. Indeed, although there is an absolute limit for all proteins, the actual limit for individual proteins varies, as mentioned, according to the antigenic epitopes within that protein.

Ensuring that a hydrolysate has no peptides greater than 3 kd, or even 1 kd, would ensure the greatest chance of eliminating any residual allergens. The expense involved in extensive hydrolysis and ultrafiltration makes this, at least for pet food manufacturers, an unrealistic objective, however. Additionally, hypersensitivity reactions in children have been identified in even the most hydrolyzed formulae [43]. Suggested explanations include the presence of an allergen within the carbohydrate component, a hapten effect, or reassembly of old or new epitopes in vivo or in vitro during or subsequent to formulation. Importantly, it should also be realized that the presence of fragments of greater than 5 kd, or even greater than 10 kd, does not guarantee allergenicity. As detailed previously, reduction of allergenic epitopes is dependent on the specificity for the proteolytic enzymes as to whether any given epitope is cleaved or disrupted and rendered nonallergenic.

Immunochemical analyses can semiquantitatively estimate hydrolysate reactivity with preformed antibody. The use of ELISAs and RAST assays to assess residual antibody binding is widespread in human medicine. The ability of hydrolysate-based products to induce an immune response can be evaluated by using animal models, such as the passive cutaneous sensitivity test or laboratory animal hyperimmunization [44,45]. It is the responsibility of the manufacturer to choose the appropriate combination of laboratory-based tests and to use them to document product consistency, thus helping to ensure consistent clinical performance.

At present, detailed in vitro analysis is only available for one of the commercially available hydrolysate diets, which limits product comparisons [6].

Ultimately, however, controlled clinical studies are necessary to demonstrate conclusively the biologic efficacy of these formulations in their target species.

PROBLEMS WITH HYDROLYSATES

The most significant problem that manufacturers of hydrolysate formulae face is persistent immunogenicity. Although a particular process may significantly reduce the allergenicity of the product, it does not abolish the risk of producing an immune-mediated reaction. In the initial stages of an enzymatic hydrolysis, it is common for previously hidden antigenic sites to become exposed and for the product to increase in allergenicity, which is only reduced with further hydrolysis. In extremely hypersensitive children, the reactions to hydrolysate formulae can be life threatening. As the number of hydrolyzed protein formulae appearing on the market for use in allergic human patients increases, so do the number and range of reported hypersensitivity reactions, even anaphylaxis [1,46 48]. It has been shown that only small amounts of intact allergenic epitopes are required to elicit significant and even fatal IgE-mediated responses in sensitized individuals [49]. The best guarantee of producing a truly nonallergenic diet resides in the production of purified amino acids and small peptides. Unfortunately, the widespread use of these elemental products is cost-prohibitive, they have poor acceptance by patients, and they are not easily fed enterally because of their exceptionally high osmolarity.

Preserving palatability for human beings is difficult with the more extensively hydrolyzed products [50]. Peptides and amino acids produce a variety of flavors. The sweet taste of some amino acids and peptides has long been known [51]. Bitterness offers the greatest hurdle to palatability, however. The bitter taste sensation of peptides is, to some degree, related to their hydrophobicity, which, in turn, is a product of their amino acid composition [52]. When a protein is hydrolyzed, the peptide fragments that contain hydrophobic side chains are exposed and can be tasted. Thus, as hydrolysis proceeds, bitterness tends to increase. The most bitter tasting peptides in soy hydrolysates occur between 4 and 2 kDa [53]. As the peptide fragments decrease in size to less than 1 kDa, or even free amino acids, bitterness declines [52]. Hydrolysates produced from more hydrophobic proteins, such as casein, are more likely to be bitter tasting than heterogeneous protein sources, such as meat proteins.

It should be noted that a variety of flavors of peptides are described by human subjects, including bitter, sweet, meaty, and yeasty [52,54]. Also, although individual amino acids and peptides may have a bitter taste, the taste of a hydrolysate is dependent on the mixtures of peptides and cannot be assumed to be any one flavor or easily predicted from the protein source of known hydrophobicity [52,53]. Finally, taste preferences among mammals vary and are not identical to human taste preferences [54–57]. For instance, leucine is a bitter tasting amino acid to human beings, but is a positive flavor enhancer to cats [54,58]. Indeed, protein hydrolysates have long been used to enhance the palatability of commercial dog and cat foods.

In a study of 63 dogs fed a commercial chicken-based hydrolysate diet, palatability was reported to be good or excellent in 48 (76%) and was described by owners of 10 dogs (16%) as being poor but was only refused by 4 dogs (6%) [59]. In another study, although palatability was not reported, 58 (97%) of 60 dogs successfully completed a 2-month feeding trial when a soy-based hydrolysate diet was prescribed, which is consistent with adequate palatability of that diet [60]. Based on data published to date, the rate of acceptance by dogs fed hydrolyzed protein diets as elimination diets is similar to that of those fed conventional select protein diets.

In addition to changes in taste and digestibility, osmolarity increases significantly with increasing hydrolysis and has been blamed for a high incidence of diarrhea in infants fed extensively hydrolyzed formulae [61]. Although the osmolarity of jejunal contents after a normal meal is mildly hyperosmolar (300–350 mOsm/L), feeding high-osmolarity enteral solutions (up to 800 mOsm/L) has been associated with diarrhea in human beings [62,63]. Even higher osmolarities can cause sloughing of enterocytes [64]. In studies of acute diarrhea in children, an osmolarity of 250 mOsm/L or less is associated with improved rehydration, lower stool volume, and less vomiting compared with a solution of 311 mOsm/L, indicating an increased sensitivity to osmolarity in enteritis [65]. However, the osmolarity of the jejunal contents following a feed of a complete hydrolyzed diet is not easily predicted, as it is affected by other ingredients and by the rate of gastric emptying. Thus a protein hydrolysate will produce a different intestinal luminal osmolarity when it is administered as a solution compared with when it is incorporated within a complex diet.

The osmolarity of one chicken-based hydrolysate diet has been determined to be 682 mOsm/L when mixed 1:1 wt/wt with water compared with 293 mOsmol/L for a standard intact protein maintenance diet [39]. Therefore, it is conceivable that hydrolyzed proteins and high food osmolarity could be detrimental in some dogs. Nevertheless, in 46 dogs fed the diet for 6 to 8 weeks as part of an evaluation for suspected food hypersensitivity, only 4 dogs developed soft feces that had been normal on their original diets [59]. Also, of the 46 dogs, 21 had gastrointestinal signs as part of their original presentation, and the feces of all 21 improved on the hydrolysate diet. These findings combine to suggest that hyperosmolar diarrhea is not a significant problem with that diet.

Finally, the use of enzymatic hydrolysis, with or without ultrafiltration, and the selection of purified carbohydrate sources, such as starch, incurs considerable cost to the manufacturer. Consequently, the protein hydrolysate diets available are at least 50% more expensive on a per-calorie basis than normal premium maintenance diets.

USE AND EVIDENCE OF EFFICACY OF HYDROLYZED PROTEIN DIETS

When considering reports of the efficacy of hydrolysate diets, it should remembered that nutritional factors other than the hydrolysis of the protein component may be responsible for reported clinical improvements. Nutritional variables that could affect clinical responses include dietary digestibility, correction of vitamin or mineral deficiencies, a lowered ω (n)-6/n-3 fatty acid ratio, and the potential for an immunomodulatory effect of soy isoflavones (eg, genistein) within the diet, especially in cases of intestinal disease. A study that would definitively demonstrate the efficacy of protein hydrolysis alone would compare two diets in which the only difference is that one of the diets has the protein component hydrolyzed.

Elimination Diets

The primary role for the use of hydrolyzed protein diets is for the diagnosis or management of food hypersensitivity in all its manifestations. Whenever the feeding of a novel protein diet is recommended, a hydrolyzed protein diet could be considered. Increasingly, feline and canine patients are being exposed to a wide variety of protein sources as the range of commercial diets increases. The identification of a truly novel protein in patients presented for evaluation of dietary hypersensitivity can be difficult. Hydrolyzed protein diets allow greater confidence in the instigation of an elimination trial when a dietary history is uncertain or reveals prior exposure to multiple proteins.

Protein hydrolysate diets have been reported to be effective and well tolerated when used as elimination diets for the diagnosis of adverse food reactions in dogs [59,60]. In those studies, owner compliance was excellent, whereby 73% and 97% of dogs completed the 6- to 8-week trial periods. The high completion rates are similar or superior to those reported by authors using home-cooked or commercial novel protein diets (64%–80%) for elimination diet trials [66–68].

The protein sources incriminated in the adverse reactions were not reported in the study by Loeffler and colleagues [59]. Therefore, it is impossible to comment on the efficacy of that diet in cases in which the patient is sensitized to the intact source protein. In the study by Biourge and coworkers [60], however, two dogs that did not improve when fed the soy- and chicken-based hydrolysate did improve when fed a home-prepared soy based diet or a commercial rabbit and rice diet. Those findings suggest sensitization to the chicken or other protein fractions within the hydrolysate diet or the creation of novel dietary antigens as the result of the food processing, as has been demonstrated to occur [32].

Finally, Jackson and colleagues [7] evaluated the efficacy of a soy-based hydrolysate diet when fed for 2 weeks to 14 cross-breed dogs that were known to be allergic to soy or corn. Of the 14 dogs, 3 reacted adversely to the hydrolyzed soy diet, all 3 of which were hypersensitive to soy and corn; thus, it is uncertain to what fraction the dogs were reacting. This study demonstrated for the first time that a commercially available hydrolysate diet can be fed to most dogs sensitized to the intact source protein without eliciting clinical signs. It also indicated that a significant proportion (21%) of dogs sensitized to the intact compounds still react adversely to the hydrolyzed diet, however. This re-emphasizes the limitations of the currently available hydrolyzed protein diets.

For maximum confidence in performing an elimination diet trial, it is still important, even when using a hydrolyzed protein diet, to obtain an accurate dietary history and to choose a diet that contains ingredients the patient is unlikely to be sensitized to.

Inflammatory Bowel Disease

Novel protein diets have been proven effective in dogs and cats with a range of small and large intestinal inflammatory bowel disease (IBD) [69–72]. Guilford and coworkers [72] reported that in 16 cats with chronic gastrointestinal signs in which elimination challenge trials had proven dietary hypersensitivity, all 16 had mild to severe inflammatory infiltrates in at least one region of the bowel. The infiltrates were lymphocytic, lymphocytic-plasmacytic (most cases), or eosinophilic (two cases). All cats responded completely to the elimination diet alone without the need for immunosuppression. In a report of 13 dogs with lymphocytic-plasmacytic colitis (LPC), clinical signs resolved in all dogs with the introduction of a novel protein diet, and 9 of 11 dogs rechallenged with their original diet relapsed [70]. In a further report of 6 cats with LPC, all responded completely to an elimination diet [69]. A complete clinical response to an elimination diet has been reported in a cat with duodenal and ileal lymphocytic infiltrates so marked that a histopathologic diagnosis of intestinal lymphosarcoma was made [73]. These reports emphasize the importance of the diet as a source of provocative antigens in a subset of cases of IBD.

Hydrolyzed protein diets have the advantage over an intact novel protein diet in the management of IBD because there is less concern about sensitization to the new diet during the initial treatment phase. The concern over newly acquired dietary hypersensitivity has led to the concept of using "sacrificial proteins" when treating intestinal disorders with loss of oral tolerance [74]. Theoretically, hydrolyzed protein diets might lead to a more rapid improvement if inappropriate immune responses directed against novel dietary antigens are contributing to ongoing enteritis. Anecdotally, hydrolyzed protein diets seem to be effective adjuncts to pharmacologic therapy, and even as the sole therapy in IBD. Clinical resolution with histopathologic improvement has been reported in four of six dogs with refractory IBD when treated with a soy-based hydrolysate diet alone [75]. Although small and uncontrolled, these results are supportive of the role of the hydrolysate, because five cases had previously failed suitably conducted elimination diet trials using intact novel proteins.

Acute Enteritis

Acute enteritis from any cause can conceivably lead to temporary sensitization to food antigens, which would be expected to prolong clinical signs. Bacterial adjuvants, such as fimbriae from enterotoxigenic *Escherichia coli*, lipo-oligosaccharide from *Campylobacter*, and cholera toxin, can induce sensitization to ingested proteins if administered concurrently [76,77]. If sensitization does occur during acute enteritis, feeding a hydrolysate diet during recovery from intestinal disease would be expected to abrogate such an effect.

The effect of feeding a hydrolyzed diet during intestinal recovery from an acute mucosal insult or intestinal resection has not been evaluated in dogs or cats. Nevertheless, it is becoming increasingly clear that the early introduction of food after severe mucosal injury can more rapidly restore normal permeability; decrease bacterial translocation; decrease time to normalization of demeanor, appetite, vomiting, and diarrhea; and decrease mortality [78,79]. It has also been shown that the form of the diet is important during recovery. Marks and colleagues [80] reported that intestinal recovery in cats after treatment with a toxic dose of methotrexate was maximized when a complex diet was fed and was impaired when a purified amino acid diet was fed.

These findings are consistent with the knowledge that intestinal recovery is dependent on the production of trophic factors, such as glucagon-like peptide-2 (GLP-2) and insulin-like growth factor-1 (IGF-1) [81]. The ileum and colon are the primary intestinal sites of synthesis and secretion of GLP-2 and IGF-1, which are released in response to the presence of nutrients, especially peptides, in the intestinal lumen. Thus, luminal nutrients are essential for maximal and rapid mucosal recovery, which is stimulated largely by enterically derived GLP-2 and IGF-1. Therefore, concerns when feeding semielemental diets are whether there is, by virtue of the hydrolysis procedure, less stimulation for intestinal recovery and whether the speculated benefit of avoiding transient or persistent food hypersensitivity outweighs a risk of impairing intestinal adaptation. Some studies have shown improved villous recovery after starvation when hydrolysates are fed compared with intact proteins or free amino acids [82,83]. In other studies, however, extensively hydrolyzed proteins have been shown to impair intestinal recovery [84].

It is likely that the degree of hydrolysis currently incorporated for the production of hydrolysate diets in veterinary medicine does not have any detrimental effect on intestinal recovery after a mucosal insult. In fact, it may be that the oligopeptide component is ideal for feeding in acute and chronic inflammatory enteropathies. This is an area that warrants further study.

Prevention of Food Hypersensitivity

Perhaps some of the most interesting work on protein hydrolysates has been the recent discovery of so-called "tolerogenic" peptides in partially hydrolyzed formulae. Fritsche and coworkers [85] investigated whether oral tolerance can be induced with protein hydrolysates. The authors investigated a partially hydrolyzed formula and an extensively hydrolyzed whey-protein formula and found that the partially hydrolyzed formula was able to induce immunologic tolerance to the intact protein when administered before and during experimental sensitization, whereas the extensively hydrolyzed formula was not. The significance of these findings is that they introduce the possibility of inducing tolerance in a sensitized patient even when the patient is sensitized to the parent protein. As long as there are no peptides large enough to induce an IgE-mediated response but there are sufficiently large fragments to be antigenic in some way, the establishment of tolerance to the parent protein may be hastened. In addition, if the feeding of a hydrolysate were to be considered as a prophylactic measure in patients "at risk" of developing a food hypersensitivity, the inclusion of some low-molecular-weight antigens might be advantageous. These findings raise the intriguing possibility that hydrolysates may have a role in preventing hypersensitivity in individuals at risk as well as for managing already sensitized individuals. In high-risk infants who are unable to be completely breast fed, there is evidence that prolonged feeding with a hydrolyzed formula compared with a cow's milk formula reduces infant and childhood allergy to cow's milk [86].

Exocrine Pancreatic Insufficiency

The benefit of hydrolyzed protein diets for the management of exocrine pancreatic insufficiency (EPI) could be argued on the basis of increased digestibility and reduced antigenicity. Predigestion of the protein seems intuitively beneficial for cases of EPI. However, there is no evidence that protein malnutrition occurs following successful treatment of EPI. It is likely that intestinal brush border endopeptidases compensate for the loss of pancreatic proteases and enable adequate protein and peptide digestion. Regardless, adverse reactions to food have been reported in up to 10% of dogs with EPI [87,88]. Biourge and Fontaine [89] reported the efficacy of a soy- and chicken-based hydrolysate diet in three German Shepherds with EPI and adverse food reactions that had been inadequately managed for a prolonged period. In all three dogs, fecal quality, dermatologic signs, and body weight improved within 3 weeks of commencing feeding. Although this was an uncontrolled study with inadequate numbers to draw firm conclusions, the results are sufficiently provocative to suggest that the hydrolyzed protein diets may be beneficial in the management of refractory cases of EPI.

SUMMARY

Although true food hypersensitivity is relatively uncommon in dogs and cats, it is an important differential diagnosis for chronic pruritic skin disease and gastrointestinal disease alike. Given the ever-increasing range of dietary proteins that our patients are exposed to, hydrolyzed protein diets offer a convenient and proven option for the diagnosis and management of food hypersensitivity. As experience with hydrolyzed protein diets in veterinary medicine increases, so should our appreciation for the range of their benefits in diseases, such as IBD, acute enteritis, and EPI. Comparing the currently available hydrolysate diets beyond basic ingredients is difficult because of the absence of standard evaluations. Determining the optimal degree of hydrolysis is even more difficult and likely differs according to protein, patient, and disease process. The degree of hydrolysis currently used in veterinary diets may be ideal from nutritional and palatability perspectives but cannot guarantee an absence of intact allergens. As such, the use of hydrolyzed protein diets does not expunge the need for a detailed dietary history when dietary hypersensitivity is suspected.

References
[1] Cantani A, Micera M. Immunogenicity of hydrolysate formulas in children (part 1). Analysis of 202 reactions. J Investig Allergol Clin Immunol 2000;10(5):261–76.
[2] Pahud JJ, Schwarz K. Research and development of infant formulae with reduced allergenic properties. Ann Allergy 1984;53(6 Pt 2):609–14.
[3] Anderson SA, Chinn HI, Fisher KD. History and current status of infant formulas. Am J Clin Nutr 1982;35(2):381–97.
[4] Cromwell O. Biochemistry of allergens. In: Kay AB, editor. Allergy and allergic diseases, vol. 2. 1st edition. Oxford: Blackwell Science; 1997. p. 797–811.
[5] Kleinman RE, Bahna SL, Powell GF, et al. Use of infant formulas in infants with cow milk allergy: a review and recommendations. Pediatr Allergy Immunol 1991;4:146–55.
[6] Cave NJ, Guilford WG. A method for in vitro evaluation of protein hydrolysates for potential inclusion in veterinary diets. Res Vet Sci 2004;77(3):231–8.
[7] Jackson HA, Jackson MW, Coblentz L, et al. Evaluation of the clinical and allergen specific serum immunoglobulin E responses to oral challenge with cornstarch, corn, soy and a soy hydrolysate diet in dogs with spontaneous food allergy. Vet Dermatol 2003;14(4):181–7.
[8] Martin A, Sierra MP, Gonzalez JI, et al. Identification of allergens responsible for canine cutaneous adverse food reactions to lamb, beef and cow's milk. Vet Dermatol 2004;15(6):349–56.
[9] Sampson HA. Food allergy. J Allergy Clin Immunol 2003;111(2 Suppl):S540–7.
[10] White SD. Food hypersensitivity in 30 dogs. J Am Vet Med Assoc 1986;188(7):695–8.
[11] Jeffers JG, Meyer EK, Sosis EJ. Responses of dogs with food allergies to single-ingredient dietary provocation. J Am Vet Med Assoc 1996;209(3):608–11.
[12] Lehrer SB, Horner WE, Reese G. Why are some proteins allergenic? Implications for biotechnology. Crit Rev Food Sci Nutr 1996;36(6):553–64.
[13] Taylor SL, Lemanske RF Jr, Bush RK, et al. Food allergens: structure and immunologic properties. Ann Allergy 1987;59(5 Pt 2):93–9.
[14] Puc M. Characterization of pollen allergens. Ann Agric Environ Med 2003;10(2):143–9.
[15] van Beresteijn EC, Meijer RJ, Schmidt DG. Residual antigenicity of hypoallergenic infant formulas and the occurrence of milk-specific IgE antibodies in patients with clinical allergy. J Allergy Clin Immunol 1995;96(3):365–74.
[16] Van Hoeyveld EM, Escalona-Monge M, de Swert LF, et al. Allergenic and antigenic activity of peptide fragments in a whey hydrolysate formula. Clin Exp Allergy 1998;28(9):1131–7.
[17] Takagi T, Naito Y, Tomatsuri N, et al. Pioglitazone, a PPAR-gamma ligand, provides protection from dextran sulfate sodium-induced colitis in mice in association with inhibition of the NF-kappaB-cytokine cascade. Redox Rep 2002;7(5):283–9.
[18] van der Klauw MM, Wilson JH, Stricker BH. Drug-associated anaphylaxis: 20 years of reporting in The Netherlands (1974–1994) and review of the literature. Clin Exp Allergy 1996;26(12):1355–63.
[19] van Ree R. Carbohydrate epitopes and their relevance for the diagnosis and treatment of allergic diseases. Int Arch Allergy Immunol 2002;129(3):189–97.
[20] Franck P, Moneret-Vautrin DA, Morisset M, et al. Anaphylactic reaction to inulin: first identification of specific IgEs to an inulin protein compound. Int Arch Allergy Immunol 2005;136(2):155–8.
[21] Foetisch K, Westphal S, Lauer I, et al. Biological activity of IgE specific for cross-reactive carbohydrate determinants. J Allergy Clin Immunol 2003;111(4):889–96.
[22] Frisner H, Rosendal A, Barkholt V. Identification of immunogenic maize proteins in a casein hydrolysate formula. Pediatr Allergy Immunol 2000;11(2):106–10.
[23] Zitouni N, Errahali Y, Metche M, et al. Influence of refining steps on trace allergenic protein content in sunflower oil. J Allergy Clin Immunol 2000;106(5):962–7.
[24] Hudson MJ. Product development horizons—a view from industry. Eur J Clin Nutr 1995;49(Suppl 1):S64–70.

[25] Lee YH. Food-processing approaches to altering allergenic potential of milk-based formula. J Pediatr 1992;121(5 Pt 2):S47–50.

[26] Purevsuren B, Davaajav Y. Thermal analysis of casein. Journal of Thermal Analysis and Calorimetry 2001;65(1):147–52.

[27] Wehbi Z, Perez MD, Sanchez L, et al. Effect of heat treatment on denaturation of bovine alpha-lactalbumin: determination of kinetic and thermodynamic parameters. J Agric Food Chem 2005;53(25):9730–6.

[28] Host A, Samuelsson EG. Allergic reactions to raw, pasteurized, and homogenized/pasteurized cow milk: a comparison. A double-blind placebo-controlled study in milk allergic children. Allergy 1988;43(2):113–8.

[29] Oobatake M, Ooi T. Hydration and heat stability effects on protein unfolding. Prog Biophys Mol Biol 1993;59(3):237–84.

[30] Otani H, Morita SI, Tokita F. Studies on the antigenicity of the browning product between beta-lactoglobulin and lactose. Japanese Journal of Zootechnical Science 1985;56:1–74.

[31] Sancho AI, Rigby NM, Zuidmeer L, et al. The effect of thermal processing on the IgE reactivity of the non-specific lipid transfer protein from apple, Mal d 3. Allergy 2005;60(10): 1262–8.

[32] Cave NJ, Marks SL. Evaluation of the immunogenicity of dietary proteins in cats and the influence of the canning process. Am J Vet Res 2004;65(10):1427–33.

[33] Astwood JD, Leach JN, Fuchs RL. Stability of food allergens to digestion in vitro. Nat Biotechnol 1996;14(10):1269–73.

[34] Barnett D, Howden ME. Partial characterization of an allergenic glycoprotein from peanut (Arachis hypogaea L.). Biochim Biophys Acta 1986;882(1):97–105.

[35] Grimble GK, Rees RG, Keohane PP, et al. Effect of peptide chain length on absorption of egg protein hydrolysates in the normal human jejunum. Gastroenterology 1987;92(1):136–42.

[36] Daenzer M, Petzke KJ, Bequette BJ, et al. Whole-body nitrogen and splanchnic amino acid metabolism differ in rats fed mixed diets containing casein or its corresponding amino acid mixture. J Nutr 2001;131(7):1965–72.

[37] Nestle-Purina. HA hypoallergenic canine formula. Nestle-Purina Petcare: St. Louis, Missouri; 2006.

[38] Clapper GM, Grieshop CM, Merchen NR, et al. Ileal and total tract nutrient digestibilities and fecal characteristics of dogs as affected by soybean protein inclusion in dry, extruded diets. J Anim Sci 2001;79(6):1523–32.

[39] Hekman M. Research into causes of diarrhoea associated with the Hill's prescription diet Canine z/d Ultra Allergen Free. Palmerston North (New Zealand): Institute of Veterinary, Animal and Biomedical Sciences, Massey University; 2003.

[40] Rigo J, Salle BL, Cavero E, et al. Plasma amino acid and protein concentrations in infants fed human milk or a whey protein hydrolysate formula during the first month of life. Acta Paediatr 1994;83(2):127–31.

[41] Karlsland Akeson PM, Axelsson IE, Raiha NC. Protein and amino acid metabolism in three- to twelve-month-old infants fed human milk or formulas with varying protein concentrations. J Pediatr Gastroenterol Nutr 1998;26(3):297–304.

[42] Leary HL Jr. Nonclinical testing of formulas containing hydrolyzed milk protein. J Pediatr 1992;121(5 Pt 2):S42–6.

[43] Ellis MH, Short JA, Heiner DC. Anaphylaxis after ingestion of a recently introduced hydrolyzed whey protein formula. J Pediatr 1991;118(1):74–7.

[44] Cordle CT, Duska-McEwen G, Janas LM, et al. Evaluation of the immunogenicity of protein hydrolysate formulas using laboratory animal hyperimmunization. Pediatr Allergy Immunol 1994;5(1):14–9.

[45] Poulsen OM, Nielsen BR, Basse A, et al. Comparison of intestinal anaphylactic reactions in sensitized mice challenged with untreated bovine milk and homogenized bovine milk. Allergy 1990;45(5):321–6.

[46] Cantani A, Micera M. Immunogenicity of hydrolysate formulas in children (Pt 2): 41 case reports. J Investig Allergol Clin Immunol 2001;11(1):21–6.

[47] Businco L, Cantani A, Longhi MA, et al. Anaphylactic reactions to a cow's milk whey protein hydrolysate (Alfa-Re, Nestle) in infants with cow's milk allergy. Ann Allergy 1989;62(4): 333–5.

[48] Saylor JD, Bahna SL. Anaphylaxis to casein hydrolysate formula. J Pediatr 1991;118(1): 71–4.

[49] Oppenheimer JJ, Nelson HS, Bock SA, et al. Treatment of peanut allergy with rush immunotherapy. J Allergy Clin Immunol 1992;90(2):256–62.

[50] Sawatzki G, Georgi G, Kohn G. Pitfalls in the design and manufacture of infant formulae. Acta Paediatr Suppl 1994;402:40–5.

[51] Iwamura H. Structure–sweetness relationship of L-aspartyl dipeptide analogues. A receptor site topology. J Med Chem 1981;24(5):572–83.

[52] Adler-Nissen J. A review of food protein hydrolysis-specific areas. Enzymic hydrolysis of food proteins. New York: Elsevier Applied Science Publishers; 1986. 427.

[53] Cho MJ, Unklesbay N, Hsieh FH, et al. Hydrophobicity of bitter peptides from soy protein hydrolysates. J Agric Food Chem 2004;52(19):5895–901.

[54] Solms J, Vuataz L, Egli RH. The taste of L- and D-amino acids. Experientia 1965;21(12): 692–4.

[55] Iwasaki K, Sato MA. Taste preferences for amino acids in the house musk shrew, Suncus murinus. Physiol Behav 1982;28(5):829–33.

[56] Ugawa T, Kurihara K. Large enhancement of canine taste responses to amino acids by salts. Am J Physiol Regul Integr Comp Physiol 1993;264:R1071–6.

[57] Bartoshuk LM, Jacobs HL, Nichols IL, et al. Taste rejection of nonnutritive sweeteners in cats. J Comp Physiol Psychol 1975;89(8):971–5.

[58] Beauchamp GK, Maller O, Rogers JG. Flavor preferences in cats (*Felis catus* and *Panthera sp.*). J Comp Physiol Psychol 1977;91:1118–27.

[59] Loeffler A, Lloyd DH, Bond R, et al. Dietary trials with a commercial chicken hydrolysate diet in 63 pruritic dogs. Vet Rec 2004;154(17):519–22.

[60] Biourge VC, Fontaine J, Vroom MW. Diagnosis of adverse reactions to food in dogs: efficacy of a soy-isolate hydrolysate-based diet. J Nutr 2004;134(8 Suppl):2062S–4S.

[61] Hyams JS, Treem WR, Etienne NL, et al. Effect of infant formula on stool characteristics of young infants. Pediatrics 1995;95(1):50–4.

[62] Ladas SD, Isaacs PE, Sladen GE. Post-prandial changes of osmolality and electrolyte concentration in the upper jejunum of normal man. Digestion 1983;26(4):218–23.

[63] Fruto LV. Current concepts: management of diarrhea in acute care. J Wound Ostomy Continence Nurs 1994;21(5):199–205.

[64] Teichberg S, Lifshitz F, Pergolizzi R, et al. Response of rat intestine to a hyperosmotic feeding. Pediatr Res 1978;12(6):720–5.

[65] Hahn S, Kim Y, Garner P. Reduced osmolarity oral rehydration solution for treating dehydration due to diarrhoea in children: systematic review. BMJ 2001;323(7304):81–5.

[66] Chesney CJ. Food sensitivity in the dog: a quantitative study. J Small Anim Pract 2002;43(5):203–7.

[67] Tapp T, Griffin C, Rosenkrantz W, et al. Comparison of a commercial limited-antigen diet versus home-prepared diets in the diagnosis of canine adverse food reaction. Vet Ther 2002;3(3):244–51.

[68] Roudebush P, Schick R. Evaluation of a commercial canned lamb and rice diet for the management of adverse reactions to food in dogs. Vet Dermatol 1994;5(2):63–7.

[69] Nelson RW, Dimperio ME, Long GG. Lymphocytic-plasmacytic colitis in the cat. J Am Vet Med Assoc 1984;184(9):1133–5.

[70] Nelson RW, Stookey LJ, Kazacos E. Nutritional management of idiopathic chronic colitis in the dog. J Vet Intern Med 1988;2(3):133–7.

[71] Hirt R, Iben C. Possible food allergy in a colony of cats. J Nutr 1998;128(12 Suppl): 2792S–4S.

[72] Guilford WG, Jones BR, Markwell PJ, et al. Food sensitivity in cats with chronic idiopathic gastrointestinal problems. J Vet Intern Med 2001;15(1):7–13.

[73] Wasmer ML, Willard MD, Helman RG, et al. Food intolerance mimicking alimentary lymphosarcoma. J Am Anim Hosp Assoc 1995;31(6):463–6.

[74] Guilford WG. Idiopathic inflammatory bowel diseases. In: Guilford WG, Center SA, Strombeck DR, et al, editors. Strombeck's small animal gastroenterology 3rd edition. Philadelphia: WB Saunders; 1996. p. 451–87.

[75] Marks SL, Laflamme DP, McCandlish AP. Dietary trial using a commercial hypoallergenic diet containing hydrolyzed protein for dogs with inflammatory bowel disease. Vet Ther 2002;3(2):109–18.

[76] Verdonck F, De Hauwere V, Bouckaert J, et al. Fimbriae of enterotoxigenic Escherichia coli function as a mucosal carrier for a coupled heterologous antigen. J Control Release 2005;104(2):243–58.

[77] Jung S, Zimmer S, Luneberg E, et al. Lipo-oligosaccharide of Campylobacter jejuni prevents myelin-specific enteral tolerance to autoimmune neuritis—a potential mechanism in Guillain-Barré syndrome? Neurosci Lett 2005;381(1–2):175–8.

[78] Mohr AJ, Leisewitz AL, Jacobson LS, et al. Effect of early enteral nutrition on intestinal permeability, intestinal protein loss, and outcome in dogs with severe parvoviral enteritis. J Vet Intern Med 2003;17(6):791–8.

[79] Dahlinger J, Marks SL, Hirsh DC. Prevalence and identity of translocating bacteria in healthy dogs. J Vet Intern Med 1997;11(6):319–22.

[80] Marks SL, Cook AK, Griffey S, et al. Dietary modulation of methotrexate-induced enteritis in cats. Am J Vet Res 1997;58(9):989–96.

[81] Strom BL, Schinnar R, Ziegler EE, et al. Exposure to soy-based formula in infancy and endocrinological and reproductive outcomes in young adulthood. JAMA 2001;286(7):807–14.

[82] Poullain MG, Cezard JP, Marche C, et al. Dietary whey proteins and their peptides or amino acids: effects on the jejunal mucosa of starved rats. Am J Clin Nutr 1989;49(1):71–6.

[83] Poullain MG, Cezard JP, Roger L, et al. Effect of whey proteins, their oligopeptide hydrolysates and free amino acid mixtures on growth and nitrogen retention in fed and starved rats. JPEN J Parenter Enteral Nutr 1989;13(4):382–6.

[84] Zarrabian S, Buts JP, Fromont G, et al. Effects of alimentary intact proteins and their oligopeptide hydrolysate on growth, nitrogen retention, and small bowel adaptation in inflammatory turpentine rat. Nutrition 1999;15(6):474–80.

[85] Fritsche R, Pahud JJ, Pecquet S, et al. Induction of systemic immunologic tolerance to beta-lactoglobulin by oral administration of a whey protein hydrolysate. J Allergy Clin Immunol 1997;100(2):266–73.

[86] Osborn DA, Sinn J. Formulas containing hydrolyzed protein for prevention of allergy and food intolerance in infants. Cochrane Database Syst Rev 2003;4:CD003664.

[87] Hall EJ, et al. A survey of the diagnosis and treatment of canine exocrine pancreatic insufficiency. J Small Anim Pract 1991;32:613–9.

[88] Wiberg ME, Lautala HM, Westermarck E. Response to long-term enzyme replacement treatment in dogs with exocrine pancreatic insufficiency. J Am Vet Med Assoc 1998;213(1): 86–90.

[89] Biourge VC, Fontaine J. Exocrine pancreatic insufficiency and adverse reaction to food in dogs: a positive response to a high-fat, soy isolate hydrolysate-based diet. J Nutr 2004;134(8 Suppl):2166S–8S.

Vet Clin Small Anim 36 (2006) 1269–1281

VETERINARY CLINICS
SMALL ANIMAL PRACTICE

Unconventional Diets for Dogs and Cats

Kathryn E. Michel, DVM, MS

Department of Clinical Studies, School of Veterinary Medicine, University of Pennsylvania,
3900 Delancey Street, Philadelphia, PA 19104–6010, USA

Tell me what you eat and I will tell you what you are.—Anthelme Brillat-Savarin, 1825 [1]

The use of diet for the promotion of good health and in the management of disease is not a new idea, but it is one that has received increasing attention in recent years by the public and the scientific and medical community. People have always sought advice about how best to feed their pets from a variety of sources, including family and acquaintances, pet food retailers, breeders, and veterinary health professionals. Today, more than ever, with the growing use of the World Wide Web, veterinary health professionals are finding themselves dealing with a clientele that, for better or worse, has access to a large body of information on small animal nutrition and medicine. Nutrition finds itself in kind of a gray area in medicine that can range from accepted conventional practices to numerous forms of alternative therapy, including manipulation of diet and using a range of dietary supplements and herbal remedies. Today's veterinary health professionals are faced with the challenge not only of staying current with emerging research on clinical nutrition, including fads and popular trends, but of being able to understand why pet owners choose certain feeding practices and how to use effective strategies to influence them to change when it is in their pet's best interest to do so.

This article explores the reasons why people might seek alternatives to conventional pet foods, describes the different categories of alternative feeding practices, and discusses approaches to communicating with pet owners about nutrition and diet for their pets. The goal is for the reader to acquire a better understanding of unconventional feeding practices being used for companion animals so that she or he is better informed on the views and concerns of the pet-owning public regarding dog and cat nutrition and better able to enter into the dialog of how these pets should best be fed.

E-mail address: michel@vet.upenn.edu

0195-5616/06/$ – see front matter
doi:10.1016/j.cvsm.2006.08.003

WHY PEOPLE SEEK ALTERNATIVES TO CONVENTIONAL PET FOODS

Perspectives on Diet and Food Consumption

As health professionals, we tend to take a nutritional science perspective when thinking about food consumption. The focus is on eating practices that promote health, and thus should be encouraged, or that impair health, and thus should be discouraged [2]. This perspective makes food habits and preferences secondary to the biologic activities of foods and views social and cultural factors surrounding food consumption as barriers to achieving a healthy diet.

For human beings, food consumption is clearly a more complex act than the nutritional science perspective takes into consideration, and for at least a subset of the pet-owning population, food selection and feeding practices for pets are influenced by the same social and cultural factors that govern the pet owners' personal eating behaviors.

Defining What Is Food

What is and is not food is defined socially and culturally. In some cultures, insects are delicacies, and in others, the idea of eating them would be viewed with disgust. This is something that resonates strongly among pet owners with concerns about the wholesomeness of commercial pet foods. The reality is that the pet food industry makes use of the byproducts of the human food industry. In most cases, animal source ingredients are offal or rendered meals from tissues that have no market as human foods. One example is pork liver, which has limited appeal in the United States, and therefore ends up in pet food, whereas in France, pork liver finds its way into paté. It should be recognized that even though many people would not find these byproducts appealing, it does not follow that they are not nutritious. People should be encouraged to disclose any concerns they may have about commercial pet food ingredients and manufacturing processes. The challenge becomes one of persuading the pet owner to focus on other indicators of commercial pet food quality, such as Association of American Feed Control Officials (AAFCO) feeding trials rather than on the label ingredient list.

Symbolism of Food

Food can be symbolic of many things. First and foremost, food is a basic necessity of life, and thus part of the shared human experience. The role that diet and nutrition play in maintaining health and preventing or treating disease is something that is usually within the grasp of most people, even if they do not understand the nutritional science involved.

Food and meals are used to symbolize and order social interactions and have ritual significance in many religions. Dietary practices can be used to maintain barriers and reinforce social order and group identity. Therefore, although substitution of one type of food with another might create a better diet from the perspective of a veterinarian, the pet owner might meet the change with resistance because it violates that person's sense of propriety. This situation often arises when a pet is overweight and a weight reduction diet is suggested.

Curtailing treating behaviors or reducing feeding portions may be resisted, in part, because these practices are seen as excluding the pet from normal family life. Furthermore, because the receiving and giving of food are construed as a way of showing affection by many, some people may fear that their pet might perceive that they no longer love it if they withhold food.

Food can be a means by which individuals define who they are in contrast to others. Thus, food and eating behaviors contribute to how an individual creates an identity. This line of thinking might influence how pet owners feed their pets in a couple of ways. If they humanize their pets, they may simply transfer their attitudes about food to how they think their pets should be fed. Alternatively, people may consider how the pet's identity is defined by diet. For example, they may focus on the dog as a carnivore and assume that cereal grains are an unsuitable ingredient in a canine diet.

For certain individuals, ideology may play a role in how they themselves eat and how they feed their pets. The most obvious example of this would be individuals who choose a vegetarian or vegan lifestyle for reasons having to do with concerns about sustainable agriculture or humane treatment of animals.

One aspect of eating behaviors that should not be overlooked is the way in which dietary habits and food selection represent empowerment and control of one's life. Eating disorders can be extreme examples of seeking control through manipulation of food intake. A person facing a serious illness, such as cancer, may embrace a new eating regimen. Obviously, this is done consciously for the potential therapeutic effects, but the feeling of empowerment that comes with taking control also has to factor into why many pet owners seek and embrace nutritional interventions for their pets, particularly those pets with serious or incurable illnesses. Furthermore, as we all know, foods can have significant effects on psychologic well-being (eg, "comfort foods"). Therefore, the use of diet in the context of preventing or treating disease is often viewed as a more holistic approach to health maintenance than conventional medical practices.

Motivation for Using Unconventional Diets

So how and what a pet is fed can be layered with meaning. It may be, in part, symbolic of inclusion of the pet in the owner's family and culture, and thus part of the bonding between human being and animal. It may be reflective of the pet owner's ideology and personal identity. Alternatively, it may be an act of empowerment in which the pet owner becomes invested in the health and well-being of her or his companion. What motivates a person to seek an alternative to conventional feeding practices for her or his pet could involve any or all of the previously mentioned factors. The first step in communicating with someone about nutrition and dietary practices is actively to seek information about her or his attitudes and beliefs regarding proper diets for her or his pet.

TYPES OF DIETS

For the purpose of this review, unconventional diets are defined rather broadly to include alternatives to what are perceived as typical commercial pet foods, such as commercially available "natural" diets, raw food diets, and vegetarian diets, in addition to the variety of home-prepared diets that exist (Box 1).

Home-Prepared Diets

Widespread feeding of commercially prepared pet foods is fairly recent practice found only in developed countries. Therefore, the home preparation of pet food has only been considered an unconventional practice in the United States for the past 50 years at most and would not be considered unconventional at all in much of the world. Many of the reasons people seek alternatives to commercial pet foods apply to people who desire to prepare food for their pets. Concerns about the wholesomeness and nutritional value of the ingredients used in commercial pet foods may be a consideration. For others, food preparation reinforces the bond they share with their pet. In some situations, people believe that their pets find commercial foods unpalatable and that they are likely to refuse to eat them. There are instances when a home-prepared diet may be indicated for diagnostic (eg, a food elimination trial) or therapeutic reasons. In cases in which a home-prepared therapeutic diet is sought, it may be because there is no commercially available diet that fits the desired nutritional profile or it may be because the patient refuses to eat the appropriate diets that are available. In addition, people may find comfort and a feeling of purpose through involvement in food preparation and feeding management for pets with chronic or terminal illness.

There are several potential drawbacks to home preparation of pet foods. The first is that it requires a greater investment of time, and likely of money, than feeding a commercially prepared pet food. The second potential drawback is that formulating a complete and balanced pet food requires specialized knowledge. The average pet owner needs to seek someone with this expertise, or at least to find a resource for a properly formulated recipe. This may not be a simple and straightforward task. Investigators reviewing recipes used for home-prepared pet foods from 116 veterinarians practicing in North America found that only 28 (65%) of 43 of the recipes used for long-term feeding of dogs and 18 (46%) of 39 of those recommended for long-term feeding for cats were nutritionally adequate (based on computer analysis) [3].

In another study, the nutritional adequacy of recipes for 49 maintenance and 36 growth diets from six published resources was reviewed using computer software [4]. Most of the diets (86%) were inadequate in various minerals, 55% were inadequate in protein (although 77% of those diets were only

---

Box 1: Alternatives to conventional commercial pet foods

- Home-prepared diets
- Natural, organic, or human food grade diets
- Vegetarian diets
- Raw food diets

deficient in taurine), and 62% were inadequate in vitamins (although 77% were only deficient in choline). That many of the ingredients in the software database had not been analyzed for taurine and choline has to be taken into consideration when interpreting these findings. Even so, based on this analysis, a number of the recipes seemed to have inadequacies.

One further concern is that even when a well-formulated recipe is provided, the overall nutritional adequacy of a home-prepared diet depends on the ingredients selected and how closely the person preparing the diet adheres to the recipe. There can be significant variation in the nutrient content of specified ingredients, for example, the fat content of ground beef. Furthermore, the person preparing the diet may have difficulty in finding one or more ingredients and opt to leave them out of the diet or may decide to substitute one item for another or even to include new ingredients in the preparation. Any of these actions could significantly change the nutrient profile of the diet and may ultimately make it unbalanced or unsuitable for the pet for which it was intended. Clearly, the likelihood of a nutritionally inadequate diet causing clinically significant adverse effects on health is more likely to occur in animals that have greater and more stringent dietary requirements: cats in general as well as growing, gestating, and lactating animals.

In situations in which a home-prepared pet food is indicated or when it is the strong preference of the pet owner, most problems can be avoided if she or he is provided with properly formulated recipes (Box 2 provides for resources for formulation of home-prepared foods) and with clear and thorough instructions on food preparation, including whether any substitutions or omissions are permissible. There should be follow-up contact with the pet owner two or more times a year (more frequently in growing animals and other pets with increased nutrient demands) to monitor for proper recipe use and to examine the patient for signs of nutrient deficiency or excess.

Natural, Organic, and Human Food Grade Diets

The types and sources of ingredients used in the manufacture of commercial pet foods are a chief concern among pet owners seeking alternative options for feeding their pets [5]. Artificial additives, particularly preservatives, colorings, and flavorings, provoke anxiety about the impact of long-term intake of these substances on health. Of special concern is the role that food additives could play in carcinogenesis and the development of dietary hypersensitivity or autoimmune disorders [6]. In addition to substances that are intentionally used in the formulation of commercial pet foods, there are potentially harmful contaminants (eg, pesticides and heavy metals) that can be found in some feed ingredients. For these reasons, pet foods free of artificial additives or those made of ingredients that are perceived to be more wholesome and safe appeal to some people.

These are reasonable concerns. There have been notable and well-publicized cases of additives that have been withdrawn from use, including examples involving pet food manufacture, such as the banning of propylene glycol in cat

Box 2: Resources for formulation of home-prepared diets

Angell Memorial: telephone consults (617) 522-7282

Michigan State University: telephone consults (517) 432-7782; diet analysis (517) 353-9312

Ohio State University: telephone consults (614) 292-1221 or (614) 292-3551

Tufts University: telephone consults (508) 839-5395 extension 84,696; VetFax 800-829-5690

University of Tennessee: telephone consults (865) 974-8387

University of California, Davis: telephone consults (530) 752-1387 (veterinarians); (530) 752-1393 (clients)

foods after it was found to cause Heinz body anemia [7,8]. In many instances, however, fears about the safety of pet food additives are unwarranted. Sometimes, an individual has simply mistaken one or more of the vitamins and minerals listed among the ingredients on a pet food label for chemical additives. Pet owners should be aware that additives are only permitted for use in pet food manufacture with oversight of the US Food and Drug Administration (FDA) and AAFCO. Sometimes, reports of health hazards attributed to an additive are anecdotal and unsubstantiated. Ethoxyquin, an artificial antioxidant, is an example of a compound that has been extensively tested in dogs. Although it has been found to be safe even when ingested at levels considerably higher than those found in commercial foods, the public perception that ethoxyquin could be harmful persists and many pet food manufacturers have turned to other types of antioxidant preservatives [6,9].

Perceived consumer preference for pet foods free of artificial ingredients has led some manufacturers to market natural products. Formulating a pet food free of artificial colorants and flavorings poses little challenge. Preservation, however, is necessary for dry foods in conventional packaging because they are exposed to air and contain ingredients (eg, fats, fat-soluble vitamins) that are subject to oxidation. Even a canned food may contain antioxidant preservatives if it was manufactured using fats and other ingredients that already contained these substances for preservation purposes. Therefore, manufacturers have turned to using naturally occurring antioxidant compounds, including mixed tocopherols and ascorbic acid, as an alternative to synthetic antioxidant preservatives. All pet foods should be tested for stability to establish each product's shelf life. In general, chemical preservatives like ethoxyquin are more effective antioxidants than natural preservatives like mixed tocopherols. Therefore, it is of particular importance that people using naturally preserved pet foods select a product that is labeled with a "best used by" date and that they do not feed food past the label date, although such labeling is not mandated by any government agency.

At the time that naturally preserved pet foods first started to be marketed, regulations for defining ingredients or labeling products as natural did not exist.

The AAFCO has since defined a natural ingredient as one that is derived solely from plant, animal, or mined sources and a natural product as one in which all ingredients meet this definition [10]. The term *natural* is not synonymous with the term *organic*. As of 2002, the US Department of Agriculture (USDA) has established standards that foods labeled organic must meet (Box 3), and although, technically, an organic pet food should meet these standards, the AAFCO has not written labeling regulations that expressly state this requirement.

Some pet foods are marketed as containing human-grade ingredients. These foods would presumably have an appeal for individuals who are leery of what they perceive to be the types and sources of ingredients found in commercial pet foods. Currently, there are no government standards for defining the term *human grade*. A pet food manufacturer is free to interpret and use this designation as it sees fit. Chances are that in many cases, the public has a different perception of what human-grade ingredients would consist of than what is actually used in the manufacture of one of these pet foods.

In summary, there are commercially available natural pet foods, and some regulatory oversight of the labeling of these foods exists. Therefore, people looking for natural alternatives to conventional pet foods do have this option, aside from home preparation of food, for feeding their pets. Although it would be possible to manufacture a pet food from certified organic ingredients, there are currently no rules for the labeling of pet foods as organic products. Currently, there are also no standards for designating pet food ingredients as human grade. Last, all pet foods should be fed in accordance with their shelf life, and, ideally, this information should be available on the product label.

Vegetarian Diets

People may choose to follow a vegetarian diet for a variety of reasons, including religious beliefs, ethical concerns, and health considerations. Some individuals are so strong in their convictions that they wish to feed their pets in a similar fashion. One investigation found that ethical concerns, followed by health considerations, were the most common reasons people stated for choosing to feed their cats a vegetarian diet [11]. In that same study, all persons interviewed who were feeding a vegetarian diet to their cats also reported being a vegetarian themselves.

Box 3: US Department of Agriculture Organic Food Standards

- Animal source ingredients come from animals that are given no antibiotics or growth hormones.
- Organically grown food is produced without using most conventional pesticides, fertilizers made with synthetic ingredients or sewage sludge, bioengineering, or ionizing radiation.
- Producers and processors of foods that are labeled organic must be inspected and certified by the USDA.

Formulating a complete and balanced vegetarian pet food can be challenging. Several nutrients that are essential in the diets of cats are only found in animal source ingredients (eg, taurine, vitamin A), in fermented foods (cobalamin), or in trace amounts in some algae (arachidonic acid). Cobalamin is also an essential nutrient for dogs. Furthermore, the protein requirement of dogs and especially cats is significantly higher than the human protein requirement, and several of the essential amino acids are limited in most vegetable sources of protein. There is a wide range of dietary practices that fall under the designation of vegetarianism, and some of them include eating animal products, such as milk and eggs. With the strictest form of vegetarianism (veganism), however, it would be necessary to use synthetic forms of some nutrients to make a complete and balanced vegan feline diet, and as such, the diet could not also be designated as natural.

Because the nutrient requirements of dogs are not as stringent as those of cats, there are a number of commercially available vegetarian and even vegan canine diets available, including some that have demonstrated nutritional adequacy through an AAFCO feeding trial. The options for vegetarian feline diets are much more limited and, with few exceptions, require home preparation of a diet with the use of special supplements. The nutritional adequacy of vegetarian pet foods has been investigated. One study analyzed 12 commercially available vegetarian dog foods and found that only 2 of them were nutritionally adequate [12]. The same investigation also reviewed home-prepared vegetarian diets that were being fed to 86 dogs and 8 cats and found many of them to be nutritionally inadequate in ways typical of home-prepared diets. In another investigation, a commercially available complete vegan cat food and a vegan feline diet prepared with a commercially available supplement according to the supplement manufacturer's directions were analyzed for several key nutrients [13]. Neither diet was found to meet the feline AAFCO nutrient profile comprehensively for any life stage. The taurine and cobalamin status of cats eating one or both of those diets were evaluated by other investigators, who found that all the cats tested had normal serum cobalamin concentrations and that 14 of 17 had whole-blood taurine concentrations within the reference range [11]. None of the cats with low blood taurine concentrations showed signs of taurine deficiency, and their blood levels were above what is considered to be the critical level for taurine status.

The findings of these two studies serve to illustrate the challenges of formulating a nutritionally adequate feline vegetarian diet. They also illustrate the pitfalls of relying simply on formulation and analysis as means of showing nutritional adequacy and the need for AAFCO feeding trials and a high level of quality assurance in manufacturing to ensure confidence in the finished product.

Because selecting this type of diet is a conscious choice on the part of these individuals, it should be relatively easy to enter into a dialog with them over the appropriateness and nutritional adequacy of these types of diets for dogs and cats. Some people may be willing to consider the ethical implications of feeding an animal a diet that can only meet its nutritional requirements through artificial manipulation and to weigh that consideration against the motives for their personal dietary choices. The same concerns and considerations that apply to home-prepared diets in general apply to home-prepared vegetarian diets, with the additional challenges of finding appropriate supplemental sources of the essential nutrients that are limited or absent in nonanimal source ingredients. Given that the nutritional adequacy of some commercially available vegetarian pet foods has been called into question, it would be prudent to advise regular follow-up with the pet owner feeding these diets, similar to what would be appropriate for an animal eating a home-prepared ration.

Raw Food Diets

Diets containing raw meat have been used for feeding animals for many years, especially by zoos and dog-racing facilities. The use of these diets for companion animals as an alternative to conventional pet foods, however, is a fairly recent development. It is difficult to gauge the popularity of raw food diets. The proponents of feeding raw food diets, some of whom are veterinary health professionals, are vocal and enthusiastic about the purported benefits of this dietary approach and promote them energetically and, at times, evangelically. A telephone survey of a random sample of pet owners from four different geographic locations across the United States and one location in Australia found that 8% of dog owners and 4% of cat owners fed raw meat with or without bones as all or part of their pet's main meal [14].

Raw food feeders can home-prepare diets or use commercially available raw products. The commercial products range from complete foods, which are generally sold frozen, to grain and supplement mixes, which are then combined with raw foods. Raw food diets have been promoted for their health benefits in terms of preventing disease and resolving or ameliorating preexisting conditions [15,16]. Objective evidence to substantiate these claims is lacking, however. Aside from their purported health benefits, one of the rationales for feeding raw food to pet dogs is that "there are no ovens in the wild," even though the domestic dog is well removed from its wild canid cousins. For some people, the raw diet becomes a symbol of the wild carnivore nature of the pet dog.

The reservations that have been expressed about raw food diets fall into two categories: nutritional adequacy and food safety issues, including public health concerns. With regard to nutritional adequacy, home-prepared raw food diets have the same drawbacks affecting any home-prepared diet. In one report, three persons feeding home-prepared raw food to their dogs provided samples of the diets for analysis of key nutrients. When the analyses were compared with the canine AAFCO nutrient profiles, all three of the diets were found to have nutrient excesses and deficiencies [17]. The consequences of feeding nutritionally inadequate diets are most likely to be serious in animals with increased nutrient demands, as is illustrated by a report of two different litters of puppies fed raw food diets, in which all the puppies developed severe nutritional osteodystrophy by 6 weeks of age [18]. Raw food diets, even those containing bones, can still be deficient in calcium, particularly when poultry bones are used [17]. Furthermore, newly weaned puppies have trouble ingesting bones unless they are finely ground.

With regard to the second concern, food safety, aside from the risk of gastrointestinal obstruction posed by feeding bones, home-prepared and commercial raw food diets have been evaluated for bacterial contamination [17,19–21]. In one investigation, 80% of home-prepared diets containing chicken were found to be contaminated with *Salmonella* spp [19]. Two investigations of commercial products found most products tested to be contaminated with *Escherichia coli* [20,21]. *Salmonella* spp were detected in 6% of the products tested in one study and in 20% of the products in the other. Protozoal contamination is of concern as well. Infection with *Toxoplasma gondii* has been reported in cats fed raw diets, and one investigation found evidence of *Cryptosporidium* spp in two commercially available raw food diets using a polymerase chain reaction (PCR) assay [21,22].

The risk of contracting an infectious disease from a raw food diet is not confined to the pets themselves [23]. People living in the same household as the pet are also at risk because they may come in contact with contaminated food through the preparation and feeding of a raw diet. Furthermore, it is documented that pets being fed raw food diets can become asymptomatic shedders of pathogens, including *Salmonella* spp and *T gondii* [19,22].

As with any dietary practice, the dialog with the pet owner must begin with an effort to understand her or his reasons for choosing to feed a raw food diet, including any concerns that she or he may have about conventional pet foods. It may be possible to address those concerns or offer alternatives that would avoid some or all of the risks inherent in feeding raw foods. Some people who are steadfast in their desire to home-prepare food for their pets may be persuaded to cook the food. As has already been discussed at length, care must be taken to ensure the nutritional adequacy of any home-prepared diet that is used for the long-term feeding of a pet. Others who insist on feeding raw food diets should be fully informed about all food safety issues and all aspects of hygiene involved in food preparation, interaction with the pet, and disposal of the pet's feces. It is incumbent on the proponents of raw food diets to produce scientific evidence of the efficacy and safety of this dietary practice. Although the pet owner ultimately decides how to feed her or his pet, she or he should be fully informed that although there are documented risks associated with raw diets, the potential health benefits are at best anecdotal.

CHANGING FEEDING PRACTICES

In recent years, there has been increasing focus on developing more effective ways for health professionals to communicate with their clients with the aim of improving compliance with prescribed treatments. Making an effort to talk with patients about their knowledge, beliefs, concerns, and expectations about their conditions has been shown to result in better adherence to treatment regimens [24]. Exploration of all these issues from a patient's perspective on her or his illness permits the attending health professional specifically to address deficiencies in knowledge or understanding of the condition and its treatment and the patient's ability and willingness to pursue a particular course of therapy.

With regard to dietary practices, despite a basic uniformity in nutritional requirements and physiologic needs, there is considerable variation in what people eat. In the case of pet dogs and cats, their owners largely determine what these animals eat on a daily basis. Yet, in many if not most cases, client education alone does not succeed in changing habits and behaviors relating to how a pet is fed. Just as a person's social and cultural context influences her or his own dietary habits, it also has an impact on how and what a pet is fed. Therefore, it is important to consider the social and cultural aspects of food consumption by people to communicate effectively with them about their pet's nutritional needs and appropriate dietary management, particularly if you are attempting to change current behaviors.

Frequently, circumstances arise in which a change in diet or feeding practices is suggested or recommended for a patient. To succeed in persuading the pet owner to follow our advice, we need some basic information, including how the pet is currently fed and an understanding of the rationale for those practices. The best way to obtain this information is to take a thorough dietary history. This can be done in an interview fashion, or you can use a standardized form that the pet owner can fill out at her or his convenience. The dietary history should consist of an accurate accounting of all foods fed to the pet on a typical day. It should include brand names of commercial pet foods and treats and specific amounts fed. Most pets get table foods, and some receive diets that are home-prepared. You should try to get the most accurate information available about the pet's consumption of table foods and, in the case of home-prepared diets, complete recipes. The pet owner may have to go home and keep a food diary for a few days before she or he can actually answer these questions. Other things to inquire about include whether the pet has access to the food fed to other pets in the household and whether there are other family members feeding the pet.

This information should greatly facilitate the process of implementing dietary therapy for the patient. It should help in making an appropriate diet selection and an accurate feeding recommendation. Most importantly, in regard to the topic at hand, the dietary history can give you some insight into the role that food plays in the interaction between the pet and the human members of its household. This insight should allow you to anticipate concerns and issues that might arise from implementing a change in feeding practices.

The diet history should be used to understand the pet owner's attitudes toward commercial pet foods, feed ingredients, and nutrition and nutritional therapy. Also seek to understand the pet owner's rationale for current feeding practices and to assess any concerns that may arise from a diet change. By anticipating problems, you should be able to craft the dietary intervention in a way that is more acceptable to the pet's household or, at the very least, to communicate more effectively with the pet owner about the rationale for the changes in feeding management. You should be in a better position to explain

> **Box 4: Negotiating a mutual plan of action for changing feeding practices**
>
> - Obtain the pet owner's beliefs and understanding about how her or his pet should be fed.
> - Obtain the pet owner's viewpoint regarding the need to change feeding practices (eg, perceived benefits, barriers, motivation to changing practices).
> - Take into consideration the pet owner's beliefs, cultural background, lifestyle, and abilities when formulating your plan for dietary modification.
> - Elicit the pet owner's reactions and concerns about the proposed dietary modifications.
>
> *Adapted from* Calgary-Cambridge guide to the medical interview-communication process. Available at: www.med.ucalgary.ca/education/learningresources/CalgaryCambridgeGuide. pdf. Accessed April 2006.

why you believe the changes you are proposing are in the pet's best interest and to look for compromise when your recommendations and the pet owner's preferences are in conflict (Box 4).

SUMMARY

To understand why some people seek alternatives to conventional commercial pet foods, we must keep in mind that food plays a far more complex role in daily life than simply serving as sustenance. How and what a pet is fed can be layered with meaning for the owner, and we must seek some understanding of that person's knowledge and beliefs about feeding pets to understand her or his motives for seeking an alternative and to be able effectively to persuade her or him to change those practices when it is in the best interest of the pet to do so.

References
  [1] Brillat-Savarin JA. The physiology of taste, or meditations on transcendental gastronomy (1825). Washington (DC): Counterpoint; 1995.
  [2] Quandt SA. Social and cultural influences on food consumption and nutritional status. In: Shils ME, Olson JA, Shine M, et al, editors. Modern nutrition in health and disease. 9th edition. Baltimore (MD): Williams & Wilkins; 1999. p. 1783–800.
  [3] Roudebush P, Cowell CS. Results of a hypoallergenic diet survey of veterinarians in North America with an evaluation of homemade diet prescription. Vet Dermatol 1992;3(1):23–8.
  [4] Lauten SD, Smith TM, Kirk CA, et al. Computer analysis of nutrient sufficiency of published home-cooked diets for dogs and cats [abstract]. J Vet Intern Med 2005;19(3):476–7.
  [5] Willoughby KN, Michel KE, Abood SK, et al. Feeding practices of dog and cat owners reflect attitudes toward pet foods [abstract]. J Anim Phys Anim Nutr 2005;89:428.
  [6] Dzanis DA. Safety of ethoxyquin in dog foods. J Nutr 1991;132(Suppl):S163–4.
  [7] Hickman MA, Rogers QR, Morris JG. Effect of diet on Heinz body formation in kittens. Am J Vet Res 1990;50(3):475–8.
  [8] Dzanis DA. Propylene glycol unsafe for use in cat foods. FDA Vet 1994;9(1):1–3.
  [9] Food and Drug Administration (FDA). FDA requests that ethoxyquin levels be reduced in dog foods. FDA Vet 1997;12(5):1.

[10] Association of American Feed Control Officials. Official publication of the Association of American Feed Control Officials; 2006.

[11] Wakefield LA, Shofer FS, Michel KE. Evaluation of cats fed vegetarian diets and attitudes of their caregivers. J Am Vet Med Assoc 2006;229:70–3.

[12] Kienzle E, Engelhard R. A field study on the nutrition of vegetarian dogs and cats in Europe. [abstract]. Compend Contin Educ Pract Vet 2001;23(9A):81.

[13] Gray CM, Sellon RK, Freeman LM. Nutritional adequacy of two vegan diets for cats. J Am Vet Med Assoc 2004;225(11):1670–5.

[14] Willoughby KN, Michel KE, Abood SK, et al. Feeding practices and attitudes about pet foods: cat vs. dog owners [abstract]. Compend Contin Educ Pract Vet 2005;27(3A):89.

[15] Billinghurst I. Give your dog a bone. The practical common sense way to feed your dog. Alexandria (Australia): Bridge Printery; 1993.

[16] Schultze KR. The ultimate diet. Descanso (CA): Affenbar Ink; 1998.

[17] Freeman LM, Michel KE. Evaluation of raw food diets for dogs. J Am Vet Med Assoc 2001;218(5):705–9.

[18] Delay J, Laing J. Nutritional osteodystrophy in puppies fed a BARF diet. AHL Newsletter 2002;6(2):23.

[19] Joffe DJ, Schlesinger DP. Preliminary assessment of the risk of *Salmonella* infection in dogs fed raw chicken diets. Can Vet J 2002;43:441–2.

[20] Strohmeyer RA, Morley PS, Hyatt DR, et al. Evaluation of bacterial and protozoal contamination of commercially available raw meat diets for dogs. J Am Vet Med Assoc 2006;228(4):537–42.

[21] Weese JS, Rousseau J, Arroya L. Bacteriological evaluation of commercial canine and feline raw diets. Can Vet J 2005;46:513–6.

[22] Lucas SRR, Hagiwara MK, Loureiro VS, et al. *Ioxoplasma gondii* infection in Brazilian domestic outpatient cats. Rev Inst Med Trop Sao Paulo 1999;41(4):221–4.

[23] Lejeune JT, Hancock DD. Public health concerns associated with feeding raw meat diets to dogs. J Am Vet Med Assoc 2001;219(9):1222–5.

[24] The 'why'a rationale for communication skills teaching and learning. In: Kurtz S, Silverman J, Draper J, editors. Teaching and learning communication skills in medicine. 2nd edition. San Francisco (CA): Radcliffe Publishing; 2005 p 13–27

[25] Calgary-Cambridge guide to the medical interview-communication process. Available at: www.med.ucalgary.ca/education/learningresources/CalgaryCambridgeGuide.pdf. Accessed April 2006.

Vet Clin Small Anim 36 (2006) 1283–1295

VETERINARY CLINICS
SMALL ANIMAL PRACTICE

Understanding and Managing Obesity in Dogs and Cats

Dottie P. Laflamme, DVM, PhD

Nestle Purina Pet Care Research, Checkerboard Square-Research South, St. Louis, MO 63164, USA

O besity is qualitatively defined as an excess of body fat sufficient to contribute to disease [1]. In human beings, this is recognized as a body weight at least 20% greater than ideal, where the excess body weight is attributable to an accumulation of adipose tissue [1]. This degree of excess body weight seems to be important in dogs as well.

Obesity is a common problem in dogs and cats. Numerous studies in developed countries suggest that between 25% and 40% of adult cats and dogs are overweight or obese [2–6]. An even higher prevalence occurs in dogs and cats between 5 and 10 years of age. Although the incidence of obesity in pets seems to be increasing, data to support this perception are currently lacking.

HEALTH RISKS OF OBESITY

Obesity has been associated with a number of diseases (Table 1) [3,5,7–19] as well as with a reduced lifespan [1,7,15]. A lifelong study in dogs showed that even moderately overweight dogs were at greater risk for earlier morbidity and a shortened lifespan [7]. Likewise, in cats, adverse effects were observed in moderately overweight cats, increasing in prevalence as the degree of obesity worsened [3,5]. In cats and dogs, the strongest associations are with diabetes mellitus and osteoarthritis. Data suggest that 31% of diabetes mellitus and 34% of lameness could be eliminated if overweight and obese cats were at optimum body weight [3].

The impact of excess body weight in dogs was best illustrated in a 14-year study by Kealy and colleagues [7]. In that study, one group of Labrador Retrievers was fed 25% less food than their sibling-pairmates throughout life. The average adult body condition scores (BCSs) for the lean-fed and control dogs were 4.6 ± 0.2 and 6.7 ± 0.2, respectively, based on a nine-point BCS system [7]. Thus, the control dogs were moderately overweight (typical of many pets) and actually weighed approximately 26% more, on average, than the lean-fed group. The lean-fed dogs were well within the ideal body condition of 4 to 5 on this nine-point scale. The difference in body condition was

E-mail address: dorothy.laflamme@rdmo.nestle.com

0195-5616/06/$ – see front matter
doi:10.1016/j.cvsm.2006.08.005

Table 1
List of diseases associated with obesity in dogs or cats

Species	Pathologic finding	Key references
Cat, dog	Insulin resistance	[8–10]
Cat	Diabetes mellitus	[3,6,8]
Cat	Lameness, no specific cause	[3]
Dog	Hip dysplasia	[7]
Dog	Osteoarthritis	[7]
Cat	Dermatopathy	[3,6]
Cat	Oral disease	[6]
Cat	Lower urinary tract diseases	[6]
Cat, dog	Increased inflammatory mediators	[10,11]
Cat, dog	Cardiovascular changes	[12–14]
Cat, dog	Reduced longevity	[7,15]
Dog	Renal pathology	[16–18]
Dog	Pancreatitis	[19]

sufficient to create significant differences between the groups in median life-span, which was 13 years for the lean-fed dogs compared with only 11.2 years for the control group, a difference of approximately 15%. An impressive correlation between the BCS at middle age and longevity in these dogs showed that even moderately overweight dogs were less likely to live beyond 12 years of age (Fig. 1) [20]. In addition, the onset and severity of hip joint and multiple joint osteoarthritis were delayed or reduced in the lean dogs. Control dogs required medication for chronic health problems or arthritis an average of 2.1 years or 3.0 years, respectively, sooner than their lean-fed siblings [7].

Recent research has suggested a mechanism for the link between excess body weight and many diseases. It seems that adipose tissue, once considered to be physiologically inert, is an active producer of hormones, such as leptin and resistin, and numerous cytokines (Fig. 2) [10,11,21,22]. Of major concern is the production of inflammatory cytokines from adipose tissue, specifically tumor necrosis factor-α (TNFα), interleukins-1β and -6, and C-reactive protein [10,11,21,22]. The persistent low-grade inflammation secondary to obesity is thought to play a causal role in chronic diseases, such as osteoarthritis, cardiovascular disease, and diabetes mellitus [21,23]. TNFα, for example, alters insulin sensitivity by blocking activation of insulin receptors [24]. In addition, obesity is associated with increased oxidative stress, which also may contribute to obesity-related diseases [25–27].

CAUSES OF OBESITY

Obesity is a result of an imbalance between energy intake and energy expenditure, with intake exceeding expenditure. Numerous risk factors that affect this

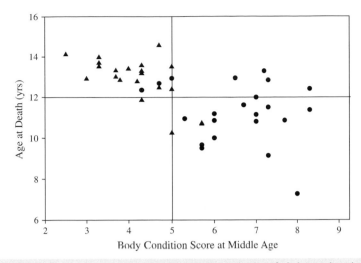

Fig. 1. Effect of body condition on longevity in dogs. The lean-fed dogs (*closed triangles*) received 25% less food than their control group littermates (*closed circles*). The BCS was determined annually using a nine-point system. Data shown are the mean BCS for ages 6 through 8 years for each dog as the independent variable for age at death: Age at Death = 15.208 − (0.589 · BCS) (R = 0.596, P < .001). Dogs with a BCS of 5 or less at middle age were more likely to live beyond 12 years of age (P < .001) compared with dogs with a BCS greater than ideal. (*Data courtesy of* Richard D. Kealy, PhD and Dennis F. Lawler, DVM, Nestle Purina Pet-Care Company, St. Louis, MO. *From* Laflamme DP. Nutrition for aging cats and dogs and the importance of body condition. Vet Clin North Am Small Anim Pract 2005;35(3):725; with permission.)

balance have been recognized. Neutering is often cited as a contributing factor in obesity [5,6,15,28–35]. Most investigations suggest that neutering results in a decrease in energy requirements [28,31,32,35,36], although some indicate that weight gain is attributable predominantly to increased food consumption [29,34].

Other recognized risk factors for feline obesity include a lack of activity, indoor housing, and feeding high-fat foods [3,5,30]. Interestingly, ad libitum feeding was not associated with an increased risk for obesity [30]. Spontaneous activity tends to decrease with age in cats, which may contribute to obesity [37]. High-fat diets and limited activity are also reported risk factors for obesity in dogs [38].

Less common factors that may play a role in some cases of obesity include endocrine dysfunction (eg, hypothyroidism) and infection-induced obesity. Canine distemper virus was the first infectious agent shown to induce obesity; it does so by downregulating genes for melanin production and disrupting hypothalamic function [39]. A number of additional viruses also have been shown to induce obesity in various laboratory animals [40]. Thus far, such an effect has not been shown to occur in companion animals.

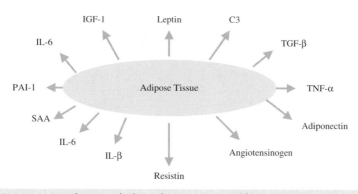

Fig. 2. Hormones, cytokines, and other substances secreted from adipose tissue. This list continues to grow as new substances are identified. [10,11,21,22]. C3, complement protein 3; IGF-1, insulin-like growth factor-1; IL, interleukin; PAI-1, plasminogen activator inhibitor-1; SAA, serum amyloid A; TNF-α, tumor necrosis factor-α; TGF-β, transforming growth factor-β.

DIAGNOSIS

Despite widespread concern about obesity among pet owners, most do not recognize that their own pet is overweight [41,42]. A study of pet cats in New Zealand suggested that owners' underestimation of body condition in their cats was a risk factor for increased prevalence of obesity [41]. Among dogs and cats seen by veterinary practices in the United States, approximately 28% were identified as overweight or obese by their BCS, yet only 2% were diagnosed as obese [4]. As noted previously, obesity is associated with significant health risks; thus, diagnosing and managing obesity are important parts of nutritional management of dogs and cats.

The first step in an effective obesity management program is recognition of the problem. Perhaps the most practical methods for in-clinic assessment of obesity are a combination of body weight and BCS. There are several BCS systems. This author prefers using validated nine-point systems for dogs and cats (a score of 5 is ideal) [43–45]. With these systems, each unit increase in BCS is approximately equivalent to 10% to 15% greater than ideal body weight; thus, a dog or cat with a BCS of 7 is approximately 20% to 30% heavier than its ideal weight. Percentage of body fat (%BF) also can be estimated, as shown in Table 2 [43,44]. By recording body weight and BCS, ideal body weight can be more easily determined. Animals that are becoming obese can be recognized sooner and managed more easily. An illustrated BCS system can provide a useful tool for client education regarding obesity prevention and management.

Other clinical options for assessing excess body weight are zoometric measures. Several such systems have been evaluated but have not been proven more effective than a BCS system for estimating %BF or for identifying overweight animals [46,47]. Zoometric measures, such as abdominal girth (AG), can vary considerably among individuals measuring the same animal [48], and thus should be considered semiquantitative. Because they are designed

Table 2
Estimation of average percent body fat by body condition score

Body condition score	Cats		Dogs	
	Male	Female	Male	Female
5	24	32	17	20
6	29	38	22	26
7	34	43	26	31
8	39	48	31	37
9	45+	54+	35+	43+

Data from Laflamme DP. Development and validation of a body condition score system for dogs: a clinical tool. Canine Pract 1997;22:10–5; and Laflamme DP. Development and validation of a body condition score system for cats: a clinical tool. Feline Pract 1997;25:13–8.

to provide a specific estimate of %BF, however, they may be of value in client communications. Some validated equations include the following:

Puppies : %BF = 38.369 − 0.064(BMI)
Cats : %BF = 66.715   0.061(BMI)
Dogs : %BF = −12.937 + 0.696(AG)

where body mass index (BMI) is measured as L^2/W; where length, L (centimeters), is measured from the nose to the base of the tail; weight (W) is measured in kilograms; and abdominal girth (AG) is measured as the circumference at the fifth to sixth lumbar vertebrae [46].

MANAGEMENT: DIETARY FACTORS

Use of an appropriate diet for weight loss is important, and there are several criteria to consider. Although it is ultimately calorie restriction that induces weight loss, it is important to avoid excessive restriction of essential nutrients. Therefore, a low-calorie product with increased nutrient/calorie ratios should be considered. Further, an important goal for weight loss is to promote fat loss while minimizing loss of lean tissue, which may be influenced by dietary composition.

Macronutrients

Fat restriction in weight loss diets reduces calorie density, which helps to reduce calorie intake. Fat contains more than twice the calories per gram of protein or carbohydrate. In a study of obese human subjects, when carbohydrate replaced dietary fat in diets fed ad libitum, weight loss was significantly enhanced [49]. Dogs fed a low-fat and high-fiber diet lost more body fat compared with dogs fed a high-fat and low-fiber diet [50]. Conversely, several human studies have shown that low-carbohydrate diets can facilitate increased short-term weight loss [51–53]. Such diets can alter the selection of foods consumed and greatly reduce intake of sugars and other highly refined carbohydrates, thus reducing calorie intake. Anecdotal reports suggest that this approach also works in overweight cats. However, feeding of a low-carbohydrate, high-protein diet did not induce weight loss in group-housed cats unless total calories also were restricted [54]. Numerous studies have shown that increasing dietary protein, often in exchange for carbohydrate, has beneficial effects for weight management [55–60]. Most "low-carbohydrate" diets are increased in protein.

Dietary protein is especially important in weight loss diets. Providing low-calorie diets with an increased protein-to-calorie ratio significantly increases the percent of fat lost and reduces the loss of lean body mass in dogs and cats undergoing weight loss [55,60]. Increasing dietary protein from 35% to 45% of energy resulted in more than 10% greater fat loss (1.2 kg versus 1.4 kg fat loss, respectively, for the lower and higher protein diets), despite nearly identical total weight loss and rate of weight loss between groups of cats. Most importantly, absolute loss of lean tissue was reduced by approximately 50% in cats fed the higher protein, low-calorie diet [60]. A similar pattern was observed in dogs, with greater preservation of lean body mass with increased dietary protein during calorie restriction [55,59].

Protein has a significant thermic effect, meaning that postprandial metabolic energy expenditure is increased more when protein is consumed compared with carbohydrates or fats [61,62]. In addition to contributing to a negative energy balance in support of weight loss directly, the thermic effect of protein may contribute to a satiety effect [63]. A higher protein diet helped to sustain weight maintenance after weight loss in human subjects [64]. This effect is likely to apply to dogs and cats as well: two studies have shown that cats fed a higher protein diet at or just below the maintenance energy requirement (MER) maintained a higher level of lean body mass [65,66]. Finally, use of a high-protein diet reduced markers of oxidative stress in obese cats undergoing weight loss compared with those fed a normal-protein diet [27].

Dietary fiber is poorly digestible; thus, it contributes little energy to the diet. Therefore, it can be used to dilute or reduce the calorie density of foods, which can aid in calorie restriction for weight loss [67–70]. Dietary fiber also provides a satiety effect, causing a voluntary reduction in total calorie consumption in dogs offered food in excess of energy needs [68,69]. Cats fed high-fiber foods also voluntarily restricted their calorie intake [67,70].

Water provides another route for diluting calories per volume of food. Thus, canned foods, which contain between 70% and 82% water, may be helpful in some obese patients. Although canned foods typically have a higher fat and calorie content on a dry matter basis, they actually have a lower calorie density per volume as fed compared with dry foods. Use of small cans may aid in portion control. In addition, the lower calories per volume may be especially beneficial when managing overweight cats. In general, animals eat to meet their energy needs. If the energy density of food is altered, they adjust the amount consumed to compensate [71,72]. This adjustment takes some time, however, and it can take many weeks for cats to adjust fully, which can provide a "head start" on weight loss [73].

Other Nutrients and Nutraceutic Agents

Nutraceutic agents and herbal compounds continue to be evaluated for use in weight loss diets. To date, published data on these have been conflicting. Carnitine seems to have received the most attention. Carnitine is produced endogenously from the amino acids lysine and methionine, and facilitates β-oxidation of fatty acids. Supplementation with this compound is likely to be of greatest benefit when the intake of dietary protein or other key nutrients is insufficient to promote adequate endogenous production [74,75]. In semistarved cats and rats undergoing rapid weight loss, L-carnitine reduced hepatic fat accumulation in cats and enhanced lipid metabolism and reduced ketogenesis in rats [76,77]. In human beings, severe calorie restriction resulted in reduced urinary and plasma carnitine, an effect that was attenuated by increased dietary protein during weight loss [78]. With a few exceptions, most studies evaluating carnitine for weight management have shown little benefit [79–82]. In one study, dogs retained more lean body mass when fed a carnitine-supplemented diet but also lost less body weight, whereas another study in dogs showed no significant difference in body composition changes with carnitine supplementation [83,84]. One clinical study in cats demonstrated an increase in the rate of weight loss in cats supplemented with carnitine compared with a control group (24% versus 20%, respectively, over an 18-week period) [48]. The carnitine-supplemented group was initially heavier, however, which may have influenced the rate of loss, and they remained heavier at the end of the weight loss study. Body composition was not analyzed; thus, the effect of carnitine on loss of lean or fat could not be determined in this study [48].

MANAGEMENT: CLIENT AND BEHAVIORAL FACTORS

Once the clinician and owner have recognized obesity in a pet, it is important to develop a management plan that fits the needs of the patient and owner. This must consider client ability and willingness to control calories and enhance exercise for the pet. Numerous options are available; thus, the keys to success are flexibility in design and regular follow up with the client. Of utmost importance is recognition that individual animals can differ greatly in their MER. Thus, the degree of calorie restriction that induces significant weight loss in one dog or cat may cause weight gain in another [85]. Adjustments in calorie allowance made on a regular basis (eg, every month) can help to address these individual differences as well as the reductions in MER that occur during weight loss [86]. Monthly rechecks also provide ongoing motivation to aid in client compliance [87].

In addition to diet, feeding management and exercise are critically important to successful weight management. Most clients provide treats for their pets. Rather than requiring that they cease this pleasurable activity, the creation of a "treat allowance" equal to 10% of the daily calories provides balance [87]. Clients may be provided with a menu of low-calorie foods or commercial treats that would be appropriate.

Increasing exercise aids in weight management by expending calories. Interactive exercise provides an alternative activity for the pet and owner to enjoy together rather than food-related activities. Increased activity can enhance weight loss in pets [88,89]. Activity in cats may be enhanced by interactive play or by environmental enrichment with climbing towers, tunnels, multiple food bowls in various locations, and cat-suitable toys. Food balls provide another option. These are plastic balls with holes that dispense kibble or treats as the cat (or dog) plays with the toy. Environmental enrichment and encouragement to play increased activity sufficiently to induce a 1% loss in body weight in overweight cats over a 4-week period without intended calorie restriction [88].

Gradual weight loss in dogs, as in people, is more likely to allow long-term maintenance of the reduced body weight [90]. Weight rebound can be minimized by providing controlled food intake and adjusting the calories fed just to meet the needs of the pet for weight maintenance. Successful long-term weight management may be achieved if clients already accustomed to measuring food and monitoring their pet's weight are encouraged to apply these behavior modifications to long-term weight management [87].

PREVENTION OF OBESITY

Currently, at least 1 in 4 dogs and cats seen by practitioners are overweight or obese [4]. Yet, many pet owners do not realize that their pets are overweight or at risk for health problems. In a survey involving 200 dogs and their owners, it was demonstrated that owners do not recognize their own dog as overweight [42]. In that survey, the mean BCS determined by trained pet experts was 6.3, whereas the mean BCS determined by the dog owners was 5.3. Approximately 27% of the owners underestimated the BCS by two units: two units on this BCS system correlates to 20% to 30% excess body weight [43]. More owners of obese cats inaccurately assessed the body condition of their pet compared with owners of normal-weight cats [41]. Even practicing veterinarians frequently overlook the diagnosis of obesity [4]. Yet, the primary way that many owners recognized their pet as overweight is based on their veterinarian's assessment [91].

Thus, veterinarians should begin or continue to evaluate the BCS of all patients and to discuss with clients the importance of maintaining an ideal BCS. Recording the BCS and body weight in the patient record during every visit allows the veterinarian to discuss trends of weight gain with the owner over time. Veterinarians may want to provide illustrated BCS charts for their clients or to post them within their clinic. A videotape teaching pet owners how to monitor and control BCS can be a valuable client education tool that practitioners may wish to provide.

Large-breed puppy owners, especially, should be taught how to assess the BCS in their puppies and advised to adjust food allowances to maintain a lean body condition while promoting a slow healthy rate of weight gain. Neutering in both genders and in cats as well as dogs is associated with a reduction in energy requirements. All pet owners should be advised to alter the feeding management of their pet after spay or castration. Ideally, all pets should be fed measured amounts individually. Owners should be advised to use a standard 8-oz measuring cup to determine the volume fed.

To ensure that all essential nutrients are provided despite energy control, it is important that the caloric density of the diet fed be appropriate to the energy needs of the individual pet. Those pets with low energy requirements should be fed products with an enhanced nutrient-to-calorie ratio, such as properly formulated "lite" or weight management diets. High-fat diets tend to be high in calories and are associated with an increased risk for obesity [5,15,38]. In addition, high-fat diets can contribute to adverse metabolic effects, such as altered glucose and insulin responses [92].

Consideration must be given to calories provided from sources other than complete and balanced pet foods so as to reduce the risk of nutrient dilution as well as calorie excess. Clients should be encouraged to develop non–food-related bonding activities, such as leash walking and interactive play, so as to reduce the intake of calories apart from meal times as well as to enhance calorie expenditure.

References

[1] National Institutes of Health. Health implications of obesity: National Institutes of Health consensus development conference statement. Ann Intern Med 1985;103:1073–7.

[2] Sloth C. Practical management of obesity in dogs and cats. J Small Anim Pract 1992;33: 178–82.

[3] Scarlett JM, Donoghue S. Associations between body condition and disease in cats. J Am Vet Med Assoc 1998;212:1725–31.

[4] Lund EM, Armstrong PJ, Kirk CK, et al. Health status and population characteristics of dogs and cats examined at private veterinary practices in the United States. J Am Vet Med Assoc 1999;214:1336–41.

[5] Lund EM, Armstrong PJ, Kirk CK, et al. Prevalence and risk factors for obesity in adult cats from private US veterinary practices. Int J Appl Res Vet Med 2005;3:88–96.

[6] McGreevy PD, Thomson PC, Price C, et al. Prevalence of obesity in dogs examined by Australian veterinary practices and the risk factors involved. Vet Rec 2005;156: 695–702.

[7] Kealy RD, Lawler DF, Ballam JM, et al. Effects of diet restriction on life span and age-related changes in dogs. J Am Vet Med Assoc 2002;220:1315–20.

[8] Rand JS, Fleeman LM, Farrow HA, et al. Canine and feline diabetes mellitus: nature or nurture? J Nutr 2004;134(Suppl):2072S–80S.

[9] Vargas AM, Barros RP, Zampieri RA, et al. Abnormal subcellular distribution of GLUT4 protein in obese and insulin-treated diabetic female dogs. Braz J Med Biol Res 2004;37:1095–101.

[10] Gayet C, Bailhache E, Dumon H, et al. Insulin resistance and changes in plasma concentration of TNFα, IGF1, and NEFA in dogs during weight gain and obesity. J Anim Physiol Anim Nutr (Berl) 2004;88:157–65.

[11] Miller D, Bartges J, Cornelius L, et al. Tumor necrosis factor-α levels in adipose tissue of lean and obese cats. J Nutr 1998;128(Suppl):2751S–2S.

[12] Litster AL, Buchanan JW. Radiographic and echocardiographic measurement of the heart of obese cats. Vet Radiol Ultrasound 2000;41:320–5.

[13] Kuruvilla A, Frankel TL. Heart rate of pet dogs: effects of overweight and exercise. Asia Pac J Clin Nutr 2003;12(Suppl):51.

[14] Knudson JD, Dincer UD, Zhang C, et al. Leptin receptors are expressed in coronary arteries, and hyperleptinemia causes significant coronary endothelial dysfunction. Am J Physiol Heart Cir Physiol 2005;289:H45–56.

[15] Scarlett JM, Donoghue S. Obesity in cats: prevalence and prognosis. Vet Clin Nutr 1996;3: 128–32.

[16] Henegar JR, Bigler SA, Henegar LK, et al. Functional and structural changes in the kidney in the early stages of obesity. J Am Soc Nephrol 2001;12:1211–7.

[17] Finco DR, Brown SA, Cooper TA. Effects of obesity on glomerular filtration rate (GFR) in dogs. Compend Contin Educ Pract Vet 2001;23(Suppl):78.

[18] Gu JW, Wang J, Stockton A, et al. Cytokine gene expression profiles in kidney medulla and cortex of obese hypertensive dogs. Kidney Int 2004;66:713–21.

[19] Hess RS, Kass PH, Shofer FS, et al. Evaluation of risk factors for fatal acute pancreatitis in dogs. J Am Vet Med Assoc 1999;214:46–51.

[20] Laflamme DP. Nutrition for aging cats and dogs and the importance of body condition. Vet Clin North Am Small Anim Pract 2005;35(3):713–42.

[21] Coppack SW. Pro-inflammatory cytokines and adipose tissue. Proc Nutr Soc 2001;60: 349–56.

[22] Trayhurn P. Inflammation in obesity: down to the fat? Compendium Cont Ed Pract Vet 2006;28(Suppl 4):33–6.

[23] Sowers M, Jannausch M, Stein E, et al. C-reactive protein as a biomarker of emergent osteoarthritis. Osteoarthritis Cartilage 2002;10:595–601.

[24] Plomgaard P, Bouzakri K, Krogh-Madsen R, et al. Tumor necrosis factor-alpha induces skeletal muscle insulin resistance in healthy human subjects via inhibition of Akt substrate 160 phosphorylation. Diabetes 2005;54:2939–45.

[25] Sonta T, Inoguchi T, Tsubouchi H, et al. Evidence for contribution of vascular NAD(P)H oxidase to increased oxidative stress in animal models of diabetes and obesity. Free Radic Biol Med 2004;37:115–23.

[26] Urakawa H, Katsuki A, Sumida Y, et al. Oxidative stress is associated with adiposity and insulin resistance in men. J Clin Endocrinol Metab 2003;88(10):4673–6.

[27] Tanner AE, Martin J, Thatcher CD, et al. Nutritional amelioration of oxidative stress induced by obesity and acute weight loss. Compendium Cont Ed Pract Vet 2006;28(Suppl 4): 72.

[28] Root MV, Johnston SD, Olson PN. Effect of prepuberal and postpuberal gonadectomy on heat production measured by indirect calorimetry in male and female domestic cats. Am J Vet Res 1996;57:371–4.

[29] Fettman MJ, Stanton CA, Banks LL, et al. Effects of neutering on bodyweight, metabolic rate and glucose tolerance of domestic cats. Res Vet Sci 1997;62:131–6.

[30] Robertson ID. The influence of diet and other factors on owner-perceived obesity in privately owned cats from metropolitan Perth, Western Australia. Prev Vet Med 1999;40: 75–85.

[31] Harper EJ, Stack DM, Watson TDG, et al. Effects of feeding regimens on bodyweight, composition and condition score in cats following ovariohysterectomy. J Small Anim Pract 2001;42:433–8.

[32] Martin L, Siliart B, Dumon H, et al. Leptin, body fat content and energy expenditure in intact and gonadectomized adult cats: a preliminary study. J Anim Physiol Anim Nutr (Berl) 2001;85:195–9.

[33] Scott KC, Levy JK, Gorman SP, et al. Body condition of feral cats and the effect of neutering. J Appl Anim Welf Sci 2002;5:203–13.

[34] Kanchuk ML, Backus RC, Calvert CC, et al. Weight gain in gonadectomized normal and lipoprotein lipase-deficient male domestic cats results from increased food intake and not decreased energy expenditure. J Nutr 2003;133:1866–74.

[35] Jeusette I, Daminet S, Nguyen P, et al. Effect of ovariectomy and ad libitum feeding on body composition, thyroid status, ghrelin and leptin plasma concentrations in female dogs. J Anim Physiol Anim Nutr (Berl) 2006;90:12–8.

[36] Hoenig M, Ferguson DC. Effects of neutering on hormonal concentrations and energy requirements in male and female cats. Am J Vet Res 2002;63:634–9.

[37] Bouthegourd JC, Jean-Philippe C, Pérez-Camargo G. Effect of age on spontaneous activity in cats—characterization of a new category: the young and active adult cat. Compendium Cont Ed Pract Vet 2006;28(Suppl 4):73.

[38] West DB, York B. Dietary fat, genetic predisposition, and obesity: lessons from animal models. Am J Clin Nutr 1998;67(Suppl):505S–12S.

[39] Verlaeten O, Griffond B, Khuth ST, et al. Down regulation of melanin concentrating hormone in virally induced obesity. Mol Cell Endocrinol 2001;181:207–19.

[40] Dhurandhar NV. Infectobesity: obesity of infectious origin. J Nutr 2001;131(Suppl): 2791S–7S.

[41] Allan FJ, Pfeiffer DU, Jones BR, et al. A cross-sectional study of risk factors for obesity in cats in New Zealand. Prev Vet Med 2000;46:183–96.

[42] Singh R, Laflamme DP, Sidebottom-Nielsen M. Owner perceptions of canine body condition score. J Vet Intern Med 2002;16:362.

[43] Laflamme DP. Development and validation of a body condition score system for dogs: a clinical tool. Canine Pract 1997;22:10–5.

[44] Laflamme DP. Development and validation of a body condition score system for cats: a clinical tool. Feline Pract 1997;25:13–8.

[45] Mawby DI, Bartges JW, d'Avignon A, et al. Comparison of various methods for estimating body fat in dogs. J Am Anim Hosp Assoc 2004;40:109–14.

[46] Laflamme DP, Hume E, Harrison J. Evaluation of zoometric measures as an assessment of body composition of dogs and cats. Compend Contin Educ Pract Vet 2001;23(Suppl 9A):88.

[47] Butterwick R. How fat is that cat? J Feline Med Surg 2000;2:91–4.

[48] Center SA, Harte J, Watrous D, et al. The clinical and metabolic effects of rapid weight loss in obese pet cats and the influence of supplemental oral L-carnitine. J Vet Intern Med 2000;14:598–608.

[49] Hays NP, Starling RD, Liu X, et al. Effects of an ad libitum low-fat, high-carbohydrate diet on body weight, body composition and fat distribution in older men and women: a randomized, controlled trial. Arch Intern Med 2004;164:210–7.

[50] Borne AT, Wolfsheimer KJ, Truett AA, et al. Differential metabolic effects of energy restriction in dogs using diets varying in fat and fiber content. Obes Res 1996;4:337–45.

[51] Volek JS, Westman EC. Very-low-carbohydrate weight-loss diets revisited. Cleve Clin J Med 2002;69:849–62.

[52] Samaha FF, Iqbal N, Seshadri P, et al. A low-carbohydrate as compared with a low-fat diet in severe obesity. N Engl J Med 2003;348:2074–81.

[53] Foster GD, Wyatt HR, Hill JO, et al. A randomized trial of a low-carbohydrate diet for obesity. N Engl J Med 2003;348:2082–90.

[54] Michel KE, Bader A, Shofer FS, et al. Impact of time-limited feeding and dietary carbohydrate content on weight loss in group-housed cats. J Feline Med Surg 2005;7: 349–55.

[55] Hannah SS, Laflamme DP. Increased dietary protein spares lean body mass during weight loss in dogs. J Vet Intern Med 1998;12:224.

[56] Skov AR, Toubro S, Ronn B, et al. Randomized trial on protein vs carbohydrate in ad libitum fat reduced diet for the treatment of obesity. Int J Obes 1999;23:528–36.

[57] Farnsworth E, Luscombe ND, Noakes M, et al. Effect of a high-protein, energy-restricted diet on body composition, glycemic control, and lipid concentrations in overweight and obese hyperinsulinemic men and women. Am J Clin Nutr 2003;78:31–9.

[58] Johnston CS, Tjonn SL, Swan PD. High-protein, low-fat diets are effective for weight loss and favorably alter biomarkers in healthy adults. J Nutr 2004;134:586–91.

[59] Bierer TL, Bui LM. High-protein low-carbohydrate diets enhance weight loss in dogs. J Nutr 2004;134(Suppl):2087S–9S.

[60] Laflamme DP, Hannah SS. Increased dietary protein promotes fat loss and reduces loss of lean body mass during weight loss in cats. Int J Appl Res Vet Med 2005;3:62–8.

[61] Karst H, Steiniger J, Noack R, et al. Diet-induced thermogenesis in man: thermic effects of single proteins, carbohydrates and fats depending on their energy amount. Ann Nutr Metab 1984;28:245–52.

[62] Hoenig M, Waldron M, Ferguson DC. Effect of high and low carbohydrate diet on respiratory exchange ratio and heat production in lean and obese cats before and after weight loss. Compendium Cont Ed Pract Vet 2006;28(Suppl 4):71.

[63] Crovetti R, Porrini M, Santangelo A, et al. The influence of thermic effect of food on satiety. Eur J Clin Nutr 1997;52:482–8.

[64] Westerterp-Plantenga MS, Lejeune MP, Nijs I, et al. High protein intake sustains weight maintenance after body weight loss in humans. Int J Obes 2004;28:57–64.

[65] Hannah SS, Laflamme DP. Effect of dietary protein on nitrogen balance and lean body mass in cats. Proceedings of the Purina Forum on Small Animal Nutrition, June 1995, St. Louis, MO. Vet Clin Nutr 1996;3:30.

[66] Nguyen P, Leray V, Dumon H, et al. High protein intake affects lean body mass but not energy expenditure in nonobese neutered cats. J Nutr 2004;134(Suppl):2084S–6S.

[67] Laflamme DP, Jackson JR. Evaluation of weight loss protocols for overweight cats. Proceedings of the 1995 Purina Forum on Small Animal Nutrition, St. Louis, MO. Vet Clin Nutr 1995;2:143.

[68] Jewell DE, Toll PW. Effects of fiber on food intake in dogs. Vet Clin Nutr 1996;3:115–8.

[69] Jackson JR, Laflamme DP, Owens SF. Effects of dietary fiber content on satiety in dogs. Vet Clin Nutr 1997;4:130–4.

[70] Fekete S, Hullar I, Andrasofszky E, et al. Reduction of the energy density of cats' foods by increasing their fibre content with a view to nutrients' digestibility. J Anim Physiol Anim Nutr (Berl) 2001;85:200–4.

[71] Owens SF. The effect of dietary fat and calorie content on the growth of puppies. Compend Contin Educ Pract Vet 2000;22(9A):111.

[72] Owens SF, Ballam JM. Effect of changes in calorie density on food intake in dogs. Compend Contin Educ Pract Vet 2002;24(9A):82.

[73] Stoll JA, Laflamme DP. Effect of dry vs. canned rations on food intake and bodyweight in cats. Proceedings of the Purina Forum on Small Animal Nutrition, June 1995, St. Louis, MO. Vet Clin Nutr 1995;2:145.

[74] Sanderson SL, Gross KL, Ogburn PN, et al. Effects of dietary fat and L-carnitine on plasma and whole blood taurine concentrations and cardiac function in healthy dogs fed protein-restricted diets. Am J Vet Res 2001;62:1616–23.

[75] Ibrahim WH, Bailey N, Sunvold GD, et al. Effects of carnitine and taurine on fatty acid metabolism and lipid accumulation in the liver of cats during weight gain and weight loss. Am J Vet Res 2003;64:1265–77.

[76] Armstrong PJ, Hardie EM, Cullen JM, et al. L-carnitine reduced hepatic fat accumulation during rapid weight loss in cats. In: Proceedings of the 1992 Meeting of the American College of Veterinary Internal Medicine. Denver (CO): American College of Veterinary Internal Medicine; 1992. p. 810.

[77] Feng Y, Guo C, Wei J, et al. Necessity of carnitine supplementation in semistarved rats fed a high-fat diet. Nutrition 2001;17:628–31.

[78] Davis AT, Davis PG, Phinney SD. Plasma and urinary carnitine of obese subjects on very-low-calorie diets. J Am Coll Nutr 1990;9:261–4.

[79] Dyck DJ. Dietary fat intake, supplements and weight loss. Can J Appl Physiol 2000;25:495–523.

[80] Villani RG, Gannon J, Self M, et al. L-carnitine supplementation combined with aerobic training does not promote weight loss in moderately obese women. Int J Sport Nutr Exerc Metab 2000;10:199–207.

[81] Brandsch C, Eder K. Effect of L-carnitine on weight loss and body composition of rats fed a hypocaloric diet. Ann Nutr Metab 2002;46:205–10.

[82] Aoki MS, Almeida ALR, Navarro F, et al. Carnitine supplementation fails to maximize fat mass loss induced by endurance training in rats. Ann Nutr Metab 2004;48:90–4.

[83] Gross KL, Wedekind KJ, Kirk CA, et al. Effect of dietary carnitine or chromium on weight loss and body composition of obese dogs. J Anim Sci 1998;76(Suppl 1):175.

[84] Sunvold GD, Vickers RJ, Kelley RL, et al. Effect of dietary carnitine during energy restriction in the canine. [abstract226.2]. FASEB J 1999;13:A268.

[85] Laflamme DP, Kuhlman G, Lawler DF. Evaluation of weight loss protocols for dogs. J Am Anim Hosp Assoc 1997;33:253–9.

[86] Saker KE, Remillard RL. Performance of a canine weight-loss program in clinical practice. Vet Ther 2005;6:291–302.

[87] Yaissle JE, Holloway C, Buffington CAT. Evaluation of owner education as a component of obesity treatment programs for dogs. J Am Vet Med Assoc 2004;224:1932–5.

[88] Clarke DL, Wrigglesworth D, Holmes K, et al. Using environmental and feeding enrichment to facilitate feline weight loss. J Anim Physiol Anim Nutr (Berl) 2005;89:427.

[89] Tripanny JR, Funk J, Buffington CAT. Effects of environmental enrichments on weight loss in cats. [abstract 208]. J Vet Intern Med 2003;17:431.

[90] Laflamme DP, Kuhlman G. The effect of weight loss regimen on subsequent weight maintenance in dogs. Nutr Res 1995;15:1019–28.

[91] Jackson M, Ballam JM, Laflamme DP. Client perceptions and canine weight loss. Compend Contin Educ Pract Vet 2001;23(Suppl):90.

[92] Thiess S, Beckskei C, Tomsa K, et al. Effects of high carbohydrate and high fat diet on plasma metabolite levels and on IV glucose tolerance test in intact and neutered male cats. J Feline Med Surg 2004;6:207–18.

Vet Clin Small Anim 36 (2006) 1297–1306

VETERINARY CLINICS
SMALL ANIMAL PRACTICE

Feline Diabetes Mellitus: Low Carbohydrates Versus High Fiber?

Claudia A. Kirk, DVM, PhD[a]

[a]Department of Small Animal Clinical Sciences, Veterinary Teaching Hospital,
College of Veterinary Medicine, The University of Tennessee, Knoxville, TN 37996-4545, USA

NUTRITIONAL GOALS

Diabetes mellitus (DM) can be classified into multiple subtypes; however, most feline diabetics are either type I (insulin-dependent DM) or type II (non–insulin-dependent DM) [1,2]. In the cat, type II DM seems to predominate, despite the need for exogenous insulin therapy. More than 80% of cats are thought to have type II DM, with the remaining cases thought to be secondary to other conditions, such as carcinoma, pancreatitis, or acromegaly. Type II DM has been referred to as a relative insulin deficiency because the amount of insulin actually secreted may be increased, decreased, or normal but is always inadequate relative to serum glucose levels. In cats, DM is characterized by peripheral insulin resistance combined with dysfunctional β cells. Cats with type II DM require oral hypoglycemic drugs or exogenous insulin coupled with nutritional management [2].

The goals of nutritional management in DM are to (1) blunt postprandial hyperglycemia, (2) control body weight, (3) support altered nutrient needs, (4) improve peripheral insulin sensitivity, (5) avoid diabetic complications (eg, hypoglycemia, ketosis, neuropathies), and (6) coordinate peak nutrient uptake with insulin activity. More recently, another goal, achieving diabetic remission, has come to the forefront of the nutritional plan. Pharmaceutic treatment combined with an appropriate food composition and feeding plan should optimize glycemic control, control weight, and result in remission in most cats.

ETIOPATHOGENESIS OF TYPE II DIABETES

The deposition of islet amylin and progressive β-cell destruction are characteristic of type II DM in people and cats [3,4]. Amylin is formed from islet amyloid polypeptide (IAPP), a peptide cosecreted with insulin. In people, chronic β-cell stimulation and increased IAPP release occur after high simple carbohydrate intake and peripheral insulin resistance. Increased pancreatic amyloid deposition is associated with impaired glucose tolerance [3–5]. This same phenomenon seems to occur in cats [3–6]. As true carnivores, evolutionary adaptations

E-mail address: ckirk4@utk.edu

0195-5616/06/$ – see front matter
doi:10.1016/j.cvsm.2006.09.004

have altered the cat's use of and tolerance to dietary carbohydrates [7]. The phenomenon of insulin resistance and carbohydrate intolerance has been referred to as the "carnivore connection" [8]. During the Ice Ages, when human beings consumed a meat-based low-carbohydrate diet, metabolic adaptations limited insulin's effect to sustain blood glucose levels [6,8]. Cats, having adapted to a meat-based diet, have also evolved to maintain blood glucose in the face of low carbohydrate intake. In the cat, these adaptations have resulted in constant hepatic glucose production from amino acids (gluconeogenesis) and delay in carbohydrate use (low glucokinase activity) [7]. Unfortunately, factors that lead to prolonged elevation of plasma glucose (ie, impaired insulin secretion, insulin resistance) can lead to diabetes. Chronic hyperglycemia and insulin resistance promote hypersecretion of insulin, which may lead to β-cell exhaustion. In addition, chronic hyperglycemia causes hydropic degeneration of the feline β cell ("glucose toxicity") [9]. Both mechanisms contribute to decreased pancreatic insulin secretion in cats.

Insulin resistance seems to be a key driving force in the development of type II DM in people and cats [10,11]. Downregulation and postreceptor defects of peripheral glucose receptors (GLUT 4 receptors) on muscle and adipose tissue result in decreased glucose disposal in response to normal levels of circulating insulin [11]. Progressively greater insulin release is required to achieve euglycemia. The process becomes a vicious cycle. Obesity promotes insulin resistance, which, in turn, increases β-cell release of insulin, cosecretion of IAPP, pancreatic amyloid accumulation, hyperglycemia, and glucose toxicity. Eventually, the triad of β-cell exhaustion, glucose toxicity, and insulin resistance progresses to overt DM [4,5,10,11].

Recent studies have described large proportions of diabetic cats in which nutritional management and pharmacologic therapy have resulted in resolution of the diabetic state [12–15]. These transient diabetics presumably have regained β-cell function following reversal of glucose toxicity and/or improved peripheral insulin resistance. The rate of transient diabetes seems to be increasing with the advent of new diet strategies and insulin therapy. Whereas transient diabetes was reported to occur in 10% to 25% of feline diabetics, DM may be transient in upward of 50% to 70% of cats [15].

DM affects cats of any age and gender but is diagnosed more commonly in neutered male cats older than 6 years of age, which is the same population most at risk for obesity (Table 1) [16,17]. In the cat, obesity has been shown to result

Table 1
Comparison of risk factors for obesity and diabetes mellitus in the cat

Obese	Diabetes mellitus
Advancing age	Advancing age
Male	Male
Neutered	Neutered
	Obesity

in abnormal glucose tolerance and peripheral insulin resistance [18–20], factors that are known to precede the development of type II DM in cats and people. The risk of developing DM increases by nearly fourfold in obese cats [17]. Weight loss reduces insulin resistance and is an important component in managing DM.

NUTRITIONAL FACTORS IN FELINE DIABETES MELLITUS

Diet composition, form, and feeding methodology can have a significant impact on diabetic regulation. When choosing a food to manage the diabetic cat, concentrations of key nutrients that may alter regulation should be considered. Traditionally, fiber-fortified foods have been recommended in the management of feline DM. The advantages include weight control and slowed glucose uptake from the intestines. Low-carbohydrate foods are now considered superior for the management of DM and have even been suggested as preventative [14,15,21]. It is important to remember that several nutrient classes vary when changing from a traditional low-fat high-fiber food to a low-carbohydrate high-protein food. Such factors as energy density, protein, and micronutrient concentration may all be affected.

Energy

Cat with DM often present with a history of significant weight loss yet are often overweight or obese [16]. Before making recommendations for daily energy requirements (DERs), it is important to emphasize that the clinical response to nutritional management of the diabetic cat is highly dependent on satisfactory medical management with insulin or oral hypoglycemic drugs and weight control. Traditional fiber-fortified foods designed for weight control (3.5 kcal/g dry matter metabolic energy [ME]) are appropriate for weight reduction and glycemic control in overweight cats. Good results can be achieved with appropriate patient compliance, which is sometime easier to achieve when feeding the larger food volume afforded by fiber-fortified foods. Recent studies suggest that cats regulate food intake by volume, and fiber-fortified foods reduce caloric intake [22].

In underweight cats or those with poor tolerance to dietary fiber, higher energy foods are more appropriate (4.0–4.5 kcal/g dry matter ME). In these cats, the low-carbohydrate foods, with their reduced fiber and increased fat and calorie content, are good alternatives.

Protein

Diabetic animals occasionally may have increased loss of amino acids in urine attributable to inappropriate or inadequate hormonal signals and glomerulonephropathies. More commonly, loss of lean body mass is attributable to inadequate insulin concentrations, with poor cellular amino acid uptake and increased protein metabolism via hepatic gluconeogenesis. Diabetic cats require high-quality protein of good biologic value. Protein content of the food should be greater than 30% dry matter of the food and greater than 85% digestible. Newer low-carbohydrate high-protein foods supply relatively similar protein levels to those of high-fiber formulas when determined as a percent of ME intake (Table 2). In the face of limited dietary carbohydrates, higher protein levels are theoretically required to support increased hepatic gluconeogenesis and normal blood glucose production. Failure to maintain blood glucose because of high glucose demands and insufficient hepatic gluconeogenesis has only been reported during gestation and lactation in the cat [23]. In adult cats, published protein requirements already account for sustained gluconeogenesis and increased protein metabolism [24]. Thus, the absolute protein requirement for the adult diabetic cat is unlikely to be significantly higher than adult maintenance requirements [24] and would certainly be less than the average protein content of most commercial feline foods. Nonetheless, when lowering the overall carbohydrate content of a diet, fat, protein, or both must increase to account for the difference. Because fat is known to increase insulin resistance and decrease glucose tolerance, it is logical to replace carbohydrates with protein as opposed to fat [25].

The total amount of protein is only modestly increased in newer low-carbohydrate foods compared with traditional high-fiber foods. Nevertheless, there are certain conditions in which this increased protein may be contraindicated. Cats with concurrent renal disease typically experience increased blood urea nitrogen when switched to a higher protein diet. It has been suggested by some that an increased glomerular filtration rate (GFR) in response to higher protein intake or alleviation of diabetic nephropathy actually improves renal function in diabetic cats. The implication is that limiting dietary protein in diabetic cats with renal disease may be unnecessary. Although protein does not promote renal failure, it is the author's experience that cats having blood urea nitrogen values greater than 50 mg/dL when eating a high-protein low-carbohydrate food often demonstrate a better attitude and appetite when switched to a lower protein renal therapeutic diet. To continue limiting carbohydrate use, adding acarbose therapy (12.5 mg/cat twice daily with a meal) to the new diet has sustained the benefit of low-carbohydrate intake.

Using low-carbohydrate diets in cats with pancreatitis is also contraindicated according to some product guides. Because cholecystokinin (CCK) is

Table 2
Nutrient comparisons for selected therapeutic foods designed to manage feline diabetes mellitus (% dry matter [g/per 100 kcal])

Food type[a]	Protein	Fat	Nitrogen free extract	Crude fiber
Hill's w/d can	40 (12)	17 (4.8)	26 (7.6)	11 (3.1)
Hill's w/d dry	39 (11)	9.6 (2.7)	38 (11)	7.4 (2.1)
Hill's m/d can	53 (13)	19 (4.8)	16 (3.9)	6.0 (1.5)
Hill's m/d dry	52 (12)	22 (5.2)	16 (3.6)	5.5 (1.4)
Royal Canin DS 44 dry	49 (12)	13 (3.2)	26 (6.4)	5.3 (1.3)
Purina DM can	57 (12)	24 (5)	8 (1.7)	3.6 (0.8)
Purina DM dry	58 (13)	18 (4)	15 (3.3)	1.3 (0.3)

[a]Hill's Pet Nutrition, Inc., Topeka, Kansas; Nestlé Purina PetCare Company, St. Louis, Missouri; Royal Canin USA, Inc., St. Charles, Missouri.

maximally secreted by proteins, amino acids, and fat, the use of moderate-protein, low-fat, and high-carbohydrate foods has been recommended. This is an area of great uncertainty. Many cats with chronic pancreatitis are well maintained on recovery type diets (high-protein, high-fat, and low-carbohydrate foods). Regardless, current food recommendations for cats with acute and/or active pancreatitis are intestinal therapeutic foods having a larger portion of the calories obtained from carbohydrates.

Finally, cats with severe liver disease and hepatoencephalopathy, or those at reasonable risk of hyperammonemia, should not be fed these high-protein foods.

Carbohydrates

The ideal composition and quantity of carbohydrates in foods for management of DM in people and cats remain controversial. Diets containing up to 85% carbohydrates have been recommended in people, with the bulk containing highly complex carbohydrates and soluble fibers [26]. Significantly lower levels of carbohydrates (<10%–20% dry matter) have been recommended for diabetic cats because of their nutritional peculiarities as an obligate carnivore [27]. The optimal level of soluble carbohydrates for feline diabetes has not been defined. Recent studies have demonstrated improved glycemic control in healthy and diabetic cats fed low-carbohydrate foods (<15% dry matter) [13–15]. By limiting dietary carbohydrates, blood glucose is maintained primarily from hepatic gluconeogenesis, which releases glucose into the circulation at a slow and steady rate. Fluctuations in blood glucose concentrations related to postprandial glucose absorption are avoided. The metabolic changes associated with feeding low-carbohydrate foods in diabetic cats have not been fully described. The shift in substrate use, from carbohydrates to fats and protein, has been called the "metabolic shift."

The concept of metabolic shift is similar to the concept used in the well-known Atkin's diet [28]. By providing foods extremely low in carbohydrates but with a surfeit of protein and fat, the metabolic drive shifts from glucose oxidation to fat metabolism for the animal's primary energy source. Low-carbohydrate intake results in lower plasma glucose concentrations and limited drive for insulin secretion from the pancreas. Purported benefits of a low-carbohydrate high-protein diet include appetite control, increased calorie loss via futile cycling and ketone loss, improved insulin sensitivity, and a shift from glucose oxidation and lipogenesis to lipolysis and weight loss [28]. Because weight control is vitally important to reversing insulin resistance that occurs in obese diabetic cats, a metabolic shift toward weight loss or weight control is of vital success to the treatment of cats with DM.

Weight control and metabolic shift

The red blood cell, kidney medulla, and central nervous system all have an absolute requirement for preformed glucose from the blood. The typical feline diet provides abundant glucose to meet essential needs. Once this "essential glucose pool" is filled, excess energy supplied as glucose is readily converted to triglycerides and stored as fat in adipocytes. When a high-carbohydrate diet is consumed, blood glucose rises, insulin requirements are increased, lipo-protein lipase activity increases, and a greater portion of glucose enters the ad-ipose cells, where it is converted to fatty acids and stored as fat. Conversely, when fed a low-carbohydrate food, blood glucose and insulin levels are low and storage of fat becomes more difficult. This metabolic shift from fat storage (lipogenesis) to fat loss (lipolysis) is attributable to several alterations in sub-strate and hormone availability. With low-carbohydrate intake, the conversion of glucose to α-glycerol phosphate (α-GP) in the adipocytes is reduced. Because α-GP is required for triglyceride formation, lipogenesis is limited. More impor-tantly, low insulin concentrations, together with relative increases in glucagon (in response to amino acid intake), increase cyclic adenosine monophosphate (cAMP) in the adipose cells. High intracellular cAMP activates hormone-sensi-tive lipase (HSL), the enzyme responsible for lipolysis. Subsequently, within the adipocytes, the rate of triglyceride hydrolysis to free fatty acids (FFAs) in-creases. FFAs are released into blood bound to albumin (nonesterified fatty acids [NEFAs]), where they serve as a preferred energy source to other tissues. In the liver, NEFAs readily undergo β-oxidation and production of ketone bod-ies. The muscles, heart, and, to some extent, central nervous system use ketones and NEFAs in preference to glucose.

Simply stated, when lipids and proteins are consumed in the absence of car-bohydrates, insulin levels remain low. The metabolic response is similar to that observed during starvation. These signals alter enzyme activities in the interme-diary pathways to conserve glucose, limit gluconeogenesis from amino acids (to conserve body proteins), and mobilize fats.

Markers of metabolic shift

The hallmark of effective metabolic shift is increased ketone body (acetoacetate, acetone, and β-hydroxybutyrate [BHBA]) production as measured in the blood and urine. Increased fat metabolism in cats favors the production of BHBA and lesser increases in acetoacetate or acetone compared with human beings, in whom ketogenesis generates high levels of acetoacetate and acetone. Recall that urine reagent strips designed to detect ketones react only with acetoacetate and acetone. Thus, these urine strips are not useful for monitoring benign dietary ketosis in cats, as in people. Only when ketone concentrations are significantly elevated (as in uncontrolled DM) does urine test positive for ketones in the cat.

Ketosis that occurs during low-carbohydrate feeding is relatively mild com-pared with ketosis that accompanies uncontrolled DM, pregnancy toxemia of ewes, or ketosis of lactating cattle. Levels of BHBA increase from approxi-mately 0.1 mmol/L in the fed state to upward of 3.0 mmol/L when feeding a low-carbohydrate food (W. Schoenherr, Hill's Pet Nutrition, Inc., unpublished data, 2004). At these levels, metabolic complications associated with ketosis are not observed. This is in contrast to DM, where BHBA levels typically exceed 15 mmol/L and are associated with metabolic acidosis and electrolyte imbalances.

What is the evidence for improved glucose regulation by feeding low-carbo-hydrate foods to diabetic cats? Three studies published over the past 5 years support the use of low-carbohydrate foods for the management of feline DM. When feeding extremely low-carbohydrate canned foods with or without acarbose (α-amylase inhibitor), blood glucose and serum fructosamine concentrations and exogenous insulin requirements were observed to decline [13]. More interestingly, Mazzaferro and colleagues [13] reported that more than 60% of cats fed low-carbohydrate foods reverted to a nondiabetic state. The proposed mechanism of diabetes reversal is improved glycemic control, lowered insulin requirements, and reversal of sustained hyperglycemia, thereby reversing glucotoxicity and allowing recovery of peripheral insulin sensitivity. Weight control and subsequent improved insulin sensitivity are critical components of the success of low-carbohydrate foods. Newer studies comparing low-carbohydrate foods with a high-fiber high-carbohydrate food in cats with naturally occurring DM also found that a large proportion of cats reverted to a non–insulin-dependent state within 4 months of diet change [15]. Approximately 68% of cats in the low-carbohydrate group and 41% of cats fed high-fiber foods were able to discontinue insulin. Calculated odds ratios indicate that cats fed a low-carbohydrate food are three times more likely to discontinue insulin and revert to a nondiabetic state. For cats that required ongoing exogenous insulin therapy, glycemic control and insulin dose were not significantly different between groups. The responders (improved glucose control and clinical signs) and nonresponders were evident in both food groups but with no clear biochemical or physical markers identified as response predictors.

Is there a "best" carbohydrate source? Carbohydrates sources suggested to have a lower glycemic index in the cat include corn, sorghum, oats, and barley. Highly processed rice (finely ground and fully gelatinized by cooking) is 100% digestible and readily absorbed in cats [29]. Fructose has been labeled a "good sugar" in people with DM. The advantage to people is a low glycemic index relative to other simple sugars. The use of fructose in foods for cats with DM should be avoided. Cats seem to lack hepatic fructokinase activity, which leads to fructose intolerance and potential renal damage [30]. Fructose is uncommon in commercial cat foods, except in semimoist foods, where the humectants may be in the form of sucrose or high-fructose corn syrup.

Ketosis and low-carbohydrate foods
Low-carbohydrate foods can improve weight loss and increase blood ketone levels. Despite possible concerns over diet-induced ketone production and the development of ketoacidosis, diet-mediated ketosis is minimal compared with that seen with poor diabetic regulation (Table 3). In nonketotic cats, the improved glycemic control and peripheral insulin activity seem to negate any complications that might be associated with the slightly increased ketone production. Based on experience, providing adequate insulin therapy is key to correcting ketosis, and low-carbohydrate foods have not been observed to worsen ketosis.

Fiber
Fiber aids in glycemic control by promoting slow and sustained gastrointestinal absorption of glucose after meals. Some studies have found improved insulin

Table 3
Ketone production in the cat

Metabolic status	β-hydroxybutyrate (mmol/L)
Fed state	0.1
Overnight fast	0.3–0.7
Metabolic shift	1–3
Diabetic ketoacidossis	>15

activity and reduced peripheral insulin resistance after fiber supplementation [31,32]. In cats, support for feeding fiber-supplemented foods comes from clinical experience and a study demonstrating that moderate fiber intake improved glycemic control in diabetic cats [32]. Cats fed fiber-supplemented foods (12% wt/wt cellulose) exhibited lower postprandial serum glucose and mean glucose concentrations compared with cats fed similar foods containing starch [32]. Although several studies in rodents and people indicate that soluble fiber is most desirable, evidence of a clear benefit of soluble over insoluble fiber is lacking in the cat. The soluble fiber may be partially fermented to short-chain fatty acids and then used as energy for enterocytes or absorbed into the blood for use by the animal. Recent studies do suggest that moderate levels of fiber suffice when feeding low-carbohydrate foods (<8%), particularly when of mixed fiber source. Not all cats tolerate fiber-enhanced foods without complications. Increase stool volume, food refusal, constipation, dry skin, and unacceptable begging behavior have been associated with high-fiber foods in some cases.

Although an ideal fiber content and source have not been established, it seems that the inclusion of moderate amounts of mixed fiber (approximately 5%–12% dry matter) aids in glycemic control and weight management of the diabetic cat. Additional studies are needed to define the effect and benefit of fiber further.

Feeding Plan

It is important to emphasize that the efficacy of dietary treatment depends on diet selection, feeding method, daily activity, and use of antidiabetic drugs or insulin. In all cases, large variations in activity or diet may alter glycemic control. Food changes or weight loss may result in the need for an insulin dose adjustment by up to 20%.

Food choice

Both high-fiber low-fat and low-carbohydrate high-protein formulas for the management of diabetes are commercially available. Low-carbohydrate foods are available from each of the major therapeutic food manufacturers (Hill's m/d, Purina DM, and Royal Canin DS 44; see Table 2), along with moderate- to high-fiber alternatives. These are good choices because they are palatable, low in protein, and fortified with vitamins and minerals that may be beneficial in DM. In addition, the products are consistent in formula and calorie content, allowing for the predictable dietary intake needed for optimal diabetic regulation. For cats reluctant to eat therapeutic foods, several gourmet type and growth formula canned foods are available in the grocery chains and have similarly low-carbohydrate levels. A quick check of the ingredient label indicates that these products contain animal meats, vitamins, minerals, and gums (but no grains or flours). Owners must be cautioned that it is only the canned form of these grocery store brands that is low in carbohydrates and that formulas can vary between flavors; thus, label reading is a must.

Studies are limited as to which food profile (high-fiber versus low-carbohydrate) provides optimal glycemic control. Feeding low-carbohydrate foods clearly increases the reversion rate of clinical diabetes to a non–insulin-dependent state (transient diabetes) by threefold compared with feeding high-fiber foods [15]. Nonetheless, transient diabetes occurs when feeding both food profiles (high-fiber or low-carbohydrate), and diabetic control is not significantly different between foods in cats that remain insulin-dependent [15]. There is individual variability in response to low-carbohydrate versus high-fiber therapeutic foods. Like the response to weight control therapy, there are no obvious clinical or biochemical indicators that predict the optimal food profile for an individual diabetic cat. Current recommendations for newly diagnosed cats are to start with a low carbohydrate food and good insulin control (typically glargine or lente insulin administered twice daily). Canned food is preferred over dry food because weight regulation seems to be better using a high-moisture product. This practice has resulted in the highest rate of diabetic remission (transient diabetes) in cats to date. Cats that are well regulated on moderate-fiber foods, or when higher protein levels are contraindicated, should continue to be fed the current diet. Cats on chronic insulin therapy were equally well controlled on the low-carbohydrate or higher fiber diet [15].

Until further studies are available, the clinician is left using diet history, personal preference, and individual food trials to determine the best food choice.

References

[1] Kirk CA, Feldman EC, Nelson RW. Diagnosis of naturally acquired type-I and type-II diabetes mellitus in cats. Am J Vet Res 1993;54:463–7.

[2] Feldman EC, Nelson RW. Diabetes mellitus. In: Canine and feline endocrinology and reproduction. Philadelphia: WB Saunders; 1996. p. 339–91.

[3] O'Brien TD, Hayden DW, Johnson KH, et al. High-dose intravenous glucose tolerance test and serum insulin and glucagon levels in diabetic and non-diabetic cats: relationships to insular amyloidosis. Vet Pathol 1985;22:250–61.

[4] Johnson KH. Impaired glucose tolerance associated with increased islet amyloid polypeptide (IAPP) immunoreactivity in pancreatic beta cells. Am J Pathol 1989;135:245–50.

[5] Henson MS, O'Brien TD. Feline models of type 2 diabetes mellitus. ILAR J 2006;47(3): 234–42.

[6] Yano BL. Feline insular amyloid: association with diabetes mellitus. Vet Pathol 1981;18: 621–7.

[7] MacDonald ML, Rogers QR, Morris JG. Nutrition of the domestic cat, a mammalian carnivore. Annu Rev Nutr 1994;4:521–62.

[8] Colagiuri S, Brand Miller J. The 'carnivore connection'—evolutionary aspects of insulin resistance. Eur J Clin Nutr 2002;56(Suppl 1):S30–5.

[9] Dohan FC, Lukens FDW. Lesions of the pancreatic islets produced in cats by administration of glucose. Science 1947;105:183.

[10] Hales CN. The pathogenesis of NIDDM. Diabetologia 1994;37(Suppl):S162–8.

[11] Brennan CL, Hoenig M, Ferguson DC. GLUT4 but not GLUT1 expression decreases early in the development of feline obesity. Domest Anim Endocrinol 2004;26(4):291–301.

[12] Nelson RW, Griffey SM, Feldman EC, et al. Transient clinical diabetes mellitus in cats: 10 cases (1989–1991). J Vet Intern Med 1999;13:28–35.

[13] Mazzaferro EM, Greco DS, Turner AS, et al. Treatment of feline diabetes mellitus using an α-glucosidase inhibitor and a low-carbohydrate diet. J Feline Med Surg 2003;5:183–9.

[14] Frank G, Anderson W, Pazak H, et al. Use of a high-protein diet in the management of feline diabetes mellitus. Vet Ther 2001;2:238–46.

[15] Bennett N, Greco DS, Peterson ME, et al. Comparison of a low-carbohydrate low-fiber diet and a moderate-carbohydrate high-fiber diet in the management of feline diabetes mellitus. J Feline Med Surg 2006;8(2):73–84.

[16] Panciera DL, Thomas CB, Eicker SW, et al. Epizootiologic patterns of diabetes mellitus in cats: 333 cases (1980–1986). J Am Vet Med Assoc 1990;197:1504–8.

[17] Scarlett JM, Donoghue S. Associations between body composition and disease in cats. J Am Vet Med Assoc 1998;212:1725–31.

[18] Nelson RW, Himsel CA, Feldman EC, et al. Glucose tolerance and insulin response in normal weight and obese cats. Am J Vet Res 1990;51:1357–62.

[19] Biourge V, Nelson RW, Feldman EC, et al. Effect of weight gain and subsequent weight loss on glucose intolerance and insulin response in healthy cats. J Vet Intern Med 1997;11:86–91.

[20] Appleton DJ, Rand JS, Sunvold GD. Insulin sensitivity decreases with obesity, and lean cats with low insulin sensitivity are at greatest risk of glucose intolerance with weight gain. J Feline Med Surg 2001;3:211–28.

[21] Rand JS, Marshall RD. Diabetes mellitus in cats. Vet Clin North Am Small Anim Pract 2005;35(1):211–24.

[22] Prola L, Dobenecker B, Kienzle E. Interaction between dietary cellulose content and food intake in cats. J Nutr 2006;136(7 Suppl):1988S–90S.

[23] Piechota TR, Rogers QR, Morris JG. Nitrogen requirement of cats during gestation and lactation. Nutr Res 1995;15:1535–46.

[24] Board on Agriculture and Natural Resources. Nutrient requirements of cats. Washington (DC): National Academy Press; 1986. p. 9–13.

[25] Thiess S, Becskei C, Tomsa K, et al. Effects of high carbohydrate and high fat diet on plasma metabolite levels and on i.v. glucose tolerance test in intact and neutered male cats. J Feline Med Surg 2004;6(4):207–18.

[26] Brunzell JD, Lerner RL, Hazzard WR, et al. Improved glucose tolerance with high carbohydrate feeding in mild diabetes. N Engl J Med 1971;284:521–5.

[27] Zoran DL. The carnivore connection to nutrition in cats. J Am Vet Med Assoc 2002;221:1559–67.

[28] Atkins RC. Dr. Atkins' new diet revolution. New York: Avon Books; 1992.

[29] Rand JS, Farrow HA, Fleeman LM, et al. Diet in the prevention of diabetes and obesity in companion animals. Asia Pac J Clin Nutr 2003;12(Suppl):S6.

[30] Kienzle E. Blood sugar levels and renal sugar excretion after the intake of high carbohydrate diets in cats. J Nutr 1994;124:S2563–7.

[31] Chandalia M, Garg A, Lutjohann D, et al. Beneficial effect of high dietary fiber intake in patients with type 2 diabetes mellitus. N Engl J Med 2000;342:1392–8.

[32] Nelson RW, Scott-Moncrieff JC, Feldman EC, et al. Effect of dietary insoluble fiber on control of glycemia in cats with naturally acquired diabetes mellitus. J Am Vet Med Assoc 2000;216:1082–8.

Vet Clin Small Anim 36 (2006) 1307–1323

VETERINARY CLINICS
SMALL ANIMAL PRACTICE

Nutrition and Osteoarthritis in Dogs: Does It Help?

Steven C. Budsberg, DVM, MS[a],*,
Joseph W. Bartges, DVM, PhD[b]

[a]Department of Small Animal Medicine and Surgery, College of Veterinary Medicine,
University of Georgia, Athens, GA 30602, USA
[b]Department of Small Animal Clinical Sciences, Veterinary Teaching Hospital,
College of Veterinary Medicine, The University of Tennessee, Knoxville, TN 37996-4544, USA

O steoarthritis (OA) is a common syndrome having multiple causes and characterized by pathologic change of the synovial or diarthrodial joint accompanied by clinical signs of pain and disability. Confusion about the definition of OA has arisen over the years; recently, the American Academy of Orthopaedic Surgeons proposed the following consensus definition: osteoarthritic diseases are a result of mechanical and biologic events that destabilize the normal coupling of degradation and synthesis of articular cartilage chondrocytes, extracellular matrix (primarily collagen and aggrecan), and subchondral bone. Although they may be initiated by multiple factors, including genetic, developmental, metabolic, and traumatic factors, osteoarthritic diseases involve all the tissues of the diarthrodial joint. Ultimately, osteoarthritic diseases are manifested by morphologic, biochemical, molecular, and biomechanical changes of cells and matrix that lead to softening, fibrillation, ulceration, articular cartilage loss, sclerosis and subchondral bone eburnation, and osteophyte production. When clinically evident, osteoarthritic diseases are characterized by joint pain, tenderness, limitation of movement, crepitus, occasional effusion, and variable degrees of inflammation without systemic effects [1]. OA has been estimated to affect as many as 20% of dogs older than 1 year of age [2]. For years, the discussion of OA and nutrition in small animal medicine has centered around nutrition and developmental orthopedic disease or the association between obesity and OA. The enormous public interest in the relation between diet supplements and OA has recently taken over center stage when discussing OA and nutrition, however. Physicians and veterinarians are constantly asked about these well-advertised supplements. Purely speculative information on nutritionally based therapies to treat OA has permeated every form of media available to the public. Unfortunately, few well-designed scientific studies have been initiated to explore these treatments in clinical

*Corresponding author. E-mail address: budsberg@vet.uga.edu (S.C. Budsberg).

0195-5616/06/$ – see front matter
doi:10.1016/j.cvsm.2006.08.007

patients. Thus, this article focuses solely on the evidence for dietary modification, including nutraceuticals formulated into diets, in patients with chronic OA.

Our initial discussion focuses on the use of evidence-based medicine. Evidence is defined as "the data on which a judgment or conclusion may be based, or by which proof or probability may be established" [3]. Evidence-based medicine is the integration of best research evidence with clinical expertise and patient values [4]. There are many ways in which to analyze and integrate evidence into the practice of veterinary medicine and several schemes by which to rank the strength of evidence. In this article, we review results of randomized placebo-controlled studies, and, where none exist, clinical trials or controlled experimental studies. Searches were performed on PubMed, setting the search limits to include only "clinical trial" and "randomized controlled trial." These searches were limited to "dogs" or "humans." The final search using "dog AND (arthritis OR osteoarthritis OR degenerative joint disease) AND (diet OR nutrition OR nutrient OR nutraceutical OR supplement)," supplemented with a search of bibliographies of articles that discussed the management of canine OA, yielded seven articles, of which five were randomized controlled studies. These studies varied in quality and type of design, limiting the strength of evidence they can provide to the clinician. The studies are briefly abstracted to give the reader some idea of the different studies done and their limitations. The most striking limitation shown here is the sheer lack of the number of studies and the number of dogs involved.

STUDY RESULTS
Study by Bui and Bierer
Bui and Bierer [5] evaluated the efficacy of green-lipped mussel (GLM; *Perna canaliculus*), added to a complete dry diet, for alleviating clinical signs of arthritis in dogs. A blind, randomized, longitudinal study design was used, with 31 dogs exhibiting varying degrees of arthritis. Each dog was evaluated by a veterinarian, and joints were individually scored for degree of pain, swelling, crepitus, and reduction in range of movement. Summation of all scores for an individual dog comprised its total score. Both groups were fed the same base dry diet, to which 0.3% GLM powder was added in the test group. The change in total score, by the end of 6 weeks, showed a significant improvement ($P < .05$) in the test group versus the control group. Significant improvements were also observed in joint pain and swelling scores in the test group. Changes in joint crepitus and range of joint movement were not significantly different between the test and control groups.

Study by Dobenecker and colleagues
The objective of the study by Dobenecker and colleagues [6] was to compare dog owners' perceptions of the effects of chondroitin sulfate (CS) or New Zealand GLM extract with a placebo in a double-blind field study in dogs with a chronic degenerative joint disease. Seventy dogs of different breeds, ages,

and genders were included in the study. Patients were randomized into three groups: the first group was given CS, the second group received mussel extract (GLM powder), and the third group was fed a placebo. The supplements were mixed into the normal diet of the patients. Changes in clinical symptoms during the 12-week oral application period were verified separately by dog owners and the attending veterinarians using standardized questionnaires at the beginning and end of the study. Fifty-eight dogs (83%) finished the trial. An important result of this study is that none of the tested substances led to a distinct improvement in the recorded symptoms or even to total recovery in general. The evaluation of the questionnaires of the attending veterinarians revealed good correspondence between the judgment of owners and experts. Both groups reported a slight improvement of the symptoms regarding the means of all three treatment groups, including that fed a placebo.

Study by Innes and colleagues

P54FP is an extract of Indian and Javanese turmeric, *Curcuma domestica* and *Curcuma xanthorrhiza*, respectively, that contains a mixture of active ingredients, including curcuminoids and essential oils. Innes and colleagues [7] conducted a randomized, blind, placebo-controlled, parallel-group clinical trial of P54FP as a treatment for OA of the canine elbow or hip. Sixty-one client-owned dogs with OA were recruited for the study at a single center. After a 2 week wash-out period, they were randomly allocated to receive P54FP or a placebo orally twice daily for 8 weeks and were re-examined after 4, 6, and 8 weeks of treatment. The effectiveness of the treatment was assessed in terms of the peak vertical force (PVz) and vertical impulse of the affected limbs, as measured with a force platform, by clinical assessments of lameness and joint pain by the investigators and overall assessment of the response to treatment by the investigators and owners. The results from 25 P54FP-treated dogs and 29 placebo-treated dogs showed that there was no statistically significant difference between the groups in terms of the PVz of the affected limb. The investigators' overall assessment showed a statistically significant treatment effect in favor of P54FP ($P = .012$), but the owners' assessment failed to reach statistical significance ($P = .063$). No serious adverse effects were recorded, but 2 P54FP-treated dogs and 4 placebo-treated dogs were withdrawn from the study because their condition deteriorated.

Study by Reichling and colleagues

Reichling and colleagues [8] conducted an open multicenter clinical trial comparing conditions before and after treatment with a natural resin extract of *Boswellia serrata*. Twenty-nine dogs with manifestations of chronic joint and spinal disease were enrolled. OA and degenerative conditions were confirmed radiologically in 25 of 29 cases. The resin extract (BSB108; Bogar AG, Wallisellen, Switzerland) was administered with the regular food at a dose of 400 mg per 10 kg of body weight once daily for 6 weeks. A statistically significant reduction of severity and resolution of typical clinical signs in individual animals, such as intermittent lameness, local pain, and stiff gait, were reported after 6 weeks. In

5 dogs, reversible brief episodes of diarrhea and flatulence occurred, but only once was a relation to the study preparation suspected.

Study by Gingerich and Strobel

Gingerich and colleagues [9] designed a questionnaire method for dog owners to monitor the orthopedic disabilities of their pets for evaluation of a nutraceutical with joint health claims. Fifty large-breed dogs presented with signs of OA were randomly allocated to placebo and active treatment groups. Degree of disability was assessed by physical examination, a standard questionnaire on daily activities, and a case-specific questionnaire that monitored specific impairments of each dog. The test product was a special milk protein concentrate (SMPC; Microlactin, Stolle Milk Biologics, Cincinnati, Ohio). Only 35 of the dogs completed the study. Overall improvement was noted in 68% and 35% of the SMPC and placebo groups, respectively. A significant $(P< .05)$ improvement in mean standardized and patient-specific questionnaire scores and in owner global assessments was detected in the SMPC group but not in the placebo group. Compared with the placebo group, the treatment response was significantly better in the SMPC group with regard to case-specific scores $(P< .001)$ and owner global assessments $(P= .004)$.

Study by Moreau and colleagues

The efficacy, tolerance, and ease of administration of a nutraceutic agent, carprofen, or meloxicam were evaluated in a prospective double-blind study by Moreau and colleagues [10] in 71 dogs with OA. The client-owned dogs were randomly assigned to one of the three treatments or to a placebo control group. The influence of OA on the dogs' gait was described by comparing the ground reaction forces of the arthritic dogs and 10 normal dogs. Additionally, subjective assessments were made by the owners and by the orthopedic surgeons. Changes in the ground reaction forces were specific to the arthritic joint and were significantly improved by carprofen and meloxicam but not by the nutraceutic agent; the values returned to normal only with meloxicam. The orthopedic surgeons assessed that there had been an improvement with carprofen and meloxicam, but the owners considered that there had been an improvement only with meloxicam. The treatments were well tolerated, except for a case of hepatopathy in a dog treated with carprofen.

Study by Impellizeri and colleagues

Impellizeri and colleagues [11] conducted a study on the effect of weight reduction on clinical signs of lameness among overweight dogs with clinical and radiographic signs of hip OA. This was a nonblind prospective clinical trial. Nine client-owned dogs with radiographic signs of hip OA that weighed 11% to 12% greater than their ideal body weight and were examined because of hind limb lameness were included in the study. Baseline body condition, hind limb lameness, and hip function scores were assigned. Severity of lameness was scored using a numeric rating scale and a visual analog scale. Dogs were fed a restricted-calorie diet, with the amount of diet fed calculated to provide 60% of the calories needed to maintain the dogs' current weight. Evaluations were repeated midway through and at the end of the weight loss period. Dogs lost between 11% and 18% of their initial body weight. Body weight, body condition score, and severity of hind limb lameness were all significantly decreased at the end of the weight loss period.

OA is the most common form of arthritis recognized in dogs [12]. Hip dysplasia, cruciate instability, and osteochondritis dissecans are common causes of canine OA (degenerative joint disease). As previously described, degenerative OA is characterized as a slowly progressive condition in which two primary pathologic processes occur: articular cartilage degeneration and subchondral bone changes. A low-grade synovitis often occurs. Inflammation is present in these joints, and steroidal or nonsteroidal anti-inflammatory drugs may modulate this inflammation. Although nutritional imbalances may result in developmental skeletal disease (see the article by Lauten elsewhere in this issue), which, in turn, may lead to degenerative joint disease, the role of nutrition in the management of degenerative joint disease is less clear. Nutrition may aid in treatment of degenerative joint disease through optimizing body condition and body weight (managing obesity), by modifying degenerative or inflammatory processes (specific nutrient effects), and by influencing pharmacologic therapy (drug-nutrient interaction).

OBESITY

Obesity can be defined as accumulation of body fat in excess of what is necessary to maintain optimum condition and health. This may be obvious in a grossly obese individual, particularly when obesity-related disease is present; however, it is less obvious in a patient that is overweight and otherwise clinically healthy but is at risk for obesity-related disease, such as degenerative OA. Quantitatively, obesity in dogs is generally defined as exceeding ideal body weight by 15% to 20% or more. One technique that is useful in the management of patients is a body condition score. The advantage of assigning a body condition score is that it uses information additional to body weight. It is a measure of the appearance of the animal, of fat stores that are identified, of muscle mass and tone, and of general health.

Obesity may result in OA as a result of excess forces placed on joints and articular cartilage, which may lead to inactivity and further development of obesity; thus, a vicious cycle ensues. Additionally, adipose tissue is recognized as being metabolically active and proinflammatory; therefore, obesity may contribute to inflammation [13–15].

Several studies have demonstrated a relation between obesity and OA [16]; however, a cause and effect mechanism has not been found [17,18]. A long-term study was performed in 48 Labrador Retrievers from seven litters divided into two dietary groups: one group was fed an adult maintenance dog food at 0.27 kJ of metabolizable energy per kilogram of body weight per day, and the second group was fed the same diet at 75% of the amount (0.2025 kJ of metabolizable energy per kilogram of body weight per day) [19,20]. Restricted fed dogs lived, on average, 2 years longer, weighed less, had better body condition scores, and had longer delay to treatment of chronic disease, including OA [21]. Therefore, maintaining an optimal or slightly lean body condition may be associated with lower risk of development of OA, development of less severe OA, and delay of onset of clinical signs of OA in dogs.

Weight reduction from an obese state is beneficial in the management of OA in human beings [22–24]. In addition to improvement in mobility, weight reduction was associated with better quality-of-life scores in human beings with knee OA [25]. Two uncontrolled clinical studies of obese dogs with OA demonstrated improvement in mobility [11,26]. In one study of 9 dogs with a body condition score of 5 of 5 and coxofemoral OA, obesity management resulted in loss of 11% to 18% of body weight, a decrease in body condition to optimal condition, and improvement in the severity of subjective hind limb lameness scores [11]. In a second study of 16 dogs with coxofemoral OA, weight loss of 13% to 29% of body weight and decrease of body condition to optimal resulted in improvement of ground reactive force as well as improvement in subjective mobility and clinical signs of OA [26]. Although these are uncontrolled clinical trials in a small number of dogs, results suggest that weight reduction may be beneficial in dogs with OA.

ω-3 FATTY ACIDS

Degenerative OA involves an inflammatory component; thus, it may be possible to modify the inflammation by nutritional components, specifically ω-3 (n3) fatty acids. Arachidonic acid (an ω-6 [n6] fatty acid) is incorporated into cell membranes; when metabolized, it yields prostaglandins, leukotrienes, and thromboxanes of the 2 and 4 series. Many drugs used to treat degenerative OA inhibit conversion of arachidonic acid to these eicosanoids. These n6-derived eicosanoids have, for the most part, vasoactive and proinflammatory effects. Substituting an n3 fatty acid in the membrane may decrease these responses. Metabolism of n3 fatty acids results in eicosanoids of the 3 and 5 series, which are less vasoactive and less proinflammatory.

Several studies have been published that demonstrate a beneficial response to n3 fatty acid incorporation into diets of human beings with rheumatoid arthritis [27–31], although other studies have not demonstrated a benefit [32]. There is a growing body of data showing positive effects of n3 fatty acids on cartilage and its metabolism in the face of degradative enzymes. Recent work has provided direct evidence that n3 fatty acid supplementation can reduce or abrogate the inflammatory and matrix degradative response elicited by chondrocytes during OA progression [33–36]. Unfortunately, there are no randomized controlled clinical trials published of n3 fatty acids and OA in dogs. An unpublished study has been performed in dogs evaluating n3 fatty acids and experimentally induced stifle arthritis [37]. Eighteen dogs were randomly assigned to one of three isocaloric diet groups containing 21.4% fat (dry matter basis) differing only in their fatty acid composition: a diet with an n6-to-n3 fatty acid ratio of 28.0:1.0 (high-n6 diet), a diet with an n6-to-n3 fatty acid ratio of

8.7:1.0 (control diet), and a diet with an n6-to-n3 fatty acid ratio of 0.7:1.0 (high-n3 diet). Diets were fed for a total of 21 months. Initially, the dogs were started on their assigned diet 3 months before surgical transection of the left cranial cruciate ligament, continued until surgical repair 6 months later, and maintained for an additional 12 months after repair. When compared with the high-n6 and control diets, consumption of the high-n3 diet was associated with lower serum concentrations of cholesterol, triglycerides, and phospholipids; lower synovial concentrations of prostaglandin E2; better ground reaction forces; and fewer radiographic changes of OA. Synovial membrane fatty acid composition mirrored the fatty acid composition of the diets consumed by the dogs. Recently, a randomized study was presented in abstract form, where 38 dogs with naturally occurring OA were placed on a commercially available therapeutic food formulated to contain an n6-to-n3 ratio of 0.7:1.0 (Prescription Diet J/d; Hill's Pet Nutrition, Topeka, Kansas) or a typical dry dog food [38]. Ground reaction forces as well as owner and veterinarian clinical evaluations were collected at days 0, 45, and 90. Ground reaction forces increased and weight bearing increased in the dogs fed the therapeutic diet when compared with the control diet. It should be noted that the two diets differed in more than just the fatty acid composition, but this was the major difference. Finally, one study in dogs reported results of observations of dog owners who perceived improvement in their pet's arthritic symptoms when treated with fatty acids for various dermatologic problems [39].

ANTIOXIDANTS

The formation of free radicals as a consequence of cellular metabolism occurs constantly, but the potential deleterious effects are minimized by antioxidants. The balance between free radicals and antioxidant defenses is a key factor in preventing development of noxious processes at the cellular and tissue levels. Recent evidence supports the theory that excessive production of free radicals or the imbalance between concentrations of free radicals and antioxidant defenses may be related to such processes as aging, cancer, diabetes mellitus, lupus, and arthritis [40]. Progressive hypoxia resulting in the production of reactive oxygen species may play a role in rheumatoid arthritis [41]. Thus, antioxidant therapy may be of benefit in the treatment of OA [42].

Most studies of antioxidant therapy for arthritis in human beings involve rheumatoid arthritis, although several studies of knee OA have been published. An early pilot study of vitamin E (tocopherol) demonstrated improvement in clinical signs and pain scores in 52% of 29 patients with knee OA compared with 4% receiving a placebo [43]. In another placebo-controlled study of human beings with OA of the coxofemoral or knee joint, high-dose tocopherol was as efficacious as diclofenac in reducing pain and improving mobility [44]. This was also found in studies of human beings with rheumatoid arthritis [45,46]. Other studies have not demonstrated a benefit of vitamin E for rheumatoid arthritis or OA [47–49]. Likewise, the efficacy of vitamin C in human beings with OA has been difficult to determine because of contradictory results of studies

[50–53] Selenium was not shown to be beneficial in human beings with rheumatoid arthritis [54]. Methyl-sulfonyl-methane (MSM) is a derivative of dimethyl sulfoxide and has been suggested as an agent for the management of pain and inflammation and as an antioxidant. The rationale for its use lies in the possibility of a dietary sulfur deficiency, with a resultant deficiency of sulfur-containing compounds in the body, such as antioxidants and CS [55]. Currently, there are no randomized controlled clinical trials evaluating MSM in human beings; however, in a recent pilot clinical trial involving a placebo control, MSM reduced the Western Ontario and McMaster University Osteoarthritis Index visual analog scale scores and pain and improved physical function when compared with placebo [56]. There are no controlled studies evaluating or documenting a benefit of vitamin C, MSM, or selenium in dogs with OA, although they may be recommended [57,58]. Dogs do not require exogenous vitamin C because they are capable of synthesizing it endogenously; therefore, its use is not encouraged.

CHONDROMODULATING AGENTS

Chondromodulating agents are purported to slow or alter the progression of OA. These agents are considered to be slow-acting drugs in osteoarthritis (SADOAs) and can be subdivided into symptomatic slow-acting drugs in osteoarthritis (SYSADOAs) and disease-modifying osteoarthritis drugs (DMOADs). Beneficial effects may include a positive effect on cartilage matrix synthesis and hyaluronan synthesis by synovial membrane as well as an inhibitory effect on catabolic enzymes in osteoarthritic joints [59]. Compounds fall into two different categories. One group is agents that are approved by the US Food and Drug Administration and can have label claims of clinical effects, such as polysulfated glycosaminoglycan (Adequan; Luitpold Pharmaceuticals, Shirley, New York). The second group comprises products that are considered to be nutritional supplements, which are not regulated and legally cannot claim any medical benefits. Examples of this group include glucosamine and CS (Glycoflex; Vetri-Science Laboratories, Essex Junction, Vermont and Cosequin; Nutramax Laboratories, Baltimore, Maryland). Although many of these products are administered as a supplement or alternative treatment, some, such as glucosamine and GLM, are incorporated into pet foods.

Glucosamine and Chondroitin Sulfate

Glucosamine is an amino sugar that is a precursor for biochemical synthesis of glycosylated proteins and lipids. D-glucosamine is made naturally in the form of glucosamine-6-phosphate and is the biochemical precursor of all nitrogen-containing sugars [60]. Specifically, glucosamine-6-phosphate is synthesized from fructose-6-phosphate and glutamine [61] as the first step of the hexosamine biosynthesis pathway. The end product of this pathway is uridine diphosphate (UDP)-N-acetylglucosamine, which is then used for making glycosaminoglycans, proteoglycans, and glycolipids. Because glucosamine is a precursor for glycosaminoglycans and glycosaminoglycans are a major component of joint cartilage, supplemental glucosamine may help to rebuild cartilage, and there are in vitro data to support this claim [62–65]. There are conflicting data on evidence of any clinical effect of glucosamine in veterinary medicine, however [10,66,67]. Commonly used forms of glucosamine include glucosamine sulfate and glucosamine hydrochloride, and it is often combined with CS and MSM. A review of studies of pharmacologic dosages of glucosamine is beyond the scope of this article; however, glucosamine, with CS, is included in dog foods at low concentrations.

When evaluating glucosamine and CS inclusion in a manufactured dog food, two questions might be asked. Are the glucosamine and CS in the food stable and bioavailable? Is the amount of glucosamine and CS in the food enough to provide a beneficial effect? It is difficult to find the amount of glucosamine and CS in pet foods. Many dog foods formulated and marketed for adult dogs, geriatric dogs, and large-breed growth contain glucosamine and CS, but the amounts are not readily available from the manufacturer or from electronic or print information. These compounds are not recognized by the American Association of Feed Control Officials, and thus are not included in dog nutrient profiles. Furthermore, they are not considered as "generally regarded as safe" (GRAS) ingredients.

New Zealand Green-Lipped Mussel

New Zealand GLM is a rich source of glycosaminoglycans, although its proposed benefit is thought to be from the anti-inflammatory effects of tetraenoic acid of the n3 series [68]. In 1986, dried mussel extracts that were stabilized with a preservative became available. The earlier studies that found no beneficial effect of GLM on arthritis all used preparations that had not been stabilized, which is a point that may help to explain some of the discrepancies in the research. A stabilized lipid extract (Lyprinol, Pharmalink International, Lancashire, England) is more effective than a nonstabilized extract at inhibiting inflammation [69]. In an uncontrolled clinical trial, Lyprinol administration resulted in an 80% improvement in human beings with rheumatoid arthritis [70]. In a randomized controlled clinical study of 31 dogs with arthritis, GLM powder (0.3%) was added to the diet during processing of one group of dogs [5]. Compared with the control group, which was fed the same diet without added GLM powder, there was significant improvement in subjective arthritis scores, joint swelling, and joint pain in the treated group. These data must not be overinterpreted, however. In a systematic review of agents used to treat canine OA, the data regarding the benefits of GLM extract in dogs were promising but uncertainties existed relating to the scientific quality of the data, and no definitive relation has been proven between clinical improvements and the therapy [71].

OTHER DIETARY COMPOUNDS

There are many other dietary supplements, including herbs and other nutraceutic agents, that are recommended. Few, if any, have been evaluated in a controlled manner. Because of limitations of space, only a few are discussed.

P54FP

P54FP is an extract of Indian and Javanese turmeric, *C domestica* and *C xanthor-rhiza*, respectively, which contains a mixture of active ingredients, including cur-cuminoids and essential oils [7]. There is evidence that these active ingredients possess anti-inflammatory activity. Specifically, curcumin has been shown to inhibit prostaglandin E2 and cyclooxygenase-2 as well as nuclear factor-κB [72–74]. One randomized blind study in dogs with OA found no difference in objective ground reaction forces but did see some improvements in certain subjective outcome measures [7].

Avocado/Soy

Avocado/soybean unsaponifiables (ASUs) are composed of the unsaponifiable fractions of avocado and soybean oils in a 1:3 to 2:3 proportion, respectively [75,76] In vitro data show that ASUs have antiosteoarthritic properties by in-hibiting interleukin-1 and stimulating collagen synthesis in cartilage cultures [77,78] In vivo, there is one report in an ovine meniscectomy model of OA pro-viding some support for disease-modifying capabilities [79]. Human clinical tri-als have shown some beneficial effects of ASUs on clinical symptoms of symptoms of OA and suggest that ASUs may have some structure modification capabilities. There are, however, some conflicting data, because one study found no long-term benefits [80–83]. ASUs have not yet been evaluated in dogs with OA.

Boron

Boron deficiency in food may be part of the cause of some arthritides [84]. Ep-idemiologic studies suggest that human beings in countries with low boron in-take (less than 1.0 mg/d) have a higher risk of development of arthritis when compared with human beings in countries in which boron intake is higher (3–10 mg/d) [85]. In a double-blind placebo/boron supplementation trial in 20 subjects with OA, a significantly favorable response to a boron supplement at 6 mg/d was found; 50% of subjects receiving supplement improved com-pared with 10% receiving placebo [85]. Whether boron deficiency occurs in pet dogs is unknown. Furthermore, whether boron supplementation and what dosage of boron would be best are unknown. Until studies are performed, supplementation cannot be recommended.

Boswellia Resin

Boswellia, also known as Boswellin or Indian frankincense, comes from the In-dian *Boswellia serrata* tree. Resin from the bark of this tree is purported to have anti-inflammatory properties. Boswellia resin has been shown to improve clin-ical signs and pain in human beings in controlled studies [86–88]. Boswellia resin has been evaluated in 24 dogs in an open multicenter study [8]. Improve-ment in clinical signs, lameness, and pain was found in 17 of 24 dogs. In 5 dogs, diarrhea and flatulence occurred. Further controlled clinical trials are needed to validate these findings.

Cat's Claw

Cat's claw, an Amazonian medicinal plant, has anti-inflammatory and antioxidant effects and has been shown to decrease clinical signs of knee arthritis and rheumatoid arthritis in human beings [89,90]. It has not been evaluated in dogs with OA.

Creatine

Creatine is used in muscle for production of ATP, which provides energy for muscle contraction. Creatine is sometimes used by body builders and people who exercise with the intent to increase muscle mass and muscular energy; however, some recommend its use with arthritis, especially rheumatoid arthritis in human beings. In rheumatoid arthritis, skeletal muscle weakness often accompanies the arthropathy. In one study, creatine supplementation in human beings with rheumatoid arthritis increased serum and skeletal muscle creatine content but failed to increase skeletal muscle creatine phosphate concentration or strength [91]. In another study of human beings undergoing total knee replacement, creatine supplementation did not improve body composition or skeletal muscle strength [92]. No randomized controlled studies have been performed in dogs with OA.

Special Milk Protein Concentrate

Milk contains a number of biologically active compounds, including immunoglobulins, cytokines, enzymes, hormones, and growth factors. These compounds impart anti-inflammatory properties that have been recognized in human breast milk [93] and milk from hyperimmunized cows [94,95]. An SMPC prepared from milk of hyperimmunized cows (Microlactin) exerts anti-inflammatory properties [96]. The anti-inflammatory properties do not seem to be caused by inhibition of arachidonic acid metabolism but by suppression of neutrophil migration from the vascular space [97]. A randomized controlled clinical trial has been performed evaluating the SMPC in dogs with naturally occurring OA [9]. In this study, dogs receiving the SMPC had improvement in subjective clinical signs of OA and owner global assessment compared with dogs receiving placebo. Further studies need to be completed to validate these findings.

CURRENTLY AVAILABLE VETERINARY DIETS

Many over-the-counter dog foods contain claims of being "joint friendly" because they contain glucosamine, CS, and perhaps other ingredients theorized to be beneficial for joint health. There are four diets specifically formulated and marketed for dogs with arthritis: CNM Joint Mobility JM (Ralston Purina, St. Louis, Missouri), Prescription Diet J/d (Hill's Pet Nutrition), Mobility Support JS 21 (Royal Canin, St. Charles, Missouri), and Mobility Support JS 21 Large Breed (Royal Canin). Nutritional characteristics are presented in Table 1. Most adult maintenance dog foods have n6-to-n3 ratios of greater than 8.0:1.0; therefore, these diets are higher in n3 fatty acids relative to maintenance adult dog foods.

Table 1
Average nutrient content for CNM Joint Mobility, Prescription Diet J/d, Mobility Support JS 21, and Mobility Support JS 21 Large Breed

Nutrient	Unit	JM dry	J/d dry	J/d canned	JS dry	JS LB dry
Protein	g/100 kcal ME	7.9	5.4	4.7	6.2	6.9
Carbohydrate	g/100 kcal ME	9.9	13.8	12.6	12.7	11.3
Fat	g/100 kcal ME	3.3	3.9	4.6	2.7	3.59
Fiber	g/100 kcal ME	0.35	2.70	0.70	0.81	0.38
Calcium	g/100 kcal ME	0.34	0.18	0.16	0.35	0.21
Phosphorous	g/100 kcal ME	0.25	0.14	0.13	0.24	0.14
Ca/P		1.4:1.0	1.3:1.0	1.2:1.0	1.5:1.0	1.5:1.0
Total n3 fatty acids	g/100 kcal ME	0.25	0.95	1.01		
Total n6 fatty acids	g/100 kcal ME	0.44	0.67	0.68		
n6/n3 fatty acid ratio		1.7:1.0	0.7:1.0	0.7:1.0	4.7:1.0	3.5:1.0
Vitamin E	mg/100 kcal ME	25.4			14.1	15.4
Glucosamine	mg/100 kcal ME	34			100	200
Other ingredients		Carnitine	Carnitine	Carnitine	Green-lipped mussel	Green-lipped mussel

Abbreviations: Ca/P, calcium-to-phosphorous ratio; J/d, Prescription diet J/d canine diet (Hill's Pet Nutrition, Topeka, Kansas); JM, CNM Joint Mobility JM canine diet (Ralston Purina, St. Louis, Missouri); JS, Mobility Support JS 21 canine diet (Royal Canin, St. Charles, Missouri); JS LB, Mobility Support JS 21 Large Breed (Royal Canin); ME, metabolizable energy.

Recent research supports a role of nutrition and nutritional modification in the management of OA in dogs. Furthermore, weight management, including weight reduction and prevention of obesity, has a positive impact on the incidence and clinical signs of OA in dogs. Feeding diets that contain increased n3 fatty acids and GLM has been shown to help dogs with OA. Whether other dietary ingredients provide benefit has yet to be determined.

References

[1] Keuttner K, Goldberg VM, editors. Osteoarthritic Disorders, American Academy of Orthopaedic Surgeons Symposium, New Horizons in Osteoarthritis, April 1995. Rosemont, IL. 1995. p. xxi-v.

[2] Johnston SA. Osteoarthritis: joint anatomy, physiology, and pathobiology. Vet Clin North Am Small Anim Pract 1997;27:699–723.

[3] American heritage dictionary of the English language. Houghton Mifflin Company: Boston; 1978.

[4] Straus SE, Richardson WS, Glasziou P, et al. Evidence based medicine: how to practice and teach EBM. 3rd edition. Edinburgh (UK): Churchill Livingstone; 2005.

[5] Bui LM, Bierer TL. Influence of green lipped mussels (Perna canaliculus) in alleviating signs of arthritis in dogs. Vet Ther 2003;4:397–407.

[6] Dobenecker B, Beetz Y, Kienzle E. A placebo-controlled double-blind study on the effect of nutraceuticals (chondroitin sulfate and mussel extract) in dogs with joint diseases as perceived by their owners. J Nutr 2002;132(Suppl):1690S–1S.

[7] Innes JF, Fuller CJ, Grover ER, et al. Randomized, double-blind, placebo-controlled parallel group study of P54FP for the treatment of dogs with osteoarthritis. Vet Rec 2003;152(15): 457–60.

[8] Reichling J, Schmokel H, Fitzi J, et al. Dietary support with Boswellia resin in canine inflammatory joint and spinal disease. Schweiz Arch Tierheilkd 2004;146:71–9.

[9] Gingerich DA, Strobel JD. Use of client-specific outcome measures to assess treatment effects in geriatric, arthritic dogs: controlled clinical evaluation of a nutraceutical. Vet Ther 2003;4: 56–66.

[10] Moreau M, Dupuis J, Bonneau NH, et al. Clinical evaluation of a nutraceutical, carprofen and meloxicam for the treatment of dogs with osteoarthritis. Vet Rec 2003;152:323–9.

[11] Impellizeri JA, Tetrick MA, Muir P. Effect of weight reduction on clinical signs of lameness in dogs with hip osteoarthritis. J Am Vet Med Assoc 2000;216:1089–91.

[12] Bennett D, May C. Joint diseases of dogs and cats. In: Ettinger SJ, Feldman EC, editors. Textbook of veterinary internal medicine. 3rd edition. Philadelphia: WB Saunders; 1995. p. 2032–77.

[13] Greenberg AS, Obin MS. Obesity and the role of adipose tissue in inflammation and metabolism. Am J Clin Nutr 2006;83(Suppl):461S–5S.

[14] Pang SS, Le YY. Role of resistin in inflammation and inflammation-related diseases. Cell Mol Immunol 2006;3:29–34.

[15] Otero M, Lago R, Gomez R, et al. Leptin: a metabolic hormone that functions like a proinflammatory adipokine. Drug News Perspect 2006;19:21–6.

[16] Edney ATB. Management of obesity in the dog. Vet Med Small Anim Clin 1974;49:46–9.

[17] Edney ATB, Smith PM. Study of obesity in dogs visiting veterinary practices in the United Kingdom. Vet Rec 1986;118:391–6.

[18] Janssen I, Mark AE. Separate and combined influence of body mass index and waist circumference on arthritis and knee osteoarthritis. Int J Obes 2006;Aug 30(8):1223–8.

[19] Larson BT, Lawler DF, Spitznagel EL Jr, et al. Improved glucose tolerance with lifetime diet restriction favorably affects disease and survival in dogs. J Nutr 2003;133:2887–92.

[20] Kealy RD, Lawler DF, Ballam JM, et al. Effects of diet restriction on life span and age-related changes in dogs. J Am Vet Med Assoc 2002;220:1315–20.

[21] Kealy RD, Lawler DF, Ballam JM, et al. Evaluation of the effect of limited food consumption on radiographic evidence of osteoarthritis in dogs. J Am Vet Med Assoc 2000;217: 1678–80.

[22] Messier SP, Gutekunst DJ, Davis C, et al. Weight loss reduces knee-joint loads in overweight and obese older adults with knee osteoarthritis. Arthritis Rheum 2005;52:2026–32.

[23] Messier SP, Loeser RF, Miller GD, et al. Exercise and dietary weight loss in overweight and obese older adults with knee osteoarthritis: the Arthritis, Diet, and Activity Promotion Trial. Arthritis Rheum 2004;50:1501–10.

[24] Huang MH, Chen CH, Chen TW, et al. The effects of weight reduction on the rehabilitation of patients with knee osteoarthritis and obesity. Arthritis Care Res 2000;13: 398–405.

[25] Rejeski WJ, Focht BC, Messier SP, et al. Obese, older adults with knee osteoarthritis: weight loss, exercise, and quality of life. Health Psychol 2002;21:419–26.

[26] Burkholder WJ, Taylor L, Hulse DA. Weight loss to optimal body condition increases ground reactive force in dogs with osteoarthritis. Compend Contin Educ Pract Vet 2000; 23(Suppl 9A):74.

[27] de Deckere EA, Korver O, Verschuren PM, et al. Health aspects of fish and n-3 polyunsaturated fatty acids from plant and marine origin. Eur J Clin Nutr 1998;52:749–53.

[28] Alexander JW. Immunonutrition: the role of omega-3 fatty acids. Nutrition 1998;147: 627–33.

[29] Skoldstam L, Borjesson O, Kjallman A, et al. Effect of six months of fish oil supplementation in stable rheumatoid arthritis. A double-blind, controlled study. Scand J Rheumatol 1992;21: 178–85.

[30] Stamp LK, James MJ, Cleland LG. Diet and rheumatoid arthritis: a review of the literature. Semin Arthritis Rheum 2005;35:77–94.

[31] Simopoulos AP. Essential fatty acids in health and chronic disease. Am J Clin Nutr 1999; 70(Suppl):560S–9S.

[32] Veale DJ, Torley HI, Richards IM, et al. A double-blind placebo controlled trial of Efamol Marine on skin and joint symptoms of psoriatic arthritis. Br J Rheumatol 1994;33: 954–8.

[33] Curtis CL, Harwood JL, Dent CM, et al. Biological basis for the benefit of nutraceutical supplementation in arthritis. Drug Discov Today 2004;9(4):165–72.

[34] Curtis CL, Rees SG, Cramp J, et al. Effects of n-3 fatty acids on cartilage metabolism. Proc Nutr Soc 2002;61(3):381–9.

[35] Curtis CL, Rees SG, Little CB, et al. Pathologic indicators of degradation and inflammation in human osteoarthritic cartilage are abrogated by exposure to n-3 fatty acids. Arthritis Rheum 2002;46(6):1544–53.

[36] Curtis CL, Hughes CE, Flannery CR, et al. n-3 Fatty acids specifically modulate catabolic factors involved in articular cartilage degradation. J Biol Chem 2000;275(2):721–4.

[37] Bartges JW, Budsberg SC, Pazak HE, et al. Effects of different n6:n3 fatty acid ratio diets on canine stifle osteoarthritis [abstract 462]. Presented at the Orthopedic Research Society 47th Annual Meeting. San Francisco, CA, 2001.

[38] Roush JK, Cross AR, Renberg WC, et al. Effects of feeding a high omega-3 fatty acid diet on serum fatty acid profiles and force plate analysis in dogs with osteoarthritis [abstract]. Vet Surg 2005;34:E21.

[39] Miller WH, Scott DW, Wellington JR. Treatment of dogs with hip arthritis with a fatty acid supplement. Canine Pract 1992;17:6–8.

[40] Bermejo-Vicedo T, Hidalgo-Correas FJ. Antioxidants: the therapy of the future? Nutr Hosp 1997;12:108–20.

[41] Mapp PL, Grootveld MC, Blake DR. Hypoxia, oxidative stress and rheumatoid arthritis. Br Med Bull 1995;51:419–36.

[42] McAlindon TE, Biggee BA. Nutritional factors and osteoarthritis: recent developments. Curr Opin Rheumatol 2005;17:647–52.

[43] Machtey I, Ouaknine L. Tocopherol in osteoarthritis: a controlled pilot study. J Am Geriatr Soc 1978;26:328–30.

[44] Scherak O, Kolarz G, Schodl C, et al. [High dosage vitamin E therapy in patients with activated arthrosis.] Z Rheumatol 1990;49:369–73 [in German].

[45] Wittenborg A, Petersen G, Lorkowski G, et al. [Effectiveness of vitamin E in comparison with diclofenac sodium in treatment of patients with chronic polyarthritis.] Z Rheumatol 1998; 57:215–21 [in German].

[46] Edmonds SE, Winyard PG, Guo R, et al. Putative analgesic activity of repeated oral doses of vitamin E in the treatment of rheumatoid arthritis. Results of a prospective placebo controlled double blind trial. Ann Rheum Dis 1997;56:649–55.

[47] Brand C, Snaddon J, Bailey M, et al. Vitamin E is ineffective for symptomatic relief of knee osteoarthritis: a six month double blind, randomized, placebo controlled study. Ann Rheum Dis 2001;60:946–9.

[48] Wluka AE, Stuckey S, Brand C, et al. Supplementary vitamin E does not affect the loss of cartilage volume in knee osteoarthritis: a 2 year double blind randomized placebo controlled study. J Rheumatol 2002;29:2585–91.

[49] Chrubasik S. Vitamin E for rheumatoid arthritis or osteoarthritis: low evidence of effectiveness [letter]. Z Rheumatol 2003;62:491.

[50] Leffler CT, Philippi AF, Leffler SG, et al. Glucosamine, chondroitin, and manganese ascorbate for degenerative joint disease of the knee or low back: a randomized, double-blind, placebo-controlled pilot study. Mil Med 1999;164:85–91.

[51] Jensen NH. [Reduced pain from osteoarthritis in hip joint or knee joint during treatment with calcium ascorbate. A randomized, placebo-controlled cross-over trial in general practice.] Ugeskr Laeger 2003;165:2563–6. [in Danish].

[52] Jaswal S, Mehta HC, Sood AK, et al. Antioxidant status in rheumatoid arthritis and role of antioxidant therapy. Clin Chim Acta 2003;338:123–9.

[53] Remans PH, Sont JK, Wagenaar LW, et al. Nutrient supplementation with polyunsaturated fatty acids and micronutrients in rheumatoid arthritis: clinical and biochemical effects. Eur J Clin Nutr 2004;58:839–45.

[54] Peretz A, Siderova V, Neve J. Selenium supplementation in rheumatoid arthritis investigated in a double blind, placebo-controlled trial. Scand J Rheumatol 2001;30:208–12.

[55] Parcell S. Sulfur in human nutrition and applications in medicine. Altern Med Rev 2002;7: 22–44.

[56] Kim LS, Axelrod LJ, Howard P, et al. Efficacy of methylsulfonylmethane (MSM) in osteoarthritis pain of the knee: a pilot clinical trial. Osteoarthritis Cartilage 2006;14:286–94.

[57] Beale BS. Orthopedic problems in geriatric dogs and cats. Vet Clin North Am Small Anim Pract 2005;35:655–74.

[58] Hastings D. Suggested treatment for polyarthritis in dogs [letter]. J Am Vet Med Assoc 2004;225:29.

[59] McNamara PS, Johnston SA, Todhunter RJ. Slow-acting, disease-modifying osteoarthritis agents. Vet Clin North Am Small Anim Pract 1997;27:863–81.

[60] Roseman S. Reflections on glycobiology. J Biol Chem 2001;276:1527–42.

[61] Ghosh S, Blumenthal HJ, Davidson E, et al. Glucosamine metabolism. V. Enzymatic synthesis of glucosamine 6-phosphate. J Biol Chem 1960;235:1265–73.

[62] Chan PS, Caron JP, Orth MW. Effect of glucosamine and chondroitin sulfate on regulation of gene expression of proteolytic enzymes and their inhibitors in interleukin-1 challenged bovine articular cartilage explants. Am J Vet Res 2005;66:1870–6.

[63] Lippiello L, Han S, Henderson T. Protective effect of the chondroprotective agent Cosequin DS on bovine articular cartilage exposed in vitro to nonsteroidal anti-inflammatory agents. Vet Ther 2002;2:128–35.

[64] Gouze JN, Bordji K, Gulberti S, et al. Interleukin-1β down regulates the expression of glucuronosyltransferase I, a key enzyme priming glycosaminoglycan biosynthesis. Arthritis Rheum 2001;44:351–60.

[65] Dodge GR, Jimenez SA. Glucosamine sulphate modulates the levels of aggrecan and matrix metalloproteinase-3 synthesized by cultured human osteoarthritis articular chondrocytes. Osteoarthritis Cartilage 2003;11:424–32.

[66] Laverty S, Sandy JD, Celeste C, et al. Synovial fluid levels and serum pharmacokinetics in a large animal model following treatment with oral glucosamine at clinically relevant doses. Arthritis Rheum 2005;52:181–91.

[67] Hanson RR, Brawner WR, Blaik MA, et al. Oral treatment with a nutraceutical (Cosequin) for ameliorating signs of navicular syndrome in horses. Vet Ther 2001;2:148–59.

[68] Gibson RG, Gibson SL, Conway V, et al. Perna canaliculus in the treatment of arthritis. Practitioner 1980;224:955–60.

[69] Butters DE, Whitehouse MW. Treating inflammation: some (needless) difficulties for gaining acceptance of effective natural products and traditional medicines. Inflammopharmacology 2003;11:97–110.

[70] Cho SH, Jung YB, Seong SC, et al. Clinical efficacy and safety of Lyprinol, a patented extract from New Zealand green-lipped mussel (Perna canaliculus) in patients with osteoarthritis of the hip and knee: a multicenter 2-month clinical trial. Allerg Immunol (Paris) 2003;35: 212–6.

[71] Aragon CL, Hofmeister EH, Budsberg SC. A systematic review of the pharmacological and nutraceutical agents currently used in the treatment of canine osteoarthritis [abstract]. Vet Surg 2006;35:E1.

[72] Singh S, Aggarwal BB. Activation of transcription factor NF-kappa B is suppressed by curcumin. J Biol Chem 1995;270(42):24995–5000.

[73] Chun KS, Keum YS, Han SS, et al. Curcumin inhibits phorbol ester-induced expression of cyclooxygenase-2 in mouse skin through suppression of extracellular signal-regulated kinase activity and NF-kappaB activation. Carcinogenesis 2003;24(9):1515–24.

[74] Surh YJ, Chun KS, Cha HH, et al. Molecular mechanisms underlying chemopreventive activities of anti-inflammatory phytochemicals: down-regulation of COX-2 and iNOS through suppression of NF-kappa B activation. Mutat Res 2001;480–1: 243–6.

[75] Verbruggen G. Chondroprotective drugs in degenerative joint diseases. Rheumatol 2006;45:129–38.

[76] Henrotin Y, Sanchez C, Balligand M. Pharmaceutical and nutraceutical management of canine osteoarthritis: present and future perspective. Vet J 2005;170:113–23.

[77] Henrotin YE, Sanchez C, Deberg MA, et al. Avocado/soybean unsaponifiables increase aggrecan synthesis and reduce catabolic and proinflammatory mediator production by human osteoarthritis chondrocytes. J Rheumatol 2003;30:1825–34.

[78] Boumediene K, Felisaz N, Bogdanowicz P, et al. Avocado/soya unsaponifiables enhance the expression of transforming growth factor beta1 and beta2 in cultured articular chondrocytes. Arthritis Rheum 1999;42(1):148–56.

[79] Cake MA, Read RA, Guillou B, et al. Modification of articular cartilage and subchondral bone pathology in an ovine meniscectomy model of osteoarthritis by avocado and soya unsaponifiables (ASU). Osteoarthritis Cartilage 2000;8(6):404–11.

[80] Appelboom T, Schuermans J, Verbruggen G, et al. Symptoms modifying effect of avocado/soybean unsaponifiables (ASU) in knee osteoarthritis. Scand J Rheumatol 2001;30(4): 242–7.

[81] Lequesne M, Maheu E, Cadet C, et al. Structural effect of avocado/soybean unsaponifiables on joint space loss in osteoarthritis of the hip. Arthritis Rheum 2002;47(1):50–8.

[82] Ernst E. Avocado-soybean unsaponifiables (ASU) for osteoarthritis—a systematic review. Clin Rheumatol 2003;22(4–5):285–8.

[83] Soeken KL. Selected CAM therapies for arthritis-related pain: the evidence from systematic reviews. Clin J Pain 2004;20(1):13–8.

[84] Newnham RE. Agricultural practices affect arthritis. Nutr Health 1991;7:89–100.

[85] Newnham RE. Essentiality of boron for healthy bones and joints. Environ Health Perspect 1994;102(Suppl 7):83–5.

[86] Kulkarni RR, Patki PS, Jog VP, et al. Treatment of osteoarthritis with a herbomineral formulation: a double-blind, placebo-controlled, cross-over study. J Ethnopharmacol 1991;33: 91–5.

[87] Sander O, Herborn G, Rau R. [Is H15 (resin extract of Boswellia serrata, "incense") a useful supplement to established drug therapy of chronic polyarthritis? Results of a double-blind pilot study.] Z Rheumatol 1998;57:11–6. [in German].

[88] Kimmatkar N, Thawani V, Hingorani L, et al. Efficacy and tolerability of Boswellia serrata extract in treatment of osteoarthritis of knee—a randomized double blind placebo controlled trial. Phytomedicine 2003;10:3–7.

[89] Piscoya J, Rodriguez Z, Bustamante SA, et al. Efficacy and safety of freeze-dried cat's claw in osteoarthritis of the knee: mechanisms of action of the species Uncaria guianensis. Inflamm Res 2001;50:442–8.

[90] Mur E, Hartig F, Eibl G, et al. Randomized double blind trial of an extract from the pentacyclic alkaloid-chemotype of uncaria tomentosa for the treatment of rheumatoid arthritis. J Rheumatol 2002;29:678–81.

[91] Willer B, Stucki G, Hoppeler H, et al. Effects of creatine supplementation on muscle weakness in patients with rheumatoid arthritis. Rheumatology (Oxford) 2000;39:293–8.

[92] Roy BD, de Beer J, Harvey D, et al. Creatine monohydrate supplementation does not improve functional recovery after total knee arthroplasty. Arch Phys Med Rehabil 2005;86: 1293–8.

[93] Goldman AS. The immunological system in human milk: the past—a pathway to the future. Adv Nutr Res 2001;10:15–37.

[94] Ormrod DJ, Miller TE. Milk from hyperimmunized dairy cows as a source of a novel biological response modifier. Agents Actions 1993;38(Spec No):C146–9.

[95] Ormrod DJ, Miller TE. The anti-inflammatory activity of a low molecular weight component derived from the milk of hyperimmunized cows. Agents Actions 1991;32:160–6.

[96] Gingerich DA, Fuhrer JP, Kiser KM, et al. Milk protein concentrate from hyperimmunized cows expresses anti-inflammatory activity and clinical utility in osteoarthritis [abstract]. J Vet Intern Med 2001;15:305.

[97] Stelwagen K, Ormrod DJ. An anti-inflammatory component derived from milk of hyperimmunised cows reduces tight junction permeability in vitro. Inflamm Res 1998;47:384–8.

Vet Clin Small Anim 36 (2006) 1325–1343

VETERINARY CLINICS
SMALL ANIMAL PRACTICE

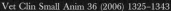

Taurine and Carnitine in Canine Cardiomyopathy

Sherry Lynn Sanderson, DVM, PhD

Department of Physiology and Pharmacology, University of Georgia, College of Veterinary
Medicine, 501 DW Brooks Drive, Athens, GA 30602, USA

Dilated cardiomyopathy (DCM) is one of the most common acquired cardiovascular diseases in dogs [1–4]. Although few studies of the prevalence of DCM in the overall population of dogs have been reported, estimates range from 0.5% to 1.1% [5,6]. Only degenerative valvular disease and, in some regions of the world, heartworm infection are more common causes of cardiac morbidity and mortality in dogs. DCM is seen most commonly in large and giant breeds of dogs, although its frequency seems to be increasing in medium-sized breeds, such as the English and American cocker spaniels [4–8]. It has been reported rarely in small and miniature breeds of dogs [9].

DCM is particularly challenging to veterinarians because the cause is often unknown and can vary among dog breeds [10]. Because most cases of DCM in dogs are classified as idiopathic, most therapies can be classified as "Band-Aid therapies" that palliate the effects of this disease for a short duration but do little to address the primary disease process. Therefore, DCM is almost always a progressive disease, and most dogs will eventually succumb to their disease. Survival times in dogs with DCM are variable and can be influenced by several factors, including breed. However, the prognosis for survival of dogs with DCM remains poor, with reported survival rates of 17.5% at 1 year and 7.5% at 2 years [11–13]. Until recently, reported cases of DCM reversal in dogs were very rare.

With advancements in echocardiology, diagnostic capabilities in canine cardiology have improved dramatically over the past 2 decades. Therapeutic advances have made surprisingly little progress. Symptomatic treatment is the standard care and outcome remains poor.

Recently, more promising therapies for dogs with DCM have resulted from a clearer understanding of the importance of biochemistry and nutrition in managing this disease. Nutrition is now widely accepted as an important adjunct to medical therapy in dogs with DCM.

E-mail address: sanderso@vet.uga.edu

0195-5616/06/$ – see front matter
doi:10.1016/j.cvsm.2006.08.010

The importance of nutrition in managing DCM has changed dramatically in the past 10 to 15 years. Historically, dietary sodium restriction was the most common nutritional recommendation for dogs with DCM. The importance of other nutrients in the origin and management of this disease was largely unknown. More recently, widely accepted beliefs about the role nutrient deficiencies could play in DCM have been proven false, further enhancing the ability to direct therapy at an underlying cause rather than just the symptoms.

This article focuses on two nutrients, taurine and carnitine, that play an important role in the cause and treatment of DCM in some dogs. Known risk factors for developing deficiencies of these nutrients are discussed, along with the use of taurine and carnitine for treating DCM in dogs.

TAURINE
What is Taurine?

Taurine is a sulfur-containing amino acid. Unlike most other amino acids, taurine is not incorporated into proteins but rather is one of the most abundant free amino acids in the body. Taurine is found in highest tissue concentrations in cardiac muscle, skeletal muscle, the central nervous system, and platelets [14].

Other than conjugation of bile acids and detoxification of xenobiotics through conjugation and excretion in bile, the function of taurine in mammals is not well understood but is highly diverse [14,15]. Since the mid-1970s, taurine has been known to be essential for normal retinal function in cats [16]. In addition, clinical and experimental evidence collected in the late 1980s documented that taurine is essential for normal myocardial function [17–20].

Taurine is involved with numerous metabolic processes, including antioxidation, retinal photoreceptor activity, development of the nervous systems, stabilization of neural membranes, reduction in platelet aggregation, and reproduction [15,16,21–26]. Although the importance of taurine for normal myocardial function is also well recognized, the mechanisms underlying its effect on the heart remain unknown. Much of the available evidence supports the theory that taurine's major effect on cellular function in the heart is modulating tissue calcium concentrations and availability [14,27,28]. In addition, taurine may inactivate free radicals and protect the heart by changing cellular osmolality [29]. Taurine may also have an effect on osmoregulation in the myocardium. Taurine is a small but highly charged osmotically active molecule, and experts have proposed that alterations in cellular osmolality induced by changes in intracellular taurine concentration are a protective mechanism in nervous tissue and myocardium [29]. Other proposed mechanisms specifically related to myocardial function include N-methylation of cell membrane phospholipids [30], direct effects on contractile proteins [31,32], and interactions with the renin–angiotensin–aldosterone system [33]. Taurine is a natural antagonist of angiotension II.

Is Taurine an Essential Amino Acid in Dogs?

Taurine is an essential amino acid in cats, and it is well known that taurine deficiency can cause DCM, retinal degeneration, and reproductive anomalies in this species [18]. However, taurine is not considered an essential amino acid in dogs. One explanation for the differences in taurine requirements between cats and dogs is that the activity of cysteine sulfinic acid decarboxylase (the rate-limiting enzyme in the synthesis of taurine from cysteine and methionine) is higher in dogs than cats [34]. However, the difference in activity of this enzyme between dogs and cats does not fully explain the difference in requirements. The activity of this enzyme in humans is even lower than in cats, and taurine is not considered an essential amino acid in healthy adult humans. Therefore, cats and dogs may have additional differences that may explain why taurine is an essential amino acid in cats and not in dogs.

A study in dogs conducted in the 1980s at the University of California at Davis showed that feeding taurine-free diets or diets found to be taurine-depleting in cats [35] did not result in taurine depletion when fed to a group of eight healthy beagles [36]. In addition, results of an early clinical study in dogs, also conducted at this University soon after the relationship between taurine deficiency and DCM was discovered in cats, were unrewarding. These studies showed that dogs could not become taurine-depleted from diet alone, and that taurine did not play a considerable role in the development of DCM in dogs.

Emergence of Taurine Deficiency in Dogs with Dilated Cardiomyopathy

The belief that taurine deficiency could not cause DCM in dogs was challenged in 1989 when taurine deficiency was linked to DCM in foxes [37]. This study reopened taurine's possible role in DCM in dogs, and a collaborative study between the University of California at Davis and the Animal Medical Center in New York City was initiated [38]. In this study, plasma taurine levels were evaluated in dogs with DCM and in those with chronic degenerative mitral valve disease. Surprisingly, results of this study showed that plasma taurine concentration was low in 17% of 75 dogs with DCM, and this deficiency occurred in breeds not commonly afflicted with DCM, such as American cocker spaniels and golden retrievers. However, because the plasma taurine concentration in breeds more commonly affected with DCM were within the reference range, experts concluded that taurine deficiency was unlikely to play an important role in the etiopathogenesis or therapy of DCM in dogs.

Multicenter Spaniel Trial (MUST) Study

Anecdotal reports emerged regarding supplementing American cocker spaniels diagnosed with DCM with taurine; however, initial reports of taurine supplementation were unrewarding. When Kittelson and colleagues [8] gave taurine and L-carnitine supplements to two American cocker spaniels with DCM, both dogs experienced response. These findings initiated the Multicenter Spaniel Trial (MUST) study. In this study, baseline plasma taurine concentrations and echocardiograms were collected in 11 American cocker spaniels diagnosed with DCM. All dogs were found to have low plasma taurine concentrations at baseline (<50 nmol/mL). After baseline information was collected, dogs were randomly assigned to receive supplementation with both taurine (500 mg by mouth every 8 hours) and L-carnitine (1000 mg by mouth every 8 hours) or a placebo for 4 months, and echocardiograms were reevaluated after 2 and 4 months of therapy. The group supplemented with both taurine and carnitine showed significant echocardiographic improvement, whereas dogs receiving the placebo did not.

After this initial 4-month period, dogs that had received the placebo initially received supplements of both taurine and carnitine, and subsequently showed echocardiographic improvement after 2 to 4 months of therapy. The magnitude of echocardiographic improvement in the American cocker spaniels was not as dramatic as that seen after taurine supplementation in cats with taurine deficiency DCM. Nonetheless, after 4 months of supplementation, the improvement in myocardial function in each dog was significant enough to allow discontinuation of cardiovascular drug therapy. Improvements were seen in not only cardiovascular function but also survival times. The mean survival time for dogs in this study was 28.3 ± 19.1 months, compared with an average life expectancy for dogs treated with conventional drug therapy of approximately 6 months. Based on results from this study, the current recommendation is to supplement American cocker spaniels diagnosed with DCM with both taurine and carnitine at the doses mentioned earlier.

University of Minnesota Study in Urolith-forming Dogs Diagnosed with Dilated Cardiomyopathy

Around the same time the MUST study was initiated, a separate clinical study was initiated at the University of Minnesota. The population of dogs studied consisted of those with either cystine or urate urolithiasis that developed DCM after long-term consumption of a protein-restricted diet that was being used to manage their stone disease (Sherry L. Sanderson, DVM, PhD, unpublished data, 1998). Dogs in group 1 underwent only conventional drug therapy for their heart disease, whereas those in group 2 underwent and taurine and/or carnitine supplementation in addition to conventional drug therapy as needed. Dogs in group 1 that were in Modified New York Heart Association (MNYHA) functional class I and II heart failure received enalapril (0.25 mg/kg by mouth every 12 hours) and digoxin (0.01–0.02 mg/kg by mouth divided twice a day), and dogs in MNYHA functional class III and IV received furosemide (dose varied depending on severity of heart disease) in addition to enalapril and digoxin. The population of dogs in group 1 (N = 6) consisted of five English bulldogs (four with cystine urolithiasis, one with urate urolithiasis) and one Dalmatian with urate urolithiasis. The population of dogs in Group 2 (N = 8) consisted of five English bulldogs (three with cystine urolithiasis, two with urate urolithiasis), two Dalmatians with urate urolithiasis, and one miniature Dachshund with cystine urolithiasis. Because when this study was initiated experts believed that dogs with DCM did not have low plasma taurine concentrations, none of the dogs in group 1 had these concentrations evaluated at baseline. Plasma taurine concentrations evaluated before supplementation in seven of eight dogs in group 2 ranged from 2 nmol/mL to 45 nmol/mL (mean, 20.9 nmol/mL). These results were below the reference range of 41 nmol/mL to 97 nmol/mL that the investigators established from healthy adult beagles. Echocardiography was performed at baseline and once every 2 months. Details from this study will be published later, but a few interesting and important results were noted:

1. The average life expectancy for dogs in group 1 was 10.5 months, and all dogs were euthanized because of progressive congestive heart failure that became refractory to therapy. The average life expectancy for dogs in group 2 was 47.1 months, and only three of eight dogs were euthanized because of progressive congestive heart failure. In addition, three of five dogs that did not succumb to their heart disease received only taurine and/or carnitine supplementation and no conventional drug therapy for the management of their heart disease.

2. DCM reversed in three of eight dogs in group 2. DCM returned in one dog after the owner discontinued taurine and carnitine supplementation on their own, and in an additional dog when the dose of carnitine was reduced because of diarrhea associated with carnitine supplementation.

3. Dogs consuming a protein-restricted diet long-term could develop taurine deficiency, in contrast to results from previous studies that concluded that a diet could not induce taurine deficiency in dogs. This finding provided an impetus for further examining the effects on plasma and whole blood taurine levels in healthy adult dogs consuming a protein-restricted diet long-term.

Diet-Induced Taurine Deficiency in Healthy Adult Dogs

Previous reports indicated that dogs could not develop diet-induced taurine deficiency, even when fed a diet devoid of taurine. However, based on the finding of University of Minnesota study that dogs developed low plasma taurine levels after consuming a protein-restricted diet long-term, a more controlled study was undertaken to determine the cause of this problem and evaluate the effects of long-term taurine deficiency on cardiac function in healthy adult dogs [39].

This study involved 17 healthy adult beagles. Baseline plasma and whole blood taurine levels were evaluated, and echocardiography was performed to assess cardiac function. Once baseline data was collected, dogs were fed one of three protein-restricted diets for 48 months. All three diets had similar levels of protein; one diet was also low in fat, a second was high in fat, and a third was high in fat and supplemented with *L*-carnitine at 200 mg/kg of diet. All diets contained methionine and cystine concentrations at or above recommended minimum requirements established by the Association of American Feed Control Officials (AAFCO) [40]. After diet assignment, plasma taurine and whole blood taurine concentrations and echocardiography were evaluated every 6 months.

All three dietary treatments caused a significant decrease in whole blood taurine concentration compared with baseline concentrations. Dogs in the high-fat group also experienced a significant decrease in plasma taurine concentration. This study was the first to show that diet could induce taurine deficiency in healthy adult dogs, in contrast to previous studies.

Another important observation was that one dog with taurine deficiency developed DCM, and that taurine supplementation resulted in almost complete reversal of the disease. This study was also the first to clearly document in dogs that taurine deficiency preceded DCM, and that taurine supplementation resulted in substantially improved cardiac function, similar to cats.

Why Did Dogs Develop Taurine Deficiency While Consuming a Protein-Restricted Diet?

The exact mechanism for this problem is unknown. However, this study showed that the AAFCO recommended minimum requirements for amino acids may need to be modified in dogs consuming a protein-restricted diet long-term. Many therapeutic diets for dogs are now supplemented with taurine.

Additional Examples of Diet-Induced Taurine Deficiency in Dogs
Soybean-based diets
Taurine deficiency was identified in two unrelated dogs fed a tofu-based diet [41]. Although the diet was low in protein, it met the National Research Council's published requirements for protein and other nutrients in dogs [42]. The authors attributed taurine deficiency to the fact that the primary protein source was soybean curd, which is low in sulfur-containing amino acids and devoid of taurine compared with meat proteins [43]. In addition, soybean curd has been shown to accelerate the loss of bile acids in cats [44].

Lamb meal and rice diets
Taurine deficiency was also identified in 12 Newfoundlands consuming two different commercially available lamb meal and rice diets [41]. Echocardiography was performed in six of the dogs, and none were diagnosed with DCM. The taurine deficiency was reversed when the diet was either changed or when the lamb meal and rice diets were supplemented with methionine. This study did not identify the exact mechanism for the development of taurine deficiency in the dogs consuming the lamb meal and rice diets.

In a study by Fascetti and colleagues [45], DCM and taurine deficiency were identified in 12 large and giant-breed dogs consuming commercially available diets that contained lamb meal, rice, or both as primary ingredients. All dogs received supplements of with taurine (1000–3000 mg by mouth every 24 hours), and significant echocardiographic improvement occurred in 9 of the 12 dogs that underwent an echocardiogram repeated after taurine supplementation. The authors hypothesized that taurine deficiency caused DCM and was caused by inadequate or unavailable dietary sulfur amino acids, which are essential precursors of taurine synthesis.

In a similar report, five related golden retrievers were diagnosed with taurine deficiency and DCM [46]. Three of five dogs were consuming lamb meal and rice or lamb and rice diets. All showed significant improvement after taurine supplementation (500 mg by mouth every 12 hours), and all five dogs survived for more than 3 years. The authors attribute the DCM to a suspected autosomal recessive mode of inheritance; however, the potential role diet played in the development of taurine deficiency warrants mentioning.

Potential Causes of Taurine Deficiency in Dogs Consuming Lamb Meal and Rice or Lamb and Rice Diets

Torres and colleagues [47] compared the effects of consuming a lamb meal and rice–based diet with effects of consuming a poultry by-product–based diet in 12 beagles aged 5 to 5.5 months. Although the differences in plasma and whole blood taurine concentrations did not differ among diet groups, dogs consuming the lamb meal and rice–based diet excreted less taurine in their urine than dogs consuming the poultry by-product–based diet. When the lamb meal and rice diet was supplemented with methionine, urinary taurine excretion increased by 54%. Because taurine homeostasis in dogs is achieved primarily through regulating renal taurine excretion, the amount of taurine excreted in urine is a sensitive indicator of the adequacy of either taurine synthesis or absorption of dietary precursor amino acids. The authors concluded that reduced bioavailability of sulfur amino acids in the lamb meal and rice diet is a likely cause of taurine deficiency. This finding is supported by the increase in urine taurine concentrations after supplementation with methionine. Johnson and colleagues [48] showed that ileal digestibility of amino acids in dogs depends on the raw material sources and the temperature used to process feeds and provides a mechanism for these specific dietary effects.

A second potential, although related, cause of taurine deficiency in dogs consuming lamb meal and rice diets was proposed [49,50]. When dietary protein is low in quality, undigested protein reaches the colon, where it serves as a substrate for bacterial growth. Some bacteria produce cholyltaurine hydrolase, an enzyme that causes release of taurine from taurocholic and other bile acids that are normally conserved in the enterohepatic circulation, resulting in increased fecal loss of taurine. Studies in dogs [49] and cats [50] have found that diets containing rice bran and whole rice products provide a source of moderately fermentable fiber and high amounts of fat. These fermentable fibers may increase the number of bacteria in the colon and result in a greater loss of taurine in the feces similar to the mechanism for undigested protein. The fat content of the diet can also affect taurine metabolism through altering intestinal bacteria and subsequent changes in the excretion of bile acids.

How Should Samples be Collected to Evaluate Plasma and Whole Blood Taurine Concentrations?

Fasting versus postprandial blood samples

Although fasting has no effect on plasma taurine concentrations in humans [51], food deprivation causes a small but significant reduction in plasma taurine concentrations in cats [52]. In a study by Torres and colleagues [47], plasma taurine concentrations were significantly reduced in food-restricted dogs compared with ad libitum–fed dogs. Whole blood taurine concentrations were also reduced, although the whole blood taurine results were not statistically significant between the two groups. Because of the potential for food intake to affect plasma and whole blood taurine concentrations in dogs, withholding food, but not water, is recommended for 8 hours before sampling.

Anticoagulant used for plasma sample collection
Paired analysis of samples comparing taurine concentrations in plasma collected in lithium heparin with those collected in sodium citrate showed that plasma taurine concentrations are higher when lithium heparin is used as the anticoagulant [38]. Because most studies have used heparinized plasma samples to evaluate plasma taurine levels in dogs, these are recommended rather than sodium citrate plasma samples.

Plasma taurine sample collection
Heparinized, nonhemolyzed blood samples should be obtained and stored on ice until they are processed. After centrifuging, the plasma should be separated immediately from the cellular components, and a small amount of plasma should be left above the buffy coat to prevent contamination of the plasma with cells. Hemolysis and platelet or white blood cell contamination falsely elevates plasma taurine concentrations. Samples should be frozen until analyzed for plasma taurine concentrations.

Whole blood taurine sample collection
Heparinized whole blood should be frozen until samples can be analyzed. Because the red blood cells are lysed before analysis, hemolyzed samples do not adversely affect whole blood taurine analysis.

Plasma and whole blood taurine samples can be sent to the Department of Molecular Biosciences at the School of Veterinary Medicine, University of California, Davis, for analysis.

Which is Better: Plasma Taurine Concentrations or Whole Blood Taurine Concentrations

Earlier studies evaluating the relationship between taurine deficiency and DCM in dogs relied primarily on plasma taurine concentrations to predict tissue taurine concentrations. Studies conducted in dogs by this author showed findings similar to those reported in cats [53]. Relying on plasma taurine concentrations alone does not reliably assess tissue taurine concentrations in dogs. Simultaneously evaluating plasma and whole blood taurine concentrations predicts skeletal and cardiac muscle taurine concentrations better than evaluating either test alone. Therefore, when evaluating taurine status in dogs with DCM, plasma and whole blood taurine concentrations should be assessed simultaneously.

Reference Ranges for Plasma and Whole Blood Taurine Concentrations in Dogs

The reference range used in earlier studies evaluating plasma and whole blood taurine concentrations in dogs was extrapolated from the reference range use in cats. However, reference ranges for plasma and whole blood taurine concentrations in dogs were published recently (Table 1).

Delaney and colleagues [49] have also suggested that plasma taurine concentrations less than 40 nmol/mL are critically low, as are whole blood taurine concentrations less than 150 nmol/mL. In addition, Sanderson and colleagues [53] found that low plasma taurine concentrations can exist without the presence of DCM.

Therefore, results showed that the onset of clinical signs in dogs, just as in cats, was variable when taurine concentrations declined markedly below the normal range [18].

Which Dogs Diagnosed with Dilated Cardiomyopathy Should Receive Taurine Supplementation?

Evaluation of plasma and whole blood taurine concentrations is recommended for all dogs diagnosed with DCM. An association between taurine deficiency and DCM was found in various breeds of dogs, including American cocker spaniels, Newfoundlands, golden retrievers, Labrador retrievers, Dalmatians, English bulldogs, and Portuguese water dogs. Taurine supplementation is highly recommended in any of these breeds that develop DCM.

Not all dogs with DCM will show dramatic improvement with taurine supplementation. However, even if plasma and whole blood taurine concentrations are within the reference range, giving taurine supplements to dogs diagnosed with DCM may still have some benefits. Because taurine is extremely safe and inexpensive, the risks and costs of supplementation are minimal, even if dogs have normal levels of plasma and whole blood. Proposed mechanisms for the beneficial actions of taurine on the myocardium include modulating tissue calcium concentrations and availability in the heart; inactivating free radicals and protecting the heart through altering cellular osmolality; osmoregulating the myocardium; directly affecting contractile proteins; and serving as a natural antagonist of angiotension II. Dogs with DCM that do not have taurine deficiency may still benefit from some of these proposed mechanisms of action for taurine.

Table 1 Normal concentrations of taurine in dogs	
Plasma (nmol/mL)	Whole blood (nmol/mL)
41–97[a]	155–347[a]
72.8–81.2[b]	255.8–276.2[b]

[a]Reference range established from 18 healthy adult beagles consuming a canned commercial maintenance diet. *Data from* Sanderson SL, Gross KL, Ogburn PN, et al. Effects of dietary fat and L-carnitine on plasma and whole blood taurine concentrations and cardiac function in healthy dogs fed protein-restricted diets. Am J Vet Res 2001;62:1616–23.
[b]Reference range established from 131 healthy adult dogs of various breeds consuming a variety of commercial adult maintenance diets. *Data from* Delaney SJ, Kass PH, Rogers QR, et al. Plasma and whole blood taurine in normal dogs of varying size fed commercially prepared food. J Anim Physiol 2003;87:236–44.

Recommended dose for taurine supplementation
This author has successfully used doses of 500 to 1000 mg of taurine administered orally two to three times per day for small dogs (<25 kg), and 1 to 2 g of taurine administered orally two to three times per day for large dogs (25–40 kg). These doses have been shown to normalize plasma and whole blood taurine levels in taurine-deficient dogs. Many other doses for taurine are reported in the literature. Whether a smaller or less frequent dose of taurine than what this author recommends can be used successfully remains to be determined. If doses are used that differ from those this author recommends, plasma and whole blood taurine concentrations must be reevaluated after taurine supplementation is initiated to determine if the dose being given is effective and appropriate. Another important point is that echocardiographic improvement in myocardial function is not usually documented before 2 months of supplementation, and often no improvement is documented before 4 months of supplementation. However, the dogs may feel better clinically and be more active before improvement in cardiac function is documented. Owners must not withdraw taurine supplementation prematurely before deciding if their dogs benefit.

Where Can Taurine be Purchased?
Taurine can be purchased through several retail outlets. If taurine is purchased through a health food store, consumers must look for a product that contains a USP certification symbol on the label. This symbol ensures that what is listed on the label is exactly what is found in the product.

LEVOCARNITINE (*L*-CARNITINE)
What is *L*-Carnitine?
L-carnitine (β-hydroxy-γ-trimethylaminobutyric acid) is a small water-soluble molecule with a molecular weight of 160. In dogs, carnitine is obtained either from dietary protein or endogenous synthesis in the liver using the essential precursor amino acids lysine and methionine. Synthesis also requires iron, vitamin C, and vitamin B_6 as cofactors [54]. Although carnitine is classified as an amino acid derivative, it is not an α-amino acid and the amino group is not free. Therefore carnitine is not used for protein synthesis [55].

Carnitine is found in the body either as free carnitine, short-chain acyl carnitine, or long-chain acylcarnitine. Acylcarnitine is carnitine bound to a fatty acid. Total carnitine is the sum of all the individual carnitine fractions. The free carnitine fraction is normally higher than either the short-chain acylcarnitine fraction or the long-chain acylcarnitine fraction.

Cardiac and skeletal muscles are significant storage sites, containing 95% to 98% of the carnitine in the body [56], and carnitine is concentrated in these tissues through an active membrane transport mechanism. The heart is unable to synthesize carnitine and depends on transport of carnitine from the circulation into cardiac muscle, which results in up to a $100\times$ gradient between extracellular and intracellular concentrations.

Only the *L*-form of carnitine exists naturally in the body. The *D*-form competitively inhibits the actions of the *L*-form, thereby inhibiting carnitine enzyme systems. In addition, mammals are unable to convert *D*-carnitine to *L*-carnitine, and therefore this discussion focuses on *L*-carnitine.

Why is *L*-Carnitine Important for Normal Myocardial Function?

The normal heart obtains approximately 60% of its total energy production from oxidation of long-chain fatty acids [57]. Long-chain fatty acids in the cytosol of myocardial cells combine with coenzyme A (CoA) as the first step toward beta oxidation. However, long-chain fatty acids must be transported across the inner mitochondrial membrane to generate energy, and the inner mitochondrial membrane is normally impermeable to such bulky polar molecules. Therefore, transport is accomplished through a "carnitine shuttle." In the carnitine shuttle, the activated fatty acid in the cytosol reacts with carnitine to form a more permeable molecule. This reaction occurs on the outer surface of the inner mitochondrial membrane and is catalyzed by the enzyme carnitine acyltransferase I. The newly formed long-chain acyl-carnitine ester molecule is permeable to the inner mitochondrial membrane and is transported across this membrane, where the enzyme acyltransferase II converts the long-chain acylcarnitine back to free carnitine and the long-chain fatty acid. Therefore, carnitine functions as a cofactor of several important enzymes necessary for transport of long-chain fatty acids from the cytosol into the mitochondrial matrix [58,59]. Once inside the mitochondria, fatty acids undergo beta oxidation to generate energy [60].

Another important function of carnitine is its buffering capacity, which modulates the intramitochondrial acyl-CoA:CoA ratio [58]. This process is important because acyl-CoA is the activated form of fatty acids used for beta oxidation and lipid synthesis. However, buildup of acyl-CoA derivatives in the mitochondria results in decreased free CoA, which inhibits oxidative metabolism. Acyl-CoA derivatives also act as detergents at high concentrations. Carnitine also facilitates removal of accumulating short- and medium-chain organic acids from the mitochondria. Therefore carnitine also has a role in detoxification in the mitochondria.

What Causes *L*-Carnitine Deficiency?

Carnitine deficiency can be a primary or secondary disorder. Primary carnitine deficiencies may arise from genetic defects in synthesis, renal transport, intestinal absorption, transmembrane uptake mechanisms, or excessive degradation of carnitine [61]. In humans, primary carnitine deficiencies have been associated with cardiomyopathies that are usually not present at birth but take 3 to 4 years to develop. *L*-carnitine therapy can prevent and reverse cardiac dysfunction in some patients.

Secondary carnitine deficiencies are believed to be much more common in humans and can have many causes [61]. In humans, carnitine deficiency can result from inborn errors of metabolism or develop in patients undergoing long-term total parenteral nutrition, vegetarians, and infants fed formulas not supplemented with carnitine. Carnitine deficiencies are recognized in dogs, but the incidence is not known.

What are the Consequences of L-Carnitine Deficiency?

Carnitine deficiency has been shown to cause or be associated with DCM in humans [62–64], hamsters [65,66], and dogs [36,67–69]. More widespread studies have not been undertaken in dogs because carnitine status is difficult to thoroughly assess.

What Types of Carnitine Deficiency Exist in Dogs?

Carnitine deficiency in dogs is classified as either (1) plasma carnitine deficiency, characterized by low concentrations of free plasma carnitine; (2) systemic carnitine deficiency, characterized by low concentrations of free plasma and tissue carnitine; or (3) myopathic carnitine deficiency, characterized by low free myocardial carnitine concentrations in the presence of normal and sometimes elevated plasma carnitine concentrations. Plasma carnitine deficiency alone is not a well-documented state and is included to account for the fact that plasma carnitine, but not tissue carnitine sampling, is often pursued in veterinary medicine.

For example, if plasma carnitine concentration is used to assess carnitine status of a dog, it can help diagnose carnitine deficiency when it is low. However, if plasma carnitine concentration is normal, it does not rule out the possibility of the myopathic form of carnitine deficiency, and the myopathic form of carnitine deficiency is estimated to occur in 17% to 60% of dogs with DCM. Evaluating cardiac muscle carnitine concentrations requires a fluoroscopy-guided endomyocardial biopsy, which is not practical to perform in most private practice situations and is not without risk. Therefore, diagnosing and determining the incidence of myopathic carnitine deficiency in dogs with cardiac disease remains elusive, but may be an underdiagnosed cause of DCM in dogs.

L-Carnitine Deficiency and Associated Myocardial Disease States in Dogs

Carnitine deficiency was associated with DCM in dogs in a limited number of clinical reports [8,9,68–70]. The first reported case of carnitine deficiency was in a family of boxers [69]. The sire, dam, and two littermates were diagnosed with DCM. One offspring had a low plasma carnitine concentration and low myocardial carnitine concentration at DCM diagnosis. After undergoing treatment with high-dose L-carnitine (220 mg/kg/d orally), this dog's fractional shortening (FS) increased from 18% to 28%. This dog's littermate had low myocardial and normal plasma carnitine concentrations and responded similarly to high-dose L-carnitine supplementation, with its FS increasing from 2% to 24%. The latter dog experienced a decline in myocardial function after L-carnitine therapy was withdrawn. Both parents of these littermates had normal plasma and low myocardial carnitine concentrations. Unfortunately, both parents died soon after beginning L-carnitine supplementation.

Costa and Labuc [70] presented another case report of two boxers with DCM. One was treated with 250 mg/kg/d of *L*-carnitine orally, and the other was not treated. The myocardial concentration of carnitine was found to be low in the dog that did not receive supplementation and elevated in the dog that did.

Concurrent supplementation with carnitine and taurine has shown benefit in American cocker spaniels with DCM [8]. An unpublished study by this author in 1998 showed beneficial effects from carnitine supplementation in urolith-forming dogs diagnosed with DCM while consuming a protein-restricted diet (Sherry Lynn Sanderson, DVM, PhD, unpublished material). Both studies showed dramatic improvement in myocardial function and survival times in dogs that received supplementation.

Which Came First: Carnitine Deficiency or Dilated Cardiomyopathy?

A common argument made against the role of carnitine deficiency in dogs diagnosed with DCM is that if carnitine deficiency is diagnosed after the onset of DCM, whether carnitine deficiency caused the DCM or DCM caused the carnitine deficiency is unclear. When myocardial cells are damaged, as may occur with DCM, carnitine can leak out of the cells, resulting in low myocardial carnitine levels. In this situation, the DCM caused the carnitine deficiency. Most published studies linking carnitine deficiency to DCM in dogs have shown this scenario when carnitine deficiency was diagnosed after the onset of DCM.

In an unpublished study conducted at the University of Minnesota, this author documented carnitine deficiency before the onset of DCM in three dogs (Sherry Lynn Sanderson, DVM, PhD, unpublished material, 1998). Therefore, the association of carnitine deficiency with DCM at diagnosis may not always imply a cause-and-effect relationship. However, this study indicates that carnitine deficiency can cause DCM in dogs.

Which Dogs with Dilated Cardiomyopathy Should Receive Carnitine Supplementation?

The importance of carnitine supplementation in the treatment and survival times of some dogs with DCM should not be overlooked. In the first reported study linking carnitine deficiency to DCM in boxers, two of four dogs experienced good response to carnitine supplementation [69]. Considering the generally poor prognosis of this disease in boxers, carnitine supplementation provides owners one additional option for treating this disease, and has made a dramatic difference in the survival times and quality of life of some dogs.

The importance of carnitine supplementation in American cocker spaniels with DCM and urolith-forming dogs with DCM should also not be overlooked. Although a few anecdotal reports exist in which American cocker spaniels with DCM experienced good response to taurine supplementation alone, most cases have shown response to combined supplementation with taurine and carnitine. In the above study by this author, a miniature Dachshund diagnosed with carnitine deficiency before the onset of DCM underwent treatment only with carnitine supplementation, and its heart disease reversed. Although DCM in many dogs is not associated with carnitine deficiency, carnitine and taurine supplementation offer the most promising hope for improved quality of life and survival times in dogs that experience response.

How is Carnitine Deficiency Diagnosed?

Because performing endomyocardial biopsies is impractical for most clinicians in private practice, most screening for carnitine deficiency relies solely on plasma carnitine levels. The method for plasma carnitine sample collection is almost identical to that used for plasma taurine sample collection. Fasting, heparinized, nonhemolyzed blood samples should be obtained and stored on ice until they are processed. The plasma should be immediately separated from the cellular components ideally in a cold-centrifuge, and a small amount of plasma should be left above the buffy coat to prevent contamination of the plasma with cells. Samples should be frozen immediately until analyzed for plasma carnitine concentrations.

What is the Recommended Dose for Carnitine Supplementation in Dogs?

The doses of carnitine being administered may contribute to the lack of favorable results with carnitine supplementation that some investigators observed. The recommended doses for carnitine supplementation in dogs with DCM vary widely in the literature. Although most authors recommend a carnitine dose of 50 to 100 mg/kg orally every 8 hours, the effective dose may depend on the form of carnitine deficiency. In a limited number of cases studied at the University of Minnesota, where pre– and post–carnitine supplemented plasma and cardiac muscle carnitine levels were obtained, this author's clinical impression was that the effective therapeutic dose in dogs with systemic carnitine deficiency was much lower than the effective dose in dogs with myopathic carnitine deficiency.

Some experts speculate that the myopathic form of carnitine deficiency may be caused by a carnitine transport defect in the heart, and much higher plasma levels of carnitine seem to be needed to overcome this defect and achieve normal concentrations of carnitine in the heart than for the systemic form of carnitine deficiency. Based on this work, the dose of carnitine recommended by this author for systemic carnitine deficiency is 100 mg/kg orally every 8 hours. However, if the myopathic form of carnitine deficiency is present or suspected, the author recommends starting carnitine supplementation at 200 mg/kg orally every 8 hours to maximize the chances that carnitine supplementation will improve myocardial function.

Carnitine is a very safe substance. Diarrhea was the only adverse effect of high doses of carnitine, reported in approximately two thirds of dogs. If diarrhea occurs, the highest dose of carnitine that the dog will tolerate without causing diarrhea should be administered. Therefore, like taurine, *L*-carnitine is a safe substance to administer, and, except for the expense, few drawbacks exist to supplementing a dog with DCM with carnitine (carnitine is much more expensive than taurine. Another important point is that the time it takes for improvement in myocardial function to occur is very similar to that for taurine supplementation. Echocardiographic improvement in myocardial function is not usually documented before 2 months of supplementation with carnitine, and often improvement is not documented for up to 4 months. However, dogs may feel better clinically and be more active before improvement in cardiac function is documented. Owners must not withdraw carnitine supplementation prematurely before determining whether their dogs benefit.

Where Can L-Carnitine Be Purchased?

Although L-carnitine can be purchased from health food stores, this source is extremely expensive. Purity of the sample is also of great importance. Therefore, only products that contain the USP certification seal should be purchased from health food stores.

L-Carnitine can also be purchased less expensively in bulk. Bulk carnitine can be purchased from Ajinamotousa, Inc (500 Frank W Burr Boulevard; Park Central West; Teaneck, New Jersey). At last check, the company required a minimum purchase of 10 kg at one time. However, the individual expense can be reduced if several owners split an order. If carnitine is purchased in bulk, owners must measure out the carnitine they are giving to their dogs. One teaspoon of carnitine is equivalent to 2 g of carnitine. Therefore, fractions of a teaspoon can be administered if necessary. Owners must be sure to purchase L-carnitine, not D- or the DL- isomers, because D-carnitine interferes with L-carnitine use.

Which Dogs with Dilated Cardiomyopathy Should be Supplemented With Carnitine?

Carnitine supplementation should be recommended for boxers, American cocker spaniels, and dogs with cystine or urate urolithiasis that are diagnosed with DCM. Even if carnitine deficiency did not cause DCM, supplementing dogs with carnitine does not hurt them, and supplementation may be beneficial even if carnitine deficiency is not present. The major drawback to supplementing dogs with carnitine is the expense and occasional gastrointestinal upset.

What are the Reference Ranges for Carnitine Concentrations in Dogs?

The reference ranges for carnitine concentrations in dogs are listed in Table 2 [69].

SUMMARY

Some newer more promising therapies for dogs with DCM do not involve drugs but rather nutritional supplements. Two of the more common nutritional supplements administered to dogs with DCM are taurine and carnitine. Deficiencies of these nutrients have been shown to cause DCM in dogs, and some breeds have been shown to experience dramatic improvement in myocardial function after supplementation with one or both nutrients. Although most dogs diagnosed with DCM do not have a documented taurine or carnitine deficiency, they may still benefit from supplementation. Both nutrients are very

Table 2
Normal concentrations of carnitine in dogs

Carnitine fraction	Plasma carnitine (nmol/mL)	Cardiac muscle carnitine (nmol/mg of NCP)
Free	8–36	4–11
Esterified	0–7	0–4
Total	12–38	5–13

Abbreviation: NCP, noncollagenous protein.

safe to administer to dogs. For some owners, the high cost of carnitine is the only deterrent to giving their dogs supplements of both nutrients.

References

[1] Cobb MA. Idiopathic dilated cardiomyopathy: advances in etiology, pathogenesis and management. J Small Anim Pract 1992;33:112–8.

[2] Keene BW. Canine cardiomyopathy. In: Kirk RW, editor. Current veterinary therapy X. Small animal practice. Philadelphia: WB Saunders Co; 1989. p. 240–51.

[3] Sisson DD, Thomas WP, Keene BW. Primary myocardial disease in the dog. In: Ettinger SJ, Feldman EC, editors. Textbook of veterinary internal medicine. Diseases of the dog and cat. 5th edition. Philadelphia: WB Saunders Co; 2000. p. 874–95.

[4] Buchanan JW. Causes and prevalence of cardiovascular disease. In: Kirk RW, Bonagura JD, editors. Kirk's current veterinary therapy XI. Philadelphia: WB Saunders Co; 1992. p. 647–55.

[5] Sisson D, Thomas WP. Myocardial diseases of dogs and cats. In: Ettinger S, editor. Textbook of veterinary internal medicine. 4th edition. Philadelphia: WB Saunders; 1995. p. 995–1032.

[6] Fioretti M, Delli CE. Epidemiological survey of dilatative cardiomyopathy in dogs [abstract]. Veterinaria 1988;2:81.

[7] Gooding JP, Robinson WF, Wyburn RS, et al. A cardiomyopathy in the English cocker spaniel: a clinico-pathological investigation. J Small Anim Pract 1982;23:133–48.

[8] Kittleson MD, Keene B, Pion PD, et al. Results of the Multicenter Spaniel Trial (MUST): taurine- and carnitine-responsive dilated cardiomyopathy in American cocker spaniels with decreased plasma taurine concentration. J Vet Intern Med 1997;11:204–11.

[9] Sanderson S, Osborne C, Ogburn P, et al. Canine cystinuria associated with carnitinuria and carnitine deficiency [abstract]. J Vet Intern Med 1995;9:212.

[10] Calvert CA. Dilated congestive cardiomyopathy in Doberman pinchers. Compend Contin Educ Pract Vet 1986;8:417–30.

[11] Monnet E, Orton C, Salman M, et al. Idiopathic dilated cardiomyopathy in dogs: survival and prognostic indicators. J Vet Intern Med 1995;9:12–7.

[12] Tidholm Am Svensson H, Sylven C. Survival and prognostic factors in 189 dogs with dilated cardiomyopathy. J Am Anim Hosp Assoc 1997;33:364–8.

[13] Tidholm A, Johsson L. A retrospective study of canine dilated cardiomyopathy (189 cases). J Am Anim Hosp Assoc 1997;33:544–50.

[14] Tenaglia A, Cody R. Evidence for a taurine-deficient cardiomyopathy. Am J Cardiol 1988;62:136–9.

[15] Hayes KC. Taurine requirement in primates. Nutr Rev 1985;43:65–70.

[16] Hayes KC, Carey RE, Schmidt SY. Retinal degeneration associated with taurine deficiency in the cat. Science 1975;188:949–51.

[17] Huxtable RJ. From heart to hypothesis: a mechanism for the calcium modulatory actions of taurine. Adv Exp Med Biol 1987;217:371–87.

[18] Pion PD, Kittleson MD, Rogers QR, et al. Myocardial failure in cats associated with low plasma taurine: a reversible cardiomyopathy. Science 1987;237:764–8.

[19] Schaffer SW, Seyed-Mozaffari M, Kramer J, et al. Effect of taurine depletion and treatment on cardiac contractility and metabolism. Prog Clin Biol Res 1985;179:167–75.

[20] Takihara K, Azuma J, Awata N, et al. Beneficial effect of taurine in rabbits with chronic congestive heart failure. Am Heart J 1986;112:1278–84.

[21] Franconi F, Bennardini F, Mattana A, et al. Taurine levels in plasma and platelets in insulin-dependent and non-insulin-dependent diabetes mellitus: correlation with platelet aggregation. Adv Exp Med Biol 1994;359:419–23.

[22] Green TR, Fellman JH. Effect of photolytically generated riboflavin radicals and oxygen on hypotaurine antioxidant free radical scavenging activity. Adv Exp Med Biol 1994;359:19–29.

[23] Rebel G, Petegnief V, Lleu P, et al. New data on the regulation of taurine uptake in cultured nervous cells. Adv Exp Med Biol 1994;359:225–32.

[24] Schmidt SY. Biochemical and functional abnormalities in retinas of taurine-deficient cats. Fed Proc 1980;39:2706–8.

[25] Sturman JA, Hayes KC. The biology of taurine in nutrition and developments. Adv Nutr Res 1980;3:231–99.

[26] Sturman JA. Dietary taurine and feline reproduction and development. J Nutr 1991;121:S166–70.

[27] Huxtable RJ, Chubb J, Asari J. Physiological and experimental regulation of taurine content in the heart. Fed Proc 1980;39:2685–90.

[28] Schaffer SW, Kramer J, Chovan JP. Regulation of calcium homeostasis in the heart by taurine. Fed Proc 1980;39:2691–4.

[29] Huxtable RJ. Physiological actions of taurine. Physiol Rev 1992;72:101–63.

[30] Hamaguchi T, Azuma J, Schaffer S. Interaction of taurine with methionine: inhibition of myocardial phospholipids methyltransferase. J Cardiovasc Pharmacol 1991;18:224–30.

[31] Lake N. Loss of cardiac myofibrils: mechanism of contractile deficits induced by taurine deficiency. Am J Physiol 1993;264(4 Part 2):H1323–6.

[32] Steele DS, Smith GL, Miller DJ. The effects of taurine on Ca^{2++} uptake by the sarcoplasmic reticulum and Ca^{2++} sensitivity of chemically skinned rat heart. J Physiol 1990;422:499–511.

[33] Gentile S, Bologna E, Terracina D, et al. Taurine-induced diuresis and natriuresis in cirrhotic patients with ascites. Life Sci 1994;54:1585–93.

[34] Jacobsen JG, Thomas LL, Smith LH Jr. Properties and distribution of mammalian L-cysteine sulfinic carboxylases. Biochim Biophys Acta 1964;85:113–6.

[35] Pion PD, Kittleson MD, Thomas WP, et al. Clinical findings in cats with dilated cardiomyopathy and relationship to finding taurine deficiency. J Am Vet Med Assoc 1992;201:267–74.

[36] Pion PD, Sanderson SL, Kittleson MD. The effectiveness of taurine and levocarnitine in dogs with heart disease. Vet Clin North Am Small Anim Pract 1998;28:1495–514.

[37] Moise NS. Cardiomyopathy in the fox and association with low dietary taurine. In: Proceedings of the Seventh American College of Veterinary Internal Medicine Forum. 1989. p. 834–5.

[38] Kramer GA, Kittleson MD, Fox PR, et al. Plasma taurine concentration in normal dogs and dogs with heart disease. J Vet Intern Med 1995;9:253–8.

[39] Sanderson SL, Gross KL, Ogburn PN, et al. Effects of dietary fat and L-carnitine on plasma and whole blood taurine concentrations and cardiac function in healthy dogs fed protein-restricted diets. Am J Vet Res 2001;62:1616–23.

[40] Association of American Feed Control Officials, Inc. Model bill and regulation. AAFCO Official Publication; 2003.

[41] Backus RC, Cohen G, Pion PD, et al. Taurine deficiency in Newfoundlands fed commercially available complete and balanced diets. J Am Vet Med Assoc 2003;223:1130–6.

[42] National Research Council. Nutrient requirements of dogs, revised 1985. Washington (DC): National Academy Press; 1985.

[43] Spitze AR, Wong DL, Rogers QR, et al. Taurine concentrations in animal feed ingredients; cooking influences taurine content. J Anim Physiol 2003;87:251–62.

[44] Kim SW, Morris JG, Rogers QR. Dietary soybean protein decreases plasma taurine in cats. J Nutr 1995;125:2831–7.

[45] Fascetti AJ, Reed JR, Rogers QR, et al. Taurine deficiency in dogs with dilated cardiomyopathy: 12 cases (1997–2001). J Am Vet Med Assoc 2003;112:1137–41.

[46] Belanger MC, Quellet M, Queney G, et al. Taurine-deficient dilated cardiomyopathy in a family of Golden Retrievers. J Am Anim Hosp Assoc 2005;41:284–91.

[47] Torres CL, Backus RC, Fascetti AJ, et al. Taurine status in normal dogs fed a commercial diet associated with taurine deficiency and dilated cardiomyopathy. J Anim Physiol 2003;87: 359–72.

[48] Johnson ML, Parsons CM, Fahey GC, et al. Effects of species raw material source, ash content and processing temperature on amino acid digestibility of animal by-product meals by cecectomized roosters and ileally cannulated dogs. J Anim Sci 1998;76: 1112–22.

[49] Delaney SJ, Kass PH, Rogers QR, et al. Plasma and whole blood taurine in normal dogs of varying size fed commercially prepared food. J Anim Physiol 2003;87:236–44.

[50] Stratton-Phelps M, Backus RB, Rogers QR, et al. Dietary rice bran decreases plasma and whole-blood taurine in cats. J Nutr 2002;132:1745S–7S.

[51] Trautwein EA, Hayes KC. Taurine concentration in plasma and whole blood in humans: estimation of error from intra- and interindividual variation and sampling technique. Am J Clin Nutr 1990;52:758–64.

[52] Pion PD, Lewis J, Greene K, et al. Effects of meal feeding and food deprivation on plasma and whole blood taurine concentration in cats. J Nutr 1991;121:S177–8.

[53] Sanderson SS, Osborne C, Gross K, et al. Reliability of canine plasma and whole blood taurine concentrations as indicators of cardiac and skeletal muscle taurine concentrations. [abstract]. J Vet Intern Med 1998;12:224.

[54] Bremer J. Carnitine-metabolism and function. Physiol Rev 1983;63:1420–80.

[55] Leibowitz BE. Carnitine. Adv Res Press 1987;2:1–13.

[56] Rebouche CJ, Engel AG. Kinetic compartmental analysis of carnitine metabolism in the dog. Arch Biochem Biophys 1983;220:60–70.

[57] Neely JR, Morgan HA. Relationship between carbohydrate metabolism and energy balance of heart muscle. Annu Rev Physiol 1974;36:413–59.

[58] Stumpt DA, Parker WD Jr, Angelini C. Carnitine deficiency, organic acidemias, and Reye's syndrome. Neurology 1985;35:1041–5.

[59] Gilbert EF. Carnitine deficiency. Pathology 1985;17:161–9.

[60] Mayes PA. Oxidation of fatty acids: ketogenesis. In: Murray RK, Granner DK, Mayes PA, et al, editors. Harper's biochemistry. 24th edition. Norwalk (CT): Appleton & Lange; 1996. p. 224–35.

[61] Paulson DJ. Carnitine deficiency-induced cardiomyopathy. Mol Cell Biochem 1998;180: 33–41.

[62] Periera RR, Scholte HR, Luyt-Houwen IEM, et al. Cardiomyopathy associated with carnitine loss in kidneys and small intestines. Eur J Pediatr 1988;148:193–7.

[63] Pierpont MEM. Carnitine and myocardial function. In: Carter AL, editor. Current concepts in carnitine research. 1st edition. Boca Raton (FL): CRC Press; 1992. p. 197–213.

[64] Paulson DJ, Sanjak M, Shug AL. Carnitine deficiency and the diabetic heart. In: Carter AL, editor. Current concepts in carnitine research. 1st edition. Boca Raton (FL): CRC Press; 1992. p. 215–30.

[65] Whitmar JT. Energy metabolism and mechanical function in perfused hearts of Syrian hamsters with dilated or hypertrophic cardiomyopathy. J Mol Cell Cardiol 1986;18:307–17.

[66] Whitmar JT. L–Carnitine treatment improves cardiac performance and restores high-energy phosphate pools in cardiomyopathic Syrian hamsters. Circ Res 1987;61:396–408.

[67] Sanderson S, Ogburn P, Osborne C. Heart disease management—Indications for nondrug therapies. Vet Forum 1996;13:36–43.

[68] McEntee K, Clercx C, Snaps F, et al. Clinical, electrocardiographic, and echocardiographic improvements after L-carnitine supplementation in a cardiomyopathic Labrador. Canine Pract 1995;20:12–5.

[69] Keene BW, Panciera DP, Atkins CE, et al. Myocardial L-carnitine deficiency in a family of dogs with dilated cardiomyopathy. J Am Vet Med Assoc 1991;198:647–50.

[70] Costa ND, Labuc RH. Case report: efficacy of oral carnitine therapy for dilated cardiomyopathy in boxer dogs. J Nutr 1995;124(supp):2687S–92S.

Vet Clin Small Anim 36 (2006) 1345–1359

VETERINARY CLINICS
SMALL ANIMAL PRACTICE

Nutritional Risks to Large-Breed Dogs: From Weaning to the Geriatric Years

Susan D. Lauten, PhD

Department of Small Animal Clinical Sciences, C247, Veterinary Teaching Hospital,
University of Tennessee, Knoxville, TN 37996–4545, USA

Large-breed puppies can be defined generally as puppies whose mature body weight exceeds 50 lb. A list of diseases associated with large- and giant-breed dogs includes those related to growth and development; however, risks inherent with breed and size persist throughout life and require specific health management. Nutrition may modify expression of genetic predisposition, influence severity of acute disease, and directly affect development of chronic disease.

The domestic dog has the greatest size diversity across mammalian species. Mature adult dogs can weigh from 2 to 200 lb. To achieve that disparity, large- and giant-breed puppies undergo an extremely rapid rate of growth. Giant-breed puppies born weighing 1 lb can easily gain 150 lb within the first 18 months of life, with the most rapid growth rate occurring between 3 and 6 months of age. With such exaggerated rates of growth, large- and giant-breed puppies are sensitive to nutrient and caloric deficiencies or excesses.

Simple overfeeding at any time of life can result in obesity, a disease that is associated with an increased risk of several inflammatory diseases (see the article by Laflamme elsewhere in this issue on understanding and managing obesity in dogs and cats). Dilated cardiomyopathy (DCM) occurs more frequently in large- and giant-breed dogs. Although a clear nutritional deficiency has not been found, low blood taurine and carnitine concentrations have been associated with some cases of DCM (see the article by Sanderson elsewhere in this issue on taurine and carnitine in canine cardiomyopathy). The risk of bloat or gastric dilatation-volvulus (GDV) is included in the list of health concerns of at least 30 purebred large- and giant-breed dogs (see the American Kennel Club web site [1]). The purpose of this article is to review nutritional factors associated with increased risk for developmental orthopedic disease (DOD) and GDV and to provide practical feeding recommendations for prevention.

E-mail address: slauten@utk.edu

0195-5616/06/$ – see front matter
doi:10.1016/j.cvsm.2006.09.003

WHAT NUTRITIONAL FACTORS ARE ASSOCIATED WITH DISEASE RISK IN LARGE- AND GIANT-BREED PUPPIES?

Few reports of general undernutrition are reported by veterinarians today. Current cases of malnutrition are more frequently associated with overnutrition, which may involve specific nutrients or an excess of food intake in general. Nutrient imbalances are also responsible for development of disease. All growing puppies can be harmed by diet imbalances and excessive food intake, but the term *developmental orthopedic disease* is used to describe those seen predominantly in large-breed dogs. This term refers to a group of diseases that occur during growth and development, including hypertrophic osteodystrophy (HOD), osteochondrosis (OC), osteochondritis dissecans (OCD), retained cartilaginous core, panosteitis, hip dysplasia (HD), and canine elbow dysplasia (CED) [2]. Briefly, the causes of OC and OCD are multifactorial, and identified factors include excess calcium intake, genetics, overnutrition, trauma, and ischemia [3]. HD, another multifactorial developmental problem, is associated with hip joint laxity, leading to incongruent and inconsistent articulation of the femoral head with the acetabulum. HD is associated with excess dietary energy and calcium [4–6]. CED is a group of elbow joint developmental disorders that includes OCD of the elbow joint, ununited anconeal process, and fractured medial coronoid process [7–10]. Breed predilections suggest a genetic component, but trauma, nutritional imbalances, and OC have been associated with this group of developmental disorders. HOD is considered an idiopathic disease that affects puppies between 2 and 8 months of age. Large- and giant-breed puppies are most frequently affected, and male dogs may be more predisposed, as are particular breeds [11–13]. Potential causes include distemper virus infection, overnutrition, genetics, and immune-mediated response to vaccination [14]. HOD has been reported in Great Dane dogs fed excess levels of calcium and phosphorus (Fig. 1) [15].

DCM affects large- and giant-breed dogs. Recent research has suggested that dietary deficiencies of taurine or carnitine, poorly available amino acid precursors in lamb meal, or ingredients like rice bran may pose an increased risk of

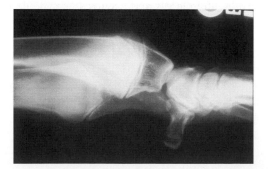

Fig. 1. Hypertrophic osteodystrophy in a growing Great Dane puppy fed higher than recommended levels of calcium, diagnosed by radiography.

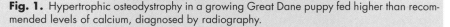

DCM in certain large and giant breeds. Dietary management of this disease is sometimes possible with supplementation of carnitine and taurine (see the article by Sanderson elsewhere in this issue for a complete discussion). Finally, a risk for obesity is present in puppies of several large breeds from weaning onward, that increases after spaying and neutering, and continues throughout the life of the dog (see the article by LaFlamme elsewhere in this issue).

HOW DOES NUTRITION INFLUENCE RISK FACTORS FOR DEVELOPMENTAL ORTHOPEDIC DISEASE AND OBESITY IN LARGE- AND GIANT-BREED PUPPIES?

Metabolic differences in large-breed dogs exist, such that rapid growth and feeding recommendations have now changed to address nutritional risks associated with feeding large-breed puppies. Fifteen years ago, commercial diets formulated for canine growth were marketed to all puppies with no distinction or formulation differences based on the puppy's anticipated mature size. These diets had evolved to nutrient-dense high-energy foods designed to encourage maximal growth, which is a risk factor for growth disorders. A variety of nutritional risk factors have been associated with DOD. Strong evidence supports the role of excess energy, calcium, phosphorus, and vitamin D in the development of DOD and subsequent osteoarthritis. Several diseases, including osteoarthritis, are associated with excess energy intake, which has been shown to decrease the life expectancy of dogs by 1.8 years compared with dogs provided restricted energy intake [16].

ENERGY

Excess energy intake can be provided to dogs by feeding high-fat nutrient-dense diets or an excess of food. When fed free choice, Great Dane puppies aged 0 to 6 months had an increase in the incidence of DOD compared with littermates that were food restricted to 70% to 80% of the amount consumed by puppies fed free choice [17]. A lifelong study of Labrador Retrievers involved restricting energy in one group of dogs, whereas the second group was fed free choice for life. Osteoarthritis occurred less frequently and occurred later in life in dogs fed a diet restricted in energy compared with dogs that were fed free choice [18].

Accordingly, large-breed puppy foods contain an energy density of approximately 3.5 to 4.0 kcal/g, which is lower than the 4.0 to 4.5 kcal/g of regular puppy foods. This reduced-energy level results in reduced fat deposition and a lower caloric intake in puppies fed free choice [19]. The dietary fat component of large-breed puppy foods has also been reduced to approximately 12% fat (compared with >20% in other foods) on a dry matter basis (DMB) in the presence of normal fiber content. Dietary fat increases caloric density, thereby increasing caloric intake. Studies in other species have shown that high-fat diets affect levels of insulin-like growth factor-1 (IGF-1), whereas diets high in saturated fats increased bone formation in chicks [20].

The recommendation for lower energy intake and requirements in large-breed puppies is supported by results of a recent study showing that large-breed puppies have greater nutrient digestibility at 11, 21, 35, and 60 weeks compared with smaller breed puppies [21].

PROTEIN

Currently, no evidence exists to suggest that high-protein intake contributes to the development of orthopedic disease in growing large-breed puppies. Previous studies suggesting a risk for high protein and DOD were confounded by higher energy intake in high-protein foods. In general, large-breed puppy diets are formulated to contain approximately 30% protein (DMB) similar to other puppy foods.

CALCIUM

The mechanism of dietary calcium absorption in puppies undergoes maturation after weaning. Several studies have shown that passive absorption of calcium from the intestine is directly proportional to dietary calcium intake in puppies from weaning (~6 weeks) until 6 months of age [22–25]. Passive absorption can represent up to 70% of total calcium uptake [26]. Absorption of calcium by active transport is also functional in weaned puppies but undergoes a maturation process, with active absorption decreasing with increasing age in young puppies fed an excess of calcium [27,28]. Active absorption is regulated by vitamin D$_3$, parathyroid hormone (PTH), growth hormone, and calcitonin [26]. Regardless of the calcium-to-phosphorus ratio, excess dietary calcium intake in large-breed puppies has been shown to increase expression of all individual DODs listed previously in this article (Fig. 2).

After puppies reach 6 months of age, calcium hormonal regulation and subsequent intestinal absorption mechanisms begin to mature and account for nearly 90% of calcium uptake [27]. Although puppies are able to "manage" dietary excesses of calcium after 6 months of age, this maturation process occurs

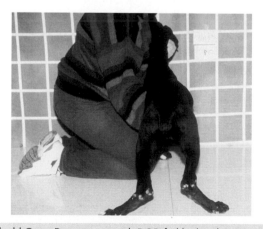

Fig. 2. Four-month-old Great Dane puppy with DOD fed higher than recommended levels of calcium.

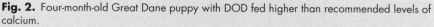

after the rapid growth phase (3–5 months) and time of highest risk for DOD. Excess dietary calcium is stored in skeletal bone of growing puppies. In overfed puppies, normal remodeling begins to reverse the excess calcium deposition at approximately 6 months of age, and the bone mineral content of overfed puppies becomes statistically identical to that of puppies fed normally from weaning by 1 year of age [15]. DOD sequelae develop before puppies are 1 year old, and diseases may be self-limiting, may result in permanent skeletal changes, or may require surgical intervention to correct. The clinical diagnosis of HD or CED may come after 1 year of age, but the joint abnormalities begin at an extremely young age. Great Dane puppies undergoing rapid growth have higher serum levels of growth hormone and IGF-1 than smaller breed puppies when fed normally, yet neither Great Danes nor Miniature Poodles showed differences in calcium handling when fed different levels of calcium [27,29].

PHOSPHORUS

This essential mineral has been not been researched as frequently as calcium in the growth of large-breed puppies. Intestinal absorption of phosphorus, in the presence of normal calcium intake, is well regulated in young puppies [28]. Digestibility or absorption of phosphorus was negatively correlated with levels of dietary calcium when puppies were overfed calcium [28,30]. Dietary deficiencies of phosphorus are not reported frequently in growing puppies, but when they are created under experimental conditions, they consist of poor weight gain and reduced growth rate [18]. The popular home-cooked and raw food diets, most of which are not balanced, usually contain sufficient or high quantities of phosphorus from the meat protein in the diet but have a low calcium content. This imbalance results in an increase in PTH levels (nutritional secondary hyperparathyroidism), but the increase is largely attributable to deficiencies in calcium content of the diet and not to excesses of phosphorus content (see section on calcium/phosphorous balance).

CALCIUM/PHOSPHORUS BALANCE

The optimum calcium/phosphorus ratio for dog foods is generally considered to be between 1.2:1 and 1.4:1 as reported by the National Research Council on Nutrient Requirements of Dogs in 2006. The American Association of Feed Control Officials (AAFCO) lists the acceptable range of ratios in commercial feeds to be between 1:1 and 2:1 [31]. These ratios can become skewed by supplementation of diets with calcium carbonate, multivitamin and/or mineral products, or top-dressing diets with various meats, for example. Weaned giant-breed puppies fed high calcium without an appropriate increase in phosphorous for 4 months developed hypercalcemia, hypophosphatemia, and DOD [29]. After normalization of the diet for a period of 2.5 months, many clinical signs of DOD resolved but OC lesions remained. Another group of giant-breed puppies was fed the same high-calcium diet for a 4-month period but in a proper ratio to phosphorus after weaning. These puppies became slightly hypophosphatemic, but their growth was retarded and DOD occurred. When the diets of these puppies were normalized for 2.5 months, the developmental disturbances improved but were not resolved. These puppies experienced the effects of high calcium and subsequent increased secretion of PTH that increased intestinal absorption of calcium through the action of vitamin D_3. The resulting asynchronous growth that occurs when mineral accretion and mineral resorption is imbalanced results in DODs, such as HD and CED, and abnormal maturation of subchondral bone resulting in OC and OCD.

VITAMIN D

Vitamin D_3, in its active forms of 1, 25-dihydroxycholecalciferol and 24,25-dihydroxycholecalciferol, regulates intestinal absorption of calcium and phosphorus and renal excretion or resorption of minerals. Hormonal regulation of vitamin D is achieved by PTH, growth hormone, and calcitonin. Dietary calcium and phosphorus intake affects serum levels of metabolites of vitamin D_3, serum levels of calcitonin, and PTH [27,32].

Vitamin D_3 is required in canine diets, because dogs do not have adequate levels of the intermediate compound 7-dehydrocholesterol in the skin that can be converted by ultraviolet radiation to previtamin D_3 [33,34]. Previtamin D_3 is converted to 25-hydroxycholecalciferol in the liver in response to regulation by negative feedback from serum levels of 25-hydroxycholecalciferol and vitamin D_3 intake [35]. The final conversion to the biologically active forms of vitamin D_3 (1, 25-dihydroxycholecalciferol and 24, 25-dihydroxycholecalciferol) occurs in the kidney. The conversion to the 1, 25 or the 24, 25 product in the kidney is controlled by plasma levels of growth hormone, IGF-1, calcitonin, PTH, and inorganic phosphate [36–39].

1, 25-Dihydroxycholecaliferol is considered to be the biologically active form, and 24, 25-dihydroxycholecalciferol is less active; its synthesis is regulated by negative feedback from 1,25-dihydroxycholecalciferol and serum calcium levels. The action of the 1, 25 product is highest in the kidney, intestine, and skeleton, and the activity of the 24, 25 product is highest in the skeleton [40–42]. Vitamin D compounds are influential in regulation of calcium homeostasis by up- and downregulating dietary calcium absorption in the intestine and by regulating resorption of calcium in the kidney. During skeletal development, mineralization is dependent on calcium and phosphorus dietary intake and the proper regulation of absorption, excretion, and resorption of vitamin D metabolites.

Levels of the 24, 25 metabolite are significantly higher in small-breed dogs, and that difference is believed to be the result of growth hormone activity and IGF-1 in the giant-breed puppy [32]. Children with growth hormone deficiencies who are treated with growth hormone experience increases in levels of 1, 25-dihydroxycholecalciferol and decreases in levels of 24, 25-dihydroxycholecalciferol [43]. The role of 24, 25-dihydroxycholecalciferol is seen at the skeletal level, and it is active in bone formation but not in bone resorption, whereas the 1, 25-dihydroxycholecalciferol metabolite is involved in osteoclast generation and related bone resorption as well as in absorption of calcium [44,45]. In giant-breed puppies, levels of 24, 25-dihydroxycholecalciferol were significantly lower, suggesting that high demand for synthesis of 1,25-deoxy-cholecalciferol may be at the expense of synthesis of 24,25-dehydroxycholecalciferol [27].

In a study using Miniature Poodles, supraphysiologic doses of growth hormone were injected to compare the metabolic effects with an untreated group. Supplementation with growth hormone rapidly increased serum levels of growth hormone, resulting in increased plasma levels of IGF-1, increases in serum levels of 1,25-dihydroxycholecalciferal, lower serum levels of 24, 25-dihydroxychole-calciferol, minimal effect on calcium and phosphate absorption in the intestine, elevated glomerular filtration rate, and no significant change in inorganic phosphate urine excretion [45]. At the skeletal level, growth hormone supplementation resulted in increased bone formation, with no bone resorption effects. Further investigation is needed into the role of vitamin metabolites in giant-breed puppies to determine how dietary levels of vitamin D_3 may affect the development of DOD by altering bone synthesis and resorption in rapidly growing large-breed puppies [45]. Commercial dog foods contain ample levels of vitamin D_3 based on the current knowledge of dietary requirements, but hormonal regulation of metabolites of vitamin D_3 can affect the skeletal development of the growing dog with adequate levels of dietary vitamin D [32,46]. Current feeding recommendations are likely to undergo further adjustment as more is understood about vitamin D metabolism in large- and giant-breed puppies.

WHAT FEEDING METHOD AND STRATEGIES SHOULD BE USED FOR LARGE-BREED PUPPIES?

Large-breed puppy foods are designed to restrict energy intake and provide more defined calcium and phosphorus levels and ratios than original puppy foods (Table 1). Clients should be urged to avoid any dietary supplementation or top dressing to diets of large-breed puppies, because commercial diets for large-breed puppies contain proper levels and balance of nutrients. Supplementation can unbalance the diet and contribute to the development of DOD by

Table 1
General nutrient contents of large-breed puppy diets compared with nonspecific puppy diets

Nutrient	Puppy diets (% DMB)	Large-breed puppy diets (% DMB)
Protein	29-36	29-34
Fat	20-23	11-16
Fiber	1.6-4.4	2.4-5.6
Calcium	1.3-1.4	0.8-1.4
Phosphorus	1.2	0.7-1.2
Ca:P ratio	1.1:1	1.1:1 to 1.3:1
Energy density[a]	3.8-4.5	3.4-4.1

Abbreviations: Ca:P ratio, calcium-to-phosphorous ratio; DMB, dry matter basis.
  [a]Energy density is provided as kilocalories per grams of diet as fed.

increasing intake of calcium or phosphorus or changing the desired 1.2:1 calcium-to-phosphorus ratio.

Regardless of careful selection of appropriate puppy foods, maintenance of the proper body weight or body condition score is critical for healthy growth. Puppies should be monitored frequently (perhaps weekly during the rapid growth phase), and managed carefully by increasing or decreasing food to maintain a trim body condition. Several of the major pet food companies have produced body condition score programs to aid in determining an ideal body condition of 3/5 measured on a five-point scale or 5/9 on a nine-point scale. A copy of scoring charts should be provided to puppy owners so that they have a reference for weekly or bimonthly weight monitoring.

Quantities of food offered should be consistently measured, divided, and offered at multiple feeding times. Free-choice feeding frequently leads to overeating and obesity as well as ingestion of higher levels of calcium and phosphorus. Timed feedings can also result in overeating, and caloric intake cannot be controlled with this feeding method. Multiple feedings may slow the rate of eating and decrease the volume of food present in the stomach. Large meal volume and infrequent feeding have been identified as risk factors for the development of GDV, which is discussed elsewhere in this article.

Meal feeding a measured amount of large-breed puppy food divided into several daily feedings is recommended. Amounts to be fed can be estimated from the formulas in Box 1, with alterations in multipliers based on the age of the puppy, where resting energy requirements are computed by the equation RER (kcal/d) = 30 (body weight$_{kg}$) + 70, where RER is resting energy expenditure. Using the age of the puppy to determine the correct multiplier results in a calculation of maintenance energy requirements.

This calculation provides a guideline to be used when estimating the proper intake for a puppy. Each puppy should be objectively compared with a body condition chart at least twice per month to avoid excess weight gain, particularly during the important rapid growth period. A healthy puppy that is maintained at ideal body weight, is being fed an appropriate large-breed puppy formula, and without additional supplementation can be assumed to be growing at a rate normal for that dog. Once the large-breed puppy approaches 12 months of age, it is recommended to change to an adult maintenance food, but feeding adult foods to large-breed puppies before 1 year of age is not recommended because the calcium-to-energy ratio is generally lower in adult foods compared with large-breed puppy food. Feeding an adult food can

---

Box 1: Energy requirements for growth in puppies

Weaning to 4 months: 3 × RER

4 months to 1 year: 2 × RER

1 year and older: 1.6 × RER (adult requirements)

actually result in greater intake of calcium than feeding puppy foods. Because the puppy must consume a larger portion of adult food to meet energy needs for growth, total calcium intake may actually be higher than with a properly formulated large-breed puppy formula.

It is also recommended that caloric intake be carefully monitored and possibly decreased once the puppy is spayed or neutered. At this time, there are contradictory reports as to the need for adjusting intake; however, it is apparent that energy needs decrease and obesity risk increases after spaying or neutering. If clients are appropriately educated about body condition scoring and have access to these tools, the incidence of obesity in all puppies can be reduced.

SUMMARY

To prevent skeletal growth disturbances and obesity in large-breed dogs, a preventive or proactive approach to managed growth of large-breed puppies is recommended. Many large-breed puppy rations are available, but not all are comparable, and adult maintenance foods are not suitable substitutes for large-breed puppy foods. Energy density, calcium, and phosphorus levels should be lower than those of standard puppy feeds. Energy density of a large-breed puppy food should be 3.5 to 4.0 kcal/g, with a fat content less than 15% (DMB). The calcium content of foods should be approximately 1%, with phosphorus levels at approximately 0.8% (DMB), with an ideal calcium-to-phosphorus ratio of 1.2:1. Vitamin D levels are usually adequate in commercial pet foods but may require supplementation when balancing home-cooked recipes. Second, feeding large-breed puppies should be accomplished by meal feeding rather than free-choice or timed feedings. Body condition should be assessed weekly or biweekly, because changes can occur quickly and adjustments to intake should be made promptly to maintain an ideal body condition. If home-cooked diets are used, recipes should be balanced by a nutritionist to ensure proper quantities of key nutrients, such as protein, fat, calcium, phosphorus, and vitamin D. The effects of skeletal disturbances and obesity can result in deformities in bones and joints that are irreversible. Any disease that affects mobility and quality of life for these large dogs can result in early death or euthanasia.

NUTRITIONAL RISKS FOR LARGE- AND GIANT- BREED DOGS: GASTRIC DILATATION AND VOLVULUS

Why Is Gastric Dilatation and Volvulus an Important Concern in Large- and Giant- Breed Dogs?

GDV is a rapidly developing syndrome that carries a mortality rate of 24%, despite surgical intervention [47]. Mortality rates have declined as medical management has improved (mortality rates of 15% to greater than 60% have been reported) [48,49]. The risk of development of GDV during a lifetime is 24% in giant-breed dogs and 21% in large-breed dogs [47]. A specific breed predilection seems to exist, as does a familial predisposition for incidence, potentially through selective breeding for physical characteristics, such as depth and width of thorax [50–52]. Great Danes and Bloodhounds are most frequently represented in reports, although more than 30 breeds are considered to be susceptible [53]. GDV is a leading cause of death in giant-breed dogs [50].

The etiology of GDV is still uncertain. It is multifactorial, and the pathophysiology is complex. Many inciting factors have been identified, such as gastric motility dysfunction, aerophagia, gastric content fermentation, gastric inflow and outflow hindrance, and rotation of the stomach. Many risk factors have been suggested. At this time, careful management of these risk factors and prophylactic surgery may be the best tools for reducing the incidence of GDV in dogs.

What Happens During Gastric Dilatation and Volvulus and How Is It a Significant Threat to Life?

The progression of this syndrome occurs quickly and can be fatal in just a few hours. During this progression, gases rapidly accumulate in a stomach, where intake and outflow are obstructed. The stomach may or may not rotate on the long axis of the esophagus, and bloat may or may not precede gastric dilatation [54–57].

What Risk Factors Have Been Identified for the Development of Gastric Dilatation and Volvulus in Dogs?

Dietary risk factors

The extrusion method of dry pet food manufacturing was introduced in 1957, and an "epidemic" of GDV was reported in the early 1960s through 1995. Naturally, an association was made between dry commercial foods and the increased incidence of this disease [58–62]. The same commercial dry dog food implication was made in 1994 with a report of a greater than doubling incidence of bloat and GDV cases in 12 veterinary hospitals between 1980 and 1989. Diet was considered to be the primary factor, and extruded foods containing cereal or soy (which were considered to be poorly digestible when compared with animal source proteins, and gas producing) were assumed to contribute to the development of GDV [63–65]. Subsequent research that measured the gastric emptying time of dogs eating canned foods or dry cereal foods, with and without added water, did not support the association between extruded dry foods and an increased risk for the development of GDV [66]. A recent study analyzing dry food ingredients did not show that animal protein sources were associated with lower risk than plant protein sources, but did find that dry diets with oil or fat among the first four ingredients were associated with a 2.4 times increase in the risk of developing GDV and that moistening dry foods before feeding also increased the risk [67,68]. Large food particle size (>30 mm) was found to decrease the risk of development of GDV [69]. Irish setters, one of the breeds with the highest susceptibility, were three times more likely to develop GDV if fed a single food type, such as dry or canned foods [59]. These data were confirmed when the addition of table scraps or canned food to a commercial dry diet reduced the risk of development of GDV by 59% and 28% in large- and giant-breed dogs, respectively [63].

Specific recommendations have been made for feeding management of susceptible animals. Feeding just one meal per day and rapid ingestion of meals

(37.8% of cases) are identified as risk factors for GDV, as is feeding a heavier meal (physical weight), which promotes gastric distention [63,70]. Once-daily feeding is associated with stretching or laxity of the hepatogastric ligaments, and rapid eating is associated with aerophagia, which is also associated with the development of GDV [59].

Results of prospective studies have shown that earlier recommendations made from retrospective study results may have been incorrect. Current research suggests that feeding from an elevated food bowl increases the risk by 51.9% despite earlier studies suggesting that a raised food bowl reduced the risk. Restricting water before and after meals was also associated with a higher risk of development of GDV, contradicting early recommendations for water restriction near meal times [67]. Exercise restriction before and after meals has also been removed from the list of potential risk factors through the results of prospective studies.

Nondietary risk factors
In addition to dietary factors, nondietary risk factors have been identified for GDV. Male dogs of less than ideal weight and with an apprehensive temperament were associated with an increased risk of GDV [50,63]. A recent stressful event (8–36 hours previously) seemed to increase the risk for development of GDV, whereas a cheerful disposition reduced the risk of development [63]. Increasing age and being of such breeds as the Great Dane, Weimaraner, St. Bernard, Gordon Setter, and Irish Setter were associated with the development of GDV as well as having a first-degree relative (sibling or offspring) that was affected by GDV [51,70].

Weather conditions and a first-quarter calendar or seasonal association with GDV were reported in a group of military working dogs [71]. A second study was unable to support the association between ambient temperature, humidity, season, or atmospheric pressure and GDV incidence [53]. Morphometric measurements of lower thoracic width, greater abdominal width, and a lower abdominal depth to width ratio were associated with a reduced risk of GDV in giant-breed dogs but not in large-breed dogs [67]. Giant-breed dogs but not large-breed dogs are more susceptible with a thin or lean body condition, postprandial abdominal distention, and a history of other medical problems. A thin body weight and a major health problem in the first year of life were factors for an increased risk of GDV [72]. A potential association between GDV and inflammatory bowel disease was reported in a study in which intestinal biopsies were collected at the time of surgery to correct GDV. Sixty-one percent of these biopsies were found to contain an identifiable inflammatory process, and 86% of the dogs in this study had prior histories of gastrointestinal disturbances [73].

How Can We Prevent Gastric Dilatation and Volvulus in Large- and Giant-Breed Dogs?
Two feeding practices that have repeatedly been identified in reported studies to reduce the risk of GDV occurrence are multiple daily feedings to reduce

food volume and slowing the rate of eating. Separation of dogs in multidog households may be required to slow the rate of meal consumption. In addition, more recent feeding recommendations include feeding from floor level (as opposed to the use of raised feeders) and management of gastrointestinal health to reduce inflammatory conditions within the gastrointestinal tract, such as management of food intolerances and other potentiators of inflammatory conditions, as well as avoiding the use of dry commercial diets with high-fat content. The addition of canned foods or meats to the diet may also reduce the incidence of GDV. Larger kibble size (>30 mm) may help to reduce the risk of GDV.

Dogs that have had GDV or have siblings, sires, or dams that have had the disease should not be bred. Selection of stable temperaments in breeding stock can also reduce the risk for the development of GDV, whereas selective breeding for particular physical traits, such as a deep chest and tight abdominal tucks, can increase the risk for development of GDV.

SUMMARY

Large- and giant-breed dogs present veterinarians and pet owners with distinct challenges throughout their lives. Among the most important are proper nutrition to ensure moderate growth rates to reduce developmental orthopedic disorders and promote proper cardiac development, maintenance of an ideal body condition to prevent diseases associated with obesity, and proper feeding techniques to reduce the risk of GDV.

References

[1] American Kennel Club. Available at: http://www.akc.org. Accessed May, 2006.

[2] Demko J, McLaughlin R. Developmental orthopedic disease. Vet Clin North Am Small Anim Pract 2005;35:1111–35.

[3] Siffert RS. Classification of osteochondroses. Clin Orthop 1981;158:10–8.

[4] Lust G, Williams AJ, Burton-Wuster N, et al. Joint laxity and its association with hip dysplasia in Labrador Retrievers. Am J Vet Res 1993;54:1990–9.

[5] Lust G, Geary JC, Sheffy BE. Development of hip dysplasia in dogs. Am J Vet Res 1973;34: 87–91.

[6] Riser WH. Canine hip dysplasia; cause and control. J Am Vet Med Assoc 1974;165: 360–2.

[7] Fox SM, Bloomberg MS, Bright RM. Developmental anomalies of the canine elbow. J Am Anim Hosp Assoc 1983;19:605–15.

[8] Goring RL, Bloomberg MS. Selected developmental abnormalities of the canine elbow: radiographic evaluation and surgical management. Compend Contin Educ Pract Vet 1983;5: 178–88.

[9] Piermattei DL, Flo GL. The elbow joint. In: Brinker WO, Piermattei DL, Flo GL, editors. Brinker, Piermattei, and Flo's handbook of small animal orthopedics and fracture repair. 3rd edition. Philadelphia: WB Saunders; 1997. p. 288–320.

[10] Kirberger RM, Fourie SL. Elbow dysplasia in the dog: pathophysiology, diagnosis and control. J S Afr Vet Assoc 1998;69(2):43–54.

[11] Alexander JW. Selected skeletal dysplasia: craniomandibular osteopathy, multiple cartilaginous exostosis, and hypertrophic osteodystrophy. Vet Clin North Am Small Anim Pract 1982;13(1):55–70.

[12] Muir P, Dubielzig RR, Johnson KA, et al. Hypertrophic osteodystrophy and calvarial hyperostosis. Compend Contin Educ Pract Vet 1996;18:143–51.

[13] Lenehan TM, Fetter AW. Hypertrophic osteodystrophy. In: Newton CD, Nunamaker DM, editors. Textbook of small animal orthopaedics. Philadelphia: JB Lippincott; 1985. p. 597–601.

[14] Munjar TA, Austin CC, Breur GJ. Comparison of risk factors for hypertrophic osteodystrophy, craniomandibular osteopathy, and canine distemper virus infection. Vet Comp Orthop Traumatol 1998;11:37–43.

[15] Lauten SD, Cox NR, Brawner WR Jr, et al. Influence of dietary calcium and phosphorus content in a fixed ratio on growth and development in Great Danes. Am J Vet Res 2002;63: 1036–47.

[16] Kealy RD, Lawler DF, Ballam JM. Effects of diet restriction on life span and age-related changes in dogs. J Am Vet Med Assoc 2002;220:1315–20.

[17] Zentek J, Meyer H, Dammrich K. The effect of a different energy supply for growing Great Danes on the body mass and skeletal development. Clinical picture and chemical studies of the skeleton. Zentralbl Veterinarmed A 1995;42(1):69–80.

[18] Smith GK, Paster ER, Powers MY, et al. Lifelong diet restriction and radiographic evidence of osteoarthritis of the hip joint in dogs. J Am Vet Med Assoc 2006;229(5):690–3.

[19] Richardson DC, Zentek J, Hazewinkel HA, et al. Developmental orthopedic disease of dogs. In: Hand MS, Thatcher CD, Remillard RL, et al, editors. Small animal clinical nutrition. Marceline (MO). Walsworth Publishing; 2000. p. 505–28.

[20] Watkins BA, Shen C-L, McMurty JP, et al. Dietary lipids modulate bone prostaglandin E_2 production, insulin-like growth factor-I concentration and formation rate in chicks. J Nutr 1997;127:1084–91.

[21] Weber M, Martin L, Beourge V, et al. Influence of age and body size on the digestibility of a dry expanded diet in dogs. J Anim Physiol Anim Nutr (Berl) 2003;87:21–31.

[22] Dobenecker B. Influence of calcium and phosphorus intake on the apparent digestibility of these minerals in growing dogs. J Nutr 2002;132(Suppl):1665S–7S.

[23] Hedhammar A, Wu F, Krook L, et al. Overnutrition and skeletal diseases, an experimental study in growing Great Dane dogs. Cornell Vet 1974;65(Suppl):1–160.

[24] Hazewinkel HAW, Goedegebuure SA, Poulos PW, et al. Influences of chronic calcium excess on the skeleton of growing Great Danes. J Am Anim Hosp Assoc 1985;21: 377–91.

[25] Goodman SA, Montgomery RD, Fitch RB, et al. Serial orthopedic examinations of growing Great Dane puppies fed three diets varying in calcium and phosphorus. In: Reinhart GA, Carey DP, editors. Recent advances in canine and feline nutrition, vol. III. Wilmington (OH): Orange Frazer Press; 1998. p. 3–12.

[26] Tryfonidou MA, Holl MS, Oosterlaken-Dijksterhuis MA, et al. Growth hormone modulates cholecalciferol metabolism with moderate effects on intestinal mineral absorption and specific effects on bone formation in growing dogs raised on balanced food. Domest Anim Endocrinol 2003;25:155–74.

[27] Tryfonidou MA, van den Broek J, van den Brom WE, et al. Intestinal calcium absorption in growing dogs is influenced by calcium intake and age but not by growth rate. J Nutr 2002;132:3363–8.

[28] Dobenecker B. Influence of calcium and phosphorus intake on the apparent digestibility of these minerals in growing dogs. J Nutr 2002;132(Suppl):1665S–7S.

[29] Schoenmakers I, Hazewinkel HAW, Voorhout G, et al. Effect of diets with different calcium and phosphorus contents on the skeletal development and blood chemistry of growing Great Danes. Vet Rec 2000;147:652–60.

[30] Jenkins KJ, Phillips PH. The mineral requirement of the dog. J Nutr 1960;70:235–40.

[31] Association of American Feed Control Officials Incorporated. Dog and cat food nutrient profiles. In: 2006 Official Publication Association of American Feed Control Officials Incorporated 2006. p. 131–46.

[32] Hazewinkel HAW, Tryfonidou MA. Vitamin D_3 metabolism in dogs. Mol Cell Endocrinol 2002;197:23–33.

[33] National Research Council (NRC). Table 15-5. In: Nutrient requirements of dogs and Cats. Washington (DC): National Academy Press; 2006. p. 359–60.

[34] How KL, Hazewinkel HAW, Mol JA. Dietary vitamin D dependence of cat and dog due to inadequate cutaneous synthesis of vitamin D. Gen Comp Endocrinol 1994;96:12–8.

[35] Rojanasathi S, Haddad JG. Hepatic accumulation of vitamin D_3 and 25-hydroxyvitamin D_3. Biochim Biophys Acta 1976;421:12–21.

[36] Nesbitt T, Drezner MK. Insulin-like growth factor-I regulation of renal 25-hydroxyvitamin D-1α-hydroxylase activity. Endocrinology 1993;132:133–8.

[37] Murayama A, Takeyama K, Kitanaka S, et al. Positive and negative regulations of the renal 25-hydroxyvitamin D_3-1α-hydroxylase gene by parathyroid hormone, calcitonin, and 1α-25(OH)$_2$D$_3$. Endocrinology 1999;140(5):2224–31.

[38] Wu S, Finch J, Zhong M, et al. Expression of the renal 25-hydroxyvitamin D-24-hydroxzy-lase gene: regulation by dietary phosphate. Am J Physiol 1996;271:F203–8.

[39] Wu S, Grieff M, Brown AJ. Regulation of renal vitamin D-24-hydroxzylase by phosphate: effects of hypophysectomy, growth hormone, and insulin-like growth factor I. Biochem Biophys Res Commun 1997;233:813–7.

[40] Brown AJ, Dusso A, Slatopolsky E. Vitamin D. Am J Physiol 1999;277:F157–75.

[41] Staal A, van den Bemd GJ, Birhenhager JC, et al. Consequences of vitamin D receptor regulation for the 1,25-dihydroxyvitamin D_3-induced 24-hydroxylase activity in osteoblast-like cells: initiation of the C24-oxidation pathway. Bone 1997;20:237–43.

[42] Boyan BD, Slyvia VL, Dean DD, et al. 24, 25-(OH)$_2$D$_3$ regulates cartilage and bone via autocrine and endocrine mechanisms. Steroids 2001;66:363–74.

[43] Wei S, Tanaka H, Kubo T, et al. Growth hormone increases serum 1,25-dihydroxy vitamin D levels and decreases 24,25-dihydroxyvitamin D levels in children with growth hormone deficiency. Eur J Endocrinol 1997;136(1):30–2.

[44] Aubin JE, Heersche JNM. Vitamin D and osteoblasts. In: Feldman D, Glorieux FH, Wesley Pike J, editors. Vitamin D. San Diego (CA): Academic Press; 1997. p. 313–28.

[45] Tryfonidou MA, Hazewinkel HAW. Different effects of physiologically and pharmacologically increased growth hormone levels on cholecalciferol metabolism at prepubertal age. J Steroid Biochem Mol Biol 2004;89–90:49–54.

[46] Kallfelz FA, Dzanis DA. Overnutrition; an epidemic problem in pet animal practice? Vet Clin North Am Small Anim Pract 1989;19:433–46.

[47] Broome CJ, Walsh VP. Gastric dilatation-volvulus in dogs. NZ Vet J 2003;51(6):275–83.

[48] Brockman DJ, Washabau RJ, Drobatz KJ. Canine gastric dilatation/volvulus syndrome in a veterinary critical care unit: 295 cases (1986–1992). J Am Vet Med Assoc 1995;207: 460–4.

[49] Matthiesen DT. Partial gastrectomy as a treatment of gastric volvulus—results in 30 dogs. Vet Surg 1985;14:185–93.

[50] Glickman LT, Glickman NW, Schellenberg DB, et al. Incidence of and breed-related risk factors for gastric dilatation-volvulus in dogs. J Am Med Vet Assoc 2000;216:40–5.

[51] Schellenberg D, Yi Q, Glickman NW, et al. Influence of thoracic conformation and genetics on the risk of gastric dilatation-volvulus in Irish setters. J Am Anim Hosp Assoc 1998;34: 64–73.

[52] Glickman LT, Emerick T, Glickman NW, et al. Radiological assessment of the relationship between thoracic conformation and the risk of gastric dilatation-volvulus in dogs. Vet Radiol Ultrasound 1996;37:174–80.

[53] Dennler R, Kock D, Hassig M, et al. Climatic conditions as a risk factor in canine gastric dilatation-volvulus. Vet J 2005;169:97–101.

[54] Rassmussen L. Stomach. In: Slatter D, editor. Textbook of small animal surgery. Philadelphia: WB Saunders; 2003. p. 592–640.

[55] Boothe HW, Ackerman N. Partial gastric torsion in two dogs. J Am Anim Hosp Assoc 1976;12:27–30.

[56] Leib MS, Martin RA. Therapy of gastric dilatation-volvulus in dogs. Compend Contin Educ Pract Vet 1987;9:1155–63.

[57] Frendin J, Funkquist B, Stavenborn M. Gastric displacement in dogs without clinical signs of acute dilatation. J Small Anim Pract 1988;29:775–9.

[58] Van Kruiningen HJ, Gergoire K, Meuten DJ. Acute gastric dilatation: a review of comparative aspects, by species, and a study in dogs and monkeys. J Am Anim Hosp Assoc 1974;10:294–324.

[59] Elwood CM. Risk factors for gastric dilatation in Irish setter dogs. J Small Anim Pract 1998;39:185–90.

[60] Cowell CS, Stout NP, Brinkmann MF, et al. Making commercial pet foods. In: Hand MS, Thatcher CD, Remillard RL, et al, editors. Small animal clinical nutrition. 4th edition. Topeka (KS): Mark Morris Institute; 2000. p. 127–46.

[61] Glickman LT. Epidemiology of gastric dilatation-volvulus in dogs. In: Proceedings of the 21st Congress of the World Small Animal Veterinary Association. Jerusalem (Israel); 1996. p. 81–3.

[62] Vankruiningen HJ, Wojan LD, Stake PE, et al. The influence of diet and feeding frequency on gastric function in the dog. J Am Anim Hosp Assoc 1987;23:145–53.

[63] Glickman LT, Glickman NW, Schellenberg DB, et al. Multiple risk factors for the gastric dilatation-volvulus syndrome in dogs: a practitioner/owner case-control study. J Am Anim Hosp Assoc 1997;33(3):197–204.

[64] Kronfeld D. Common questions about the nutrition of dogs and cats. Compend Contin Educ Pract Vet 1979;1:33–42.

[65] Morgan RV. Acute gastric dilatation-volvulus syndrome. Compend Contin Educ Pract Vet 1982;4:677–82.

[66] Burrows CF, Bright RM, Spencer CP. Influence of dietary composition on gastric emptying and motility in dogs: potential involvement in acute gastric dilatation. Am J Vet Res 1985;46(12):2609–12.

[67] Raghavan M, Glickman NW, Glickman LT. The effect of ingredients in dry dog foods on the risk of gastric dilatation-volvulus in dogs. J Am Anim Hosp Assoc 2006;42:28–36.

[68] Raghaven M, Glickman NW, McCabe G, et al. Diet related risk factors for gastric dilatation-volvulus in dogs of high risk breeds. J Am Anim Hosp Assoc 2004;40:192–203.

[69] Theyse LFW, Brom WE, Sluijs FJ. Small size of food particles and age as risk factors for gastric dilatation-volvulus. Vet Rec 1998;143:48–50.

[70] Glickman LT, Glickman NW, Perez CM, et al. Analysis of risk factors for gastric dilatation and dilatation volvulus in dogs. J Am Vet Med Assoc 1994;204(9):1165–71.

[71] Herbold JR, Moore GE, Gosch TL, et al. Relationship between incidence of gastric dilatation-volvulus and biometeorologic events in a population of military working dogs. Am J Vet Res 2002;63:47–52.

[72] Glickman LT, Glickman NW, Schellenberg DB, et al. Non-dietary risk factors for gastric dilatation-volvulus in large and giant breed dogs. J Am Med Vet Assoc 2000;217:1492–9.

[73] Braun L, Lester S, Kuzma AB, et al. Gastric dilatation-volvulus in the dog with histological evidence of pre-existing inflammatory bowel disease: a retrospective study of 23 cases. J Am Anim Hosp Assoc 1996;32:287–90.

Vet Clin Small Anim 36 (2006) 1361–1376

VETERINARY CLINICS
SMALL ANIMAL PRACTICE

Nutrition and Lower Urinary Tract Disease in Cats

Joseph W. Bartges, DVM, PhD*, Claudia A. Kirk, DVM, PhD

Department of Small Animal Clinical Sciences, Veterinary Teaching Hospital,
College of Veterinary Medicine, The University of Tennessee, Knoxville, TN 37996–4544, USA

INCIDENCE

Lower urinary tract disease occurs commonly in cats, but the incidence is unknown. Previous estimates of the incidence in the United States and United Kingdom have been 0.85% to 1.0% per year [1,2]. These estimates were based on the presence of clinical signs only, and therefore did not consider actual diagnoses. The proportional morbidity rate, defined as the frequency with which cases are seen at veterinary hospitals, has been reported to be 10% [3], although 1% to 6% is more commonly reported [3,4]. In a cross-sectional study of 15,226 cats examined at 52 private practices, cats were likely to be examined because of renal disease, cystitis, feline urologic syndrome, and inappetence [5].

FELINE LOWER URINARY TRACT DISEASE

Any disorder of the lower urinary tract may cause signs of lower urinary tract disease. In two prospective studies, 1 of 143 cats [6] and 1 of 109 cats [7] with lower urinary tract disease, idiopathic cystitis was diagnosed most commonly (Fig. 1). In a retrospective study performed at the University of Georgia and University of Tennessee of 110 cats older than 10 years of age with lower urinary tract disease, bacterial cystitis was diagnosed most commonly [8]. Thus, causes of lower urinary tract disease seem to be different in cats of different ages, although clinical signs are similar.

IDIOPATHIC CYSTITIS

The most common cause of lower urinary tract disease in cats younger than 10 years of age is idiopathic cystitis. Idiopathic cystitis is characterized by signs of lower urinary tract disease (hematuria, stranguria, pollakiuria, and inappropriate urination) without identifiable cause(s) for the clinical signs. Often, the clinical signs resolve in 3 to 7 days; however, recurrence is variable and unpredictable. Because no specific cause has been identified, no specific treatment is available that works consistently in all cats.

*Corresponding author. E-mail address: jbartges@utk.edu (J.W. Bartges).

0195-5616/06/$ – see front matter
doi:10.1016/j.cvsm.2006.08.006

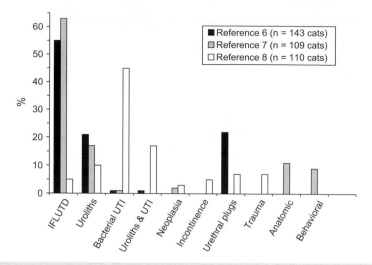

Fig. 1. Percentage of cats evaluated with lower urinary tract disease in two prospective [6,7] and one retrospective [8] studies. Cats in the retrospective study were older than 10 years of age.

The role of a canned diet in managing cats with idiopathic cystitis has been evaluated in two studies. In one nonrandomized prospective study of cats with idiopathic cystitis, recurrence of clinical signs occurred in 11% of cats consuming a canned food when compared with 39% of cats consuming a dry food [9]. The diets evaluated in this study were acidifying and formulated to prevent struvite crystalluria and urolithiasis. In another study, clinical improvement and decreased recurrence of clinical signs in cats with idiopathic cystitis were associated with the owners feeding canned foods [10]. Results of these studies have resulted in the recommendation to feed canned food to cats with idiopathic cystitis: however, these studies were not randomized controlled trials. Furthermore, specific dietary ingredients have not been evaluated in cats with idiopathic cystitis.

CRYSTAL-RELATED LOWER URINARY TRACT DISEASE

Of the various causes of feline lower urinary tract disease, crystal-related disease accounts for 15% to 45% of cases. There are many minerals that may precipitate in the urinary tract to form crystals and stones; however, more than 90% of uroliths from cats are composed of struvite (magnesium ammonium phosphate hexahydrate) or calcium oxalate monohydrate or dihydrate (Fig. 2). Struvite is the most common mineral observed to occur in matrix-crystalline urethral plugs (Fig. 3).

Urolith and matrix-crystalline plug formation involves complex physiochemical processes. Major factors include (1) urine supersaturation resulting in crystal formation (nucleation); (2) effect of inhibitors of mineral nucleation, crystal

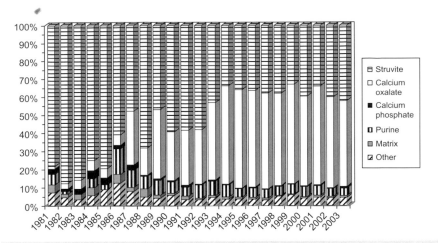

Fig. 2. Mineral composition of 55,418 uroliths retrieved from cats and analyzed at the Minnesota Urolith Center between 1981 and 2003. (*From* Kirk CA, Bartges JW. Dietary considerations for calcium oxalate urolithiasis. In: August JR, editor. Consultations in feline medicine, vol. 5. St. Louis (MO): Elsevier; 2005. p. 425; with permission.)

aggregation, and crystal growth; (3) crystalloid complexors; (4) effects of promoters of crystal aggregation and growth; (5) effects of noncrystalline matrix; (6) and urine retention or slowed transit for the process to occur [11,12]. Urethral matrix-crystalline plugs have only been identified in male cats and may represent an intermediate phase between lower urinary tract inflammation without crystals and urolith formation [13]. The most important driving force

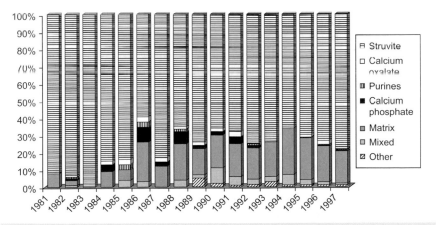

Fig. 3. Mineral composition of 1901 matrix-crystalline urethral plugs retrieved from male cats and analyzed at the Minnesota Urolith Center between 1981 and 1997. (*From* Osborne CA, Lulich JP, Albansan H, et al. Mineral composition of feline uroliths and urethral plugs: current status. In: Managing urolithiasis in cats: recent updates and practice guidelines. Topeka (KS): Hill's Pet Nutrition Inc.; 2003. p. 26; with permission.)

behind urolith formation is urinary supersaturation with calculogenic substances [14]; however, as mentioned previously, other factors are important. The goal of urinary crystal-related disease is to promote a reduced state of urinary saturation.

Urolithiasis

Calcium oxalate

Calcium oxalate urolith formation occurs when urine is oversaturated with calcium and oxalate [14]. In addition to these alterations in activities of ions, large-molecular-weight proteins occurring in urine, such as nephrocalcin, uropontin, and Tamm-Horsfall mucoprotein, influence calcium oxalate formation [15]. We have a limited understanding of the role of these macromolecular and ionic inhibitors of calcium oxalate formation in cats. Certain metabolic factors are known to increase the risk of calcium oxalate urolith formation in several species, including cats. Medical and nutritional strategies for stone prevention have focused on amelioration of these factors.

Hypercalcemia is associated with an increased risk of calcium oxalate urolith formation. In cats with calcium oxalate uroliths, hypercalcemia was observed in 35% of the cases [16]. Conversely, uroliths developed in 35% of cats with idiopathic hypercalcemia [17]. Hypercalcemia results in increased calcium fractional excretion and hypercalciuria when severe.

Hypercalciuria is a significant risk factor but not necessarily the cause of calcium oxalate urolith formation in human beings, dogs, and cats [18]. Hypercalciuria can result from excessive intestinal absorption of calcium (gastrointestinal [GI] hyperabsorption), impaired renal reabsorption of calcium (renal leak), or excessive skeletal mobilization of calcium (resorptive) [12]. In Miniature Schnauzers, GI hyperabsorption seems to occur most commonly, although renal leak hypercalciuria has also been observed [19]. Hypercalciuria has not been well defined in normocalcemic cats with calcium oxalate uroliths but is thought to occur.

Metabolic acidosis promotes hypercalciuria by promoting bone turnover (release of calcium with buffers from bone); increasing serum ionized calcium concentration, resulting in increased urinary calcium excretion; and decreased renal tubular reabsorption of calcium. Consumption of diets supplemented with the urinary acidifier ammonium chloride by cats has been associated with increased urinary calcium excretion [20]. Significant aciduria (urine pH <6.2) may represent a risk factor for calcium oxalate formation because of acidemia and hypercalciuria. In addition, acidic urine alters the function and concentration of crystal inhibitors. Low urine pH decreases the urinary citrate concentration by increasing renal proximal tubular citrate reabsorption. Acidic urine is known to impair the function of macromolecular protein inhibitors.

Inhibitors, such as citrate, magnesium, and pyrophosphate, form soluble salts with calcium or oxalic acid and reduce the availability of calcium or oxalic acid for precipitation. Other inhibitors, such as Tamm-Horsfall glycoprotein and nephrocalcin, interfere with the ability of calcium and oxalic acid to combine, minimizing crystal formation, aggregation, and growth.

Oxalic acid is a metabolic end product of ascorbic acid (vitamin C) and several amino acids, such as glycine and serine, derived from dietary sources. Oxalic acid forms soluble salts with sodium and potassium ions but a relatively insoluble salt with calcium ions. Therefore, any increased urinary concentration of oxalic acid may promote calcium oxalate formation. Dietary increases of oxalate and vitamin B_6 deficiency are known factors increasing urinary oxalate. Hyperoxaluria has been observed experimentally in kittens consuming vitamin B_6–deficient diets [11] but has not been associated with naturally occurring calcium oxalate urolith formation. Genetic anomalies may increase urine oxalic acid concentration. Hyperoxaluria has also been recognized in a group of related cats with reduced quantities of hepatic D-glycerate dehydrogenase, an enzyme involved in the metabolism of oxalic acid precursors (primary hyperoxaluria type II) [21]. Hyperoxaluria has also been associated with defective peroxisomal alanine/glyoxylate aminotransferase activity (primary hyperoxaluria type I) and intestinal disease in human beings (enteric hyperoxaluria). These have not been evaluated in cats.

Decreased urine volume results in increased calcium and oxalic acid saturation and an increased risk for urolith formation. Cats can achieve urine specific gravities in excess of 1.065, indicating a marked ability to produce concentrated urine. Many cats affected with calcium oxalate uroliths have a urine specific gravity greater than 1.040 unless there is some impairment of renal function or concentrating ability [18].

Detection of calcium oxalate crystals indicates that urine is supersaturated with calcium oxalate and, if persistent, represents an increased risk for calcium oxalate urolith formation. Calcium oxalate crystalluria is present in less than 50% of feline cases at the time of diagnosis of urolithiasis, however [18].

Medical protocols that promote dissolution of calcium oxalate uroliths are not currently available; therefore, uroliths must be removed physically, surgically or by voiding urohydropropulsion [22].

Nutritional or medical protocols should be considered to minimize urolith recurrence or prevent further growth of uroliths remaining in the urinary tract. A significant number of cats develop recurrent uroliths within 2 years of their initial episode if prevention protocols are not initiated [23]. If possible, metabolic factors known to increase calcium oxalate risk should be corrected or minimized. Goals of dietary prevention include (1) reducing urine calcium and oxalate concentration, (2) promoting high concentrations and activity of urolith inhibitors, (3) reducing urine acidity, and (4) promoting dilute urine.

Increasing urine volume is a mainstay of preventative therapy for calcium oxalate urolithiasis in human beings. By increasing water intake, urinary concentrations of calculogenic minerals are reduced. In addition, larger urine volumes typically increase urine transit time and voiding frequency, thereby reducing retention time for crystal formation and growth. Feeding cats a canned food is the most practical means of increasing water intake and lowering calcium oxalate urine saturation. The goal is to dilute urine to a specific gravity of 1.030 or lower [24]. Flavoring water, enhancing water access, and adding water to dry foods may be used in cats that refuse to eat canned foods. Sodium chloride should not routinely be added to the diet in an effort to stimulate thirst. Although cats increase water intake and dilute urine in response to salt, the consequence of high-sodium foods in cats prone to oxalate uroliths is unknown. Increased dietary sodium may increase urinary calcium excretion and can contribute to ongoing renal damage in cats with marginal renal function [24].

The solubility of calcium oxalate in urine is minimally influenced by pH; however, epidemiologic studies consistently identify acidifying diets among the most prominent risk factors for calcium oxalate urolithiasis [25–27]. Persistent aciduria may be associated with low-grade metabolic acidosis, which promotes bone mobilization and increases urinary calcium excretion. In a case series of five cats with hypercalcemia and calcium oxalate uroliths, discontinuation of acidifying diets or urinary acidifiers was associated with normalization of the serum calcium concentration [26]. Furthermore, aciduria promotes hypocitraturia and functional impairment of endogenous urolith inhibitors. Thus, feeding an acidifying diet or administering urinary acidifiers to cats at risk for calcium oxalate is contraindicated. A target urine pH of 6.6 to 7.5 is suggested in cats at risk for recurrence of calcium oxalate uroliths [24].

Although reduction of urine calcium and oxalic acid concentrations by restriction of dietary calcium and oxalic acid seems logical, it is not without risk. Reducing consumption of only one of these constituents may increase availability and intestinal absorption of the other, resulting in increased urinary excretion. Conversely, increasing dietary calcium levels in normal cats contributes directly to an increased urine calcium concentration. Because epidemiologic data in cats suggest that marked dietary calcium restriction increases urolith risk, moderate levels of dietary calcium are advised in nonhypercalcemic cats [24].

Urinary oxalate is derived from the endogenous metabolism of oxalate precursors (ie, glycine, ascorbic acid) and dietary oxalic acid. Most pet food ingredients are low in oxalic acid, with the exception of vegetables, legumes, and several vegetable-based fermentable fibers (ie, beet pulp, soybean fiber). Dietary oxalic acid concentrations in foods for cats should be reduced to the lowest possible level. Suggested levels are less than 20 mg of oxalic acid per 100 g of food (dry matter basis) [25].

Excess intake of vitamin C, a metabolic oxalate precursor, should similarly be avoided [24]. Although normal dietary vitamin C levels are not considered a risk in human beings, extremely small increases in urinary oxalate are a concern in urolith formers. Because cats do not have a dietary vitamin C requirement, supplementation should be avoided in foods fed to cats at risk for calcium oxalate uroliths. Cranberry concentrate tablets are also contraindicated. They provide mild acidification and are high in oxalate as well as vitamin C [28].

Potassium citrate is often included in diets designed for calcium oxalate prevention. In urine, citric acid combines with calcium to form soluble complexes, thereby reducing the ionic calcium concentration. Citric acid also directly inhibits nucleation of calcium and oxalate crystals. When oxidized within the tricarboxylic acid cycle, supplemental citrate results in urine alkalinization because of the production of bicarbonate. The metabolic alkalinization increases endogenous renal citrate excretion and reduces calcium absorption and urinary excretion [24]. Commercial products that add citrate but continue to acidify the urine (pH < 6.5) negate the benefit of citrate therapy.

Consumption of high levels of sodium may augment renal calcium excretion in human beings. Recent studies in healthy cats did not find increased urine calcium excretion in response to high dietary salt intake [24]. In cats with marginal renal function and increased calciuria, sodium exacerbated calcium excretion. No studies have evaluated the effect of sodium in cats prone to calcium oxalate stones. Epidemiologic evidence suggests that low dietary sodium levels in cat foods increase the risk for calcium oxalate urolithiasis [29]. Nonetheless, when fed a food lower in sodium, cats with naturally occurring calcium oxalate uroliths excreted less urine calcium [23]. Until further data are available, orally administered sodium chloride or loop diuretics, which promote renal sodium excretion, for diuresis should be used cautiously and with careful monitoring because they may increase the risk of calcium oxalate urolith formation in some patients. Recommended levels of sodium in foods for cats predisposed to calcium oxalate formation are between 0.3% and 0.5% sodium on a dry matter basis.

Dietary phosphorus should not be restricted in cats with calcium oxalate urolithiasis. Low dietary phosphorus is a risk factor for calcium oxalate urolith formation in cats [29]. Reduction in dietary phosphorus may be associated with activation of vitamin D, which, in turn, promotes intestinal calcium absorption and hypercalciuria. Additionally, phosphate status determines pyrophosphate urinary concentrations, an inhibitor of calcium oxalate urolith formation in human beings and rodents. If calcium oxalate urolithiasis is associated with hypophosphatemia and normal calcium concentration, oral phosphorus supplementation may be considered. Caution should be used, however, because excessive dietary phosphorus may predispose to formation of calcium phosphate uroliths. Whether this occurs in cats is unknown. Phosphorus levels in the foods for cats predisposed to calcium oxalate formation should not be excessive. Levels from 0.5% to 0.8% have been recommended [24].

Urinary magnesium forms complexes with oxalic acid, reducing the amount of oxalic acid available to form calcium oxalate. Studies in cats associate low dietary magnesium with calcium oxalate risk [26,27,29–32]. In human beings, supplemental magnesium has been used to minimize the recurrence of calcium oxalate uroliths; however, supplemental magnesium may increase the risk of struvite formation in cats. At this time, the risks and benefits of magnesium supplementation to cats with calcium oxalate urolithiasis have not been evaluated, and it is not advised. It seems logical that magnesium should not be highly restricted in diets that are consumed by cats with calcium oxalate urolithiasis. Many diets that claim to benefit feline "urinary tract health" are reduced in magnesium and promote urinary acidification. These foods are designed for struvite prevention and are not appropriate for cats at risk for calcium oxalate urolithiasis. Prudent levels of dietary magnesium are from 0.08% to 0.10% dry matter, or approximately 20 mg of magnesium per 100 kcal [24,29].

Consumption of high amounts of animal protein by human beings is associated with an increased risk of calcium oxalate formation. Dietary protein of animal origin may increase urinary calcium and oxalic acid excretion, decrease urinary citrate excretion, and promote bone mobilization to buffer the acid intake from metabolism of animal proteins. A case-control study showed that higher protein concentration in cat foods seemed to be protective against calcium oxalate uroliths, however [29]. Protein levels between 8 and 9 g of protein per 100 kcal seemed most protective. Although several coassociations (eg, higher protein in canned foods) might explain this finding, cats are obligatory carnivores and dietary protein restriction in the management of calcium oxalate urolithiasis is not advised.

Excessive levels of vitamin D (which promotes intestinal absorption of calcium) and vitamin C (which is a precursor of oxalic acid) should be avoided. Diets with vitamin D levels between 500 and 2000 IU/kg should suffice. As discussed previously, vitamin C is an oxalate precursor as well as a weak urinary acidifier. Both features may increase the likelihood of urolith recurrence.

The diet should be adequately fortified with vitamin B_6 because vitamin B_6 deficiency promotes endogenous production and subsequent urinary excretion of oxalic acid [33]. There is no evidence that providing increased vitamin B_6 beyond meeting the nutritional requirement provides a benefit in cats. Because most commercial diets designed for cats are well fortified with vitamin B_6, it is unlikely that additional supplementation is beneficial, except in homemade diets. Regardless, vitamin B_6 is reasonably safe and sometimes provided to cats with persistent calcium oxalate crystalluria or frequent recurrences.

Increased dietary fiber intake is associated with a decreasing risk of calcium oxalate recurrence in some human beings but not in cats unless they are hypercalcemic. Certain types of fiber (soy or rice bran) decrease calcium absorption from the GI tract, which may decrease urinary calcium excretion. Also, higher fiber diets tend to be less acidifying. In five cats with idiopathic hypercalcemia and calcium oxalate uroliths, feeding a high-fiber diet with supplemental potassium citrate resulted in normalization of serum calcium concentrations [34]; however, the efficacy of increased fiber intake is unproved at this time.

Although the relation of obesity to urolith formation is not understood, it remains a consistent risk factor in all studies to date. Restricting food intake to obtain an ideal weight and body condition is encouraged.

Cats that are meal fed, on average, have a more alkaline urinary pH, controlled food intake for obesity prevention, and a lower risk of calcium oxalate urolith formation. This method of feeding is also the preferred choice for canned foods. This is a relatively simple step that owners can take to improve preventative measures.

At the time of writing, there are three therapeutic foods that are formulated and marketed for the prevention of calcium oxalate uroliths in cats (Table 1). These diets contain potassium citrate (as an alkalinizing agent and a source of citrate) and are designed to induce a higher urine pH compared with standard foods or are designed to promote a significant increase in water intake. Consumption of Prescription Diet Feline x/d (Hill's Pet Nutrition, Topeka, Kansas) and Urinary SO (Royal Canin, St. Charles, Missouri) by healthy cats results in

Table 1
Comparison of diets formulated for prevention of calcium oxalate urolithiasis in cats

Component	x/d dry[a]	x/d canned[a]	pH/O dry[b]	pH/O canned[b]	S/O dry[c]	S/O canned[c]
Moisture As fed (%)	8	76	10	78	7	79
Protein						
As fed (%)	31.3	10.5	32.4	10.6	32.2	8.5
Dry matter (%)	34.0	42.9	36.0	48.3	34.6	40.5
G/100 kcal ME	8.3	8.8	7.7	9.2	7.8	8.3
Fat						
As fed (%)	15.3	4.8	16.5	6.9	17.5	9.1
Dry matter (%)	16.6	19.6	18.3	31.2	18.0	43.1
G/100 kcal ME	4.1	4.0	3.9	5.9	4.2	8.8
Fiber						
As fed (%)	0.8	0.6	1.7	0.2	3.0	0.51
Dry matter (%)	0.9	2.4	1.9	1.0	3.2	2.4
G/100 kcal ME	0.2	0.5	0.4	0.2	0.7	0.5
Sodium						
As fed (%)	0.33	0.09	0.44	0.11	1.3	0.2
Dry matter (%)	0.36	0.37	0.49	0.5	1.4	1.0
G/100 kcal ME	0.09	0.08	.10	0.10	0.32	0.20
Calcium						
As fed (%)	0.70	0.17	1.01	0.27	1.0	0.21
Dry matter (%)	0.76	0.69	1.12	1.23	1.1	1.0
G/100 kcal ME	0.19	0.14	0.24	0.23	0.24	0.20
Phosphorus						
As fed (%)	0.61	0.13	0.87	0.20	0.8	0.28
Dry matter (%)	0.66	0.53	0.97	0.91	0.86	1.33
G/100 kcal ME	0.16	0.11	0.21	0.17	0.19	0.27
Magnesium						
As fed (%)	0.07	0.02	0.08	0.02	0.07	0.02
Dry matter (%)	0.08	0.08	0.09	0.14	0.08	0.09
G/100 kcal ME	0.02	0.02	0.02	0.02	0.02	0.02

Dry matter indicates percentage of nutrient in product after moisture is removed. G/100 kcal ME indicates intake for every 100 kcal of metabolizable energy consumed.

[a]Prescription Diet Feline x/d: nutrient information for diets as of November 2004; manufactured by Hill's Pet Nutrition, (Topeka, Kansas).

[b]Moderate pH/O/Feline: nutrient information for diets as of July 2003; manufactured by Iams Company (Dayton, Ohio).

[c]Urinary S/O: nutrient information for diets as of November 2004; manufactured by Royal Canin (St. Charles, Missouri).

From Kirk CA, Bartges JW. Dietary considerations for calcium oxalate urolithiasis. In: August JR, editor. Consultations in feline medicine, vol. 5. St. Louis (MO): Elsevier; 2005. p. 431.

low urine saturation with calcium oxalate. Clinical trials using Prescription Diet Feline x/d in cats with naturally occurring calcium oxalate urolithiasis reduced calcium oxalate supersaturation by 59% [23]. The reduction in calcium oxalate formation production seemed to be a function of its ability to lower urine calcium. We have had some success in reducing mild hypercalcemia in certain calcium oxalate urolith-forming cats by feeding a high-fiber diet (Prescription Diet Feline w/d; Hill's Pet Nutrition) and administering potassium citrate.

Struvite

Struvite is another name for crystals or uroliths composed of magnesium ammonium phosphate hexahydrate. The chemical composition of struvite is $Mg^{2+} NH_4^+ PO_4 [3-]*6H_2O$. For uroliths to form, urine must be oversaturated with respect to the minerals that precipitate to form that type of urolith. For struvite uroliths to form, urine must be oversaturated with magnesium, ammonium, and phosphate ions. Urinary oversaturation with struvite may occur as a consequence of a urinary tract infection with a urease-producing microbe (infection-induced struvite) or without the presence of a urinary tract infection (sterile struvite) in cats [35].

Sterile struvite. Sterile struvite uroliths typically form in cats between 1 and 10 years of age. The risk for struvite urolith formation decreases after approximately 6 to 8 years of age in cats [32]. They occur with equal frequency in male and female cats. Sterile struvite uroliths form because of dietary composition as well as innate risks for urolith formation. Experimentally, magnesium phosphate and struvite uroliths formed in healthy cats consuming calculogenic diets containing 0.15% to 1.0% magnesium (dry matter basis) [36–38]. These data are difficult to interpret, however, because the amount of magnesium consumption by cats in these studies may be different than that by cats consuming commercial diets and spontaneously forming sterile struvite uroliths because of differences in caloric density, palatability, and digestibility [39]. The influence of magnesium on struvite formation depends on urine pH [40] and the influence of ions, minerals, and other components in urine [41]. Alkaluria is associated with an increased risk for struvite formation [42,43]. In a clinical study including 20 cats with naturally occurring struvite urocystoliths and no detectable bacterial urinary tract infection, the mean urinary pH at the time of diagnosis was 6.9 ± 0.4 [35]. An additional factor is water intake and urine volume. Consumption of increased quantities of water may result in lowering concentrations of calculogenic substances in urine, thus decreasing the risk of urolith formation [44]. Consumption of small quantities of food frequently rather than one or two large meals per day is associated with the production of more acidic urine and a lesser degree of struvite crystalluria by cats [45,46].

Sterile struvite uroliths can be dissolved by feeding a diet that is restricted in magnesium, phosphorous, and protein and that induces aciduria relative to maintenance adult cat foods [35]. In a clinical study including 22 cats with sterile struvite urocystoliths, urocystoliths dissolved in 20 cats in a mean of 36.2 ± 26.6 days (range: 14–141 days) [35]. The cats were fed a high-moisture (canned) calorically dense diet containing 0.058% magnesium (dry matter basis) and increased sodium chloride (0.79% dry matter basis). The diet (Prescription Diet Feline s/d; Hill's Pet Nutrition) induced a urine pH of approximately 6.0.

Prevention of sterile struvite uroliths involves inducing a urine pH less than approximately 6.8; increasing urine volume; and decreasing excretion of magnesium, ammonium, and phosphorous. There are many diets available that are formulated to be "struvite preventative."

Infection-induced struvite. Infection-induced struvite uroliths occur more commonly in cats less than 1 year and greater than 10 years of age. There is no published information on gender predilection for infection-induced struvite uroliths in cats. Infection induced-struvite uroliths form because of an infection with a urease-producing microbe in a fashion similar to that in dogs and human beings [38]. In this situation, dietary composition is not important, because the production of the enzyme urease by the microbial organism is the driving force behind struvite urolith formation.

Infection-induced struvite uroliths can be dissolved by feeding a "struvite dissolution" diet and administering an appropriate antimicrobial agent based on bacteriologic culture and sensitivity testing. The average dissolution time for infection-induced struvite uroliths was 79 days (range: 64–92 days) in three cats reported on in a study [35]. It is important that the cat receives an appropriate antimicrobial agent during the entire time of medical dissolution, because bacteria become trapped in the matrix of the urolith and are released into urine as the urolith dissolves. If therapeutic levels of an appropriate antimicrobial agent are not present in urine, an infection may recur and dissolution ceases.

Prevention of infection-induced struvite does not require feeding a special diet, because the infection causes these struvite uroliths to form. It involves preventing a bacterial urinary tract infection from recurring and treating bacterial infections as they arise. Dietary manipulation does not prevent infection-induced struvite uroliths from recurring, because diet does not prevent the recurrence of a bacterial urinary tract infection.

Purines

Uric acid is one of several biodegradation products of purine nucleotide metabolism [47]. In most dogs and cats, allantoin is the major metabolic end product; it is the most soluble of the purine metabolic products excreted in urine. Purine accounted for approximately 5% to 8% of feline uroliths submitted to the Minnesota Urolith Center from 1981 to 2002: 64 (0.14%) were composed of xanthine and the rest were composed of urate. Ammonium urate is the monobasic ammonium salt of uric acid, and it is the most common form of naturally occurring purine uroliths observed to occur in dogs and cats [48]. Other naturally occurring purine uroliths include sodium urate, sodium calcium urate, potassium urate, uric acid dihydrate, and xanthine.

Urate. Urate uroliths have been observed in several breeds of cats; male cats seem to be affected as frequently as female cats. Most urate uroliths occur in cats younger than 4 years of age. Urate uroliths may occur as a consequence of liver disease, specifically a portal vascular anomaly, or without the presence of liver disease, termed *idiopathic urate urolithiasis*. Urate uroliths occurring in association with portal vascular anomalies are most commonly composed of ammonium urate and are often diagnosed in cats younger than 1 year of age.

Apparently, there have been few studies of the biologic behavior of ammonium urate uroliths in dogs with portal vascular anomalies [49–52] and none in cats. It is logical to hypothesize that elimination of hyperuricuria and reduction of urine ammonium concentration after surgical correction of anomalous shunts would result in spontaneous dissolution of uroliths composed primarily of ammonium urate. Appropriate clinical studies are needed to prove or disprove this hypothesis. We have occasionally been successful in medically dissolving urate uroliths in dogs with portal vascular anomalies but have not attempted dissolution in cats with ammonium urate uroliths and portal vascular anomalies. Additional clinical studies are needed to evaluate the relative value of calculolytic diets, allopurinol, or alkalinization of urine in dissolving ammonium urate uroliths in cats with portal vascular anomalies. The pharmacokinetics and efficacy of allopurinol may be altered in cats with portal vascular anomalies, because biotransformation of this drug, which has a short half-life, to oxypurinol, which has a longer half-life, requires adequate hepatic function. Xanthine uroliths have been observed to form in dogs with portal vascular anomalies given allopurinol; therefore, allopurinol had an effect on xanthine oxidase conversion of xanthine to uric acid.

Although no studies have been performed evaluating the efficacy or safety of medical dissolution of urate uroliths in cats with idiopathic urate urolithiasis, we have successfully dissolved urate uroliths in cats using a low-protein diet (Prescription Diet k/d; Hill's Pet Products) and allopurinol (7.5 mg/kg administered orally every 12 hours). Until further studies are performed to confirm the safety and efficacy of medical dissolution, surgical removal remains the treatment of choice for urate uroliths in cats. Prevention of urate urolith recurrence in cats has been greater than 90% successful when using a protein-restricted alkalinizing diet (Prescription Diet k/d).

Xanthine. Xanthine uroliths retrieved and analyzed from cats contain pure xanthine, although a few contain small quantities of uric acid. Of 64 cats that formed xanthine uroliths in one report [53], none of the cats had been treated with the xanthine oxidase inhibitor, allopurinol. Sixty-one xanthine uroliths were obtained from the lower urinary tract, whereas xanthine uroliths from 3 cats came from the upper urinary tract. Xanthine uroliths occurred in 30 neutered and 8 nonneutered male cats and in 25 neutered female cats (the gender of 1 cat was not specified). The mean age of the cats at the time of diagnosis of xanthine uroliths was 2.8 ± 2.3 years (range: 4 months to 10 years). Eight of the 64 cats were less than 1 year of age. Urinary uric acid excretion was similar between 8 xanthine urolith-forming cats and healthy cats (2.09 ± 0.8 mg/kg/d versus 1.46 ± 0.56 mg/kg/d); however, urinary xanthine excretion ($2.46 \pm$

1.17 mg/kg/d) and urinary hypoxanthine excretion (0.65 ± 0.17 mg/kg/d) were higher (neither are detectable in urine from healthy cats).

No medical dissolution protocol for feline xanthine uroliths exists. Prevention involves feeding a protein-restricted alkalinizing diet. Without preventative measures, xanthine uroliths often recur within 3 to 12 months after removal. In 10 cats consuming the protein-restricted alkalinizing diet and followed for at least 2 years, only 1 has had a recurrence.

Cystine

Cystine accounts for less than 1% of feline uroliths. Cysteine uroliths occur with equal frequency in male and female cats. The mean age at diagnosis of cats with cystine uroliths is 4.1 years (range: 10 months to 11 years) [39]. Most cats affected with cystine uroliths are domestic short-hair cats.

Cystine uroliths occur when urine is oversaturated with cystine. Cystine is a disulfide-containing amino acid that is normally filtered and reabsorbed by proximal renal tubular cells. Therefore, cystinuria occurs when there is a defect in proximal renal tubular absorption and must be present for cystine uroliths to form. Evaluation of urine amino acid profiles from four cats with cystine uroliths revealed increased concentrations of the amino acids cystine, arginine, lysine, and ornithine [39,54].

Medical protocols exist for dissolution of cystine uroliths in dogs using thiol-containing drugs, such as N-(2-mercaptopropionyl)-glycine (2-MPG), with or without dietary modification [55] or urinary alkalinization. Reducing dietary protein has the potential of minimizing the formation of cystine uroliths by decreasing intake and excretion of sulfur-containing amino acids and by decreasing renal medullary tonicity, resulting in a larger urine volume. Many feline protein-restricted diets are formulated for use with renal failure and have an added advantage of containing a urinary alkalinizing agent. Solubility of cystine increases exponentially when the urine pH is greater than 7.2 [56]. If necessary or if dietary modification cannot be implemented, potassium citrate may be administered to induce alkaluria. Although thiol-containing drugs are used in dogs and human beings, their use has not been evaluated adequately in cats.

Matrix-Crystalline Urethral Plugs

Urethral matrix-crystalline plugs occur in approximately 20% of male cats younger than 10 years of age that are presented with obstructive lower urinary tract disease [6]. Urethral plugs have only been observed to occur in male cats. They are composed of at least 45% to 50% matrix and variable amounts of mineral; they may be composed entirely of matrix [57]. Struvite is the most common mineral found in urethral plugs. Multiple factors are thought to be associated with urethral plug formation. If a mineral is present in the urethral plug, risk factors associated with that crystal formation, as discussed previously, are involved, at least in part. Compared with uroliths, urethral plugs contain large quantities of matrix. Components of matrix that may be important in urethral plug formation include Tamm-Horsfall mucoprotein, serum proteins, cellular debris, and virus-like particles [13,58].

Management of urethral matrix-crystalline plugs involves relieving the obstructive uropathy [59]. Modifying urine composition by feeding a therapeutic diet may be beneficial if mineral is present in the urethral plug. Increasing urine volume may help to decrease the concentration of minerals and matrix components in urine. Successful prevention of recurrent urethral obstruction using diets designed to reduce urine pH and urine magnesium and phosphorous concentrations has been reported [60]. Perineal urethrostomy may be considered in cats with recurrent urethral plug formation; however, it is associated with complications, including recurrent bacterial urinary tract infections and lower urinary tract disease [60].

Not all feline urinary tract disorders are associated with dietary factors; however, most benefit from nutritional management. It is important to understand the pathophysiology of feline lower urinary tract disease and the physiologic effects of foods and feeding so as to formulate the best nutritional and treatment plan.

References

[1] Lawler DF, Sjolin DW, Collins JE. Incidence rates of feline lower urinary tract disease in the United States. Feline Pract 1985;15:13–6.

[2] Willeberg P. Epidemiology of naturally occurring feline urologic syndrome. Vet Clin North Am Small Anim Pract 1984;14:455–69.

[3] Foster SJ. The "urolithiasis" syndrome in male cats; a statistical analysis of the problems, with clinical observations. J Small Anim Pract 1967;8:207–14.

[4] Osborne CA, Kruger JM, Johnston GR, et al. Feline lower urinary tract disorders. In: Textbook of Veterinary Internal Medicine. Ettinger SJ, editor. Philadelphia: WB Saunders; 1989. p. 2057–82.

[5] Lund EM, Armstrong PJ, Kirk CA, et al. Health status and population characteristics of dogs and cats examined at private veterinary practices in the United States. J Am Vet Med Assoc 1999;214:1336–41.

[6] Kruger JM, Osborne CA, Goyal SM, et al. Clinical evaluation of cats with lower urinary tract disease. J Am Vet Med Assoc 1991;199:211–6.

[7] Buffington CA, Chew DJ, Kendall MS, et al. Clinical evaluation of cats with nonobstructive urinary tract diseases. J Am Vet Med Assoc 1997;210:46–50.

[8] Bartges JW. Lower urinary tract disease in older cats: what's common, what's not? In: Health and nutrition of geriatric cats and dogs. North American Veterinary Conference, Orlando FL, 1996.

[9] Markwell PJ, Buffington CA, Chew DJ, et al. Clinical evaluation of commercially available urinary acidification diets in the management of idiopathic cystitis in cats. J Am Vet Med Assoc 1999;214:361–5.

[10] Gunn-Moore DA, Shenoy CM. Oral glucosamine and the management of feline idiopathic cystitis. J Feline Med Surg 2004;6:219–25.

[11] Brown C, Purich D. Physical-chemical processes in kidney stone formation. In: Coe F, Favus M, editors. Disorders of bone and mineral metabolism. New York: Raven Press; 1992. p. 613–24.

[12] Coe FL, Parks JH, Asplin JR. The pathogenesis and treatment of kidney stones. N Engl J Med 1992;327:1141–52.

[13] Osborne CA, Lulich JP, Kruger JM, et al. Feline urethral plugs. Etiology and pathophysiology. Vet Clin North Am Small Anim Pract 1996;26:233–53.

[14] Bartges JW, Osborne CA, Lulich JP, et al. Methods for evaluating treatment of uroliths. Vet Clin North Am Small Anim Pract 1999;29:45–57.

[15] Balaji KC, Menon M. Mechanism of stone formation. Urol Clin North Am 1997;24:1–11.

[16] Bartges JW. Calcium oxalate urolithiasis. In: August JR, editor. Consultations in feline internal medicine. 4th edition. Philadelphia: WB Saunders; 2001. p. 352–64.

[17] Midkiff AM, Chew DJ, Randolph JF, et al. Idiopathic hypercalcemia in cats. J Vet Intern Med 2000;14:619–26.

[18] Bartges JW, Kirk C, Lane IF. Update: management of calcium oxalate uroliths in dogs and cats. Vet Clin North Am Small Anim Pract 2004;34:969–87.

[19] Lulich JP, Osborne CA, Nagode LA, et al. Evaluation of urine and serum metabolites in miniature schnauzers with calcium oxalate urolithiasis. Am J Vet Res 1991;52:1583–90.

[20] Ching SV, Fettman MJ, Hamar DW, et al. The effect of chronic dietary acidification using ammonium chloride on acid-base and mineral metabolism in the adult cat. J Nutr 1989;119:902–15.

[21] McKerrell RE, Blakemore WF, Heath MF, et al. Primary hyperoxaluria (L-glyceric aciduria) in the cat: a newly recognised inherited disease. Vet Rec 1989;125:31–4.

[22] Lulich JP, Osborne CA, Sanderson SL, et al. Voiding urohydropropulsion: lessons from 5 years of experience. Vet Clin North Am Small Anim Pract 1999;29:283–92.

[23] Lulich JP, Osborne CA, Lekcharoensuk C, et al. Effects of diet on urine composition of cats with calcium oxalate urolithiasis. J Am Anim Hosp Assoc 2004;40:185–91.

[24] Kirk CA, Ling GV, Osborne CA, et al. Clinical guidelines for managing calcium oxalate uroliths in cats: medical therapy, hydration, and dietary therapy. In: Managing urolithiasis in cats: recent updates and practice guidelines. Topeka (KS): Hill's Pet Nutrition; 2003. p. 10–9.

[25] Kirk CA, Ling GV, Franti CE, et al. Evaluation of factors associated with development of calcium oxalate urolithiasis in cats. J Am Vet Med Assoc 1995;207:1429–34.

[26] Thumchai R, Lulich J, Osborne CA, et al. Epizootiologic evaluation of urolithiasis in cats. 3,498 cases (1982–1992). J Am Vet Med Assoc 1996;208:547–51.

[27] Lekcharoensuk C, Lulich JP, Osborne CA, et al. Association between patient-related factors and risk of calcium oxalate and magnesium ammonium phosphate urolithiasis in cats. J Am Vet Med Assoc 2000;217:520–5.

[28] Terris MK, Issa MM, Tacker JR. Dietary supplementation with cranberry concentrate tablets may increase the risk of nephrolithiasis. Urology 2001;57:26–9.

[29] Lekcharoensuk C, Osborne CA, Lulich JP, et al. Association between dietary factors and calcium oxalate and magnesium ammonium phosphate urolithiasis in cats. J Am Vet Med Assoc 2001;219:1228–37.

[30] Robertson WG. Urinary calculi. In: Nordin BEC, Need AG, Morris HA, editors. Metabolic bone and stone disease. Edinburgh (UK): Churchill Livingstone; 1993. p. 249–311.

[31] Lulich JP, Osborne CA, Bartges JW, et al. Canine lower urinary tract disorders. In: Ettinger SJ, Feldman EC, editors. Textbook of veterinary internal medicine. 5th edition. Philadelphia: WB Saunders; 1999. p. 1747–83.

[32] Smith BHE, Moodie SJ, Wensley S, et al. Differences in urinary pH and relative supersaturation values between senior and young adult cats. In: Proceedings of the 15th American College of Veterinary Internal Medicine Forum. Lake Buena Vista, FL, 1997. p. 674.

[33] Bai SC, Sampson DA, Morris JG, et al. Vitamin B6 requirement of growing kittens. J Nutr 1989;119:1020–7.

[34] McClain HM, Barsanti JA, Bartges JW. Hypercalcemia and calcium oxalate urolithiasis in cats: a report of five cases. J Am Anim Hosp Assoc 1999;35:297–301.

[35] Osborne CA, Lulich JP, Kruger JM, et al. Medical dissolution of feline struvite urocystoliths. J Am Vet Med Assoc 1990;196:1053–63.

[36] Buffington T. Struvite urolithiasis in cats. J Am Vet Med Assoc 1989;194:7–8.

[37] Finco DR, Barsanti JA, Crowell WA. Characterization of magnesium-induced urinary disease in the cat and comparison with feline urologic syndrome. Am J Vet Res 1985;46:391–400.

[38] Osborne CA, Polzin DJ, Abdullahi SU, et al. Struvite urolithiasis in animals and man: formation, detection, and dissolution. Adv Vet Sci Comp Med 1985;29:1–101.

[39] Osborne CA, Kruger JM, Lulich JP, et al. Feline lower urinary tract diseases. In: Ettinger SJ, Feldman EC, editors. Textbook of veterinary internal medicine. 5th edition. Philadelphia: WB Saunders, 1999. p. 1710–46.

[40] Buffington CA, Rogers QR, Morris JG. Effect of diet on struvite activity product in feline urine. Am J Vet Res 1990;51:2025–30.

[41] Buffington CA, Blaisdell JL, Sako T. Effects of Tamm-Horsfall glycoprotein and albumin on struvite crystal growth in urine of cats. Am J Vet Res 1994;55:965–71.

[42] Tarttelin MF. Feline struvite urolithiasis: factors affecting urine pH may be more important than magnesium levels in food. Vet Rec 1987;121:227–30.

[43] Bartges JW, Tarver SL, Schneider C. Comparison of struvite activity product ratios and relative supersaturations in urine collected from healthy cats consuming four struvite management diets. Presented at the Ralston Purina Nutrition Symposium, St. Louis, MO. 1998.

[44] Smith BH, Stevenson AE, Markwell PJ. Urinary relative supersaturations of calcium oxalate and struvite in cats are influenced by diet. J Nutr 1998;128(Suppl):2763S–4S.

[45] Finke MD, Litzenberger BA. Effect of food intake on urine pH in cats. J Small Anim Pract 1992;33:261–5.

[46] Tarttelin MF. Feline struvite urolithiasis: fasting reduced the effectiveness of a urinary acidifier (ammonium chloride) and increased the intake of a low magnesium diet. Vet Rec 1987;121:245–8.

[47] Bartges JW, Osborne CA, Lulich JP, et al. Canine urate urolithiasis. Etiopathogenesis, diagnosis, and management. Vet Clin North Am Small Anim Pract 1999;29:161–91.

[48] Osborne CA, Bartges JW, Lulich JP, et al. Canine urolithiasis. In: Hand MS, Thatcher CD, Remillard RL, et al, editors. Small animal clinical nutrition. 4th edition. Marceline (MO): Wadsworth Publishing Company; 2000. p. 605–88.

[49] Marretta SM, Pask AJ, Greene RW, et al. Urinary calculi associated with portosystemic shunts in six dogs. J Am Vet Med Assoc 1981;178:133–7.

[50] Hardy RM, Klausner JS. Urate calculi associated with portal vascular anomalies. In: Kirk RW, editor. Current veterinary therapy VIII. Philadelphia: WB Saunders; 1983. p. 1073–8.

[51] Brain PH. Portosystemic shunts—urate calculi as a guide to diagnosis. Aust Vet Pract 1988;18:3–4.

[52] Johnson CA, Armstrong PJ, Hauptman JG. Congenital portosystemic shunts in dogs: 46 cases (1979–1986). J Am Vet Med Assoc 1987;19:1478–83.

[53] Osborne CA, Bartges JW, Lulich JP. Feline xanthine urolithiasis: a newly recognized cause of urinary tract disease. [abstract]. Urol Res 2004;32:171.

[54] DiBartola SP, Chew DJ, Horton ML. Cystinuria in a cat. J Am Vet Med Assoc 1991;198:102–4.

[55] Osborne CA, Sanderson SL, Lulich JP, et al. Canine cystine urolithiasis. Cause, detection, treatment, and prevention. Vet Clin North Am Small Anim Pract 1999;29:193–211.

[56] Milliner DS. Cystinuria. Endocrinol Metab Clin North Am 1990;19:889–907.

[57] Osborne CA, Lulich JP, Albansan H, et al. Mineral composition of feline uroliths and urethral plugs: current status. In: Managing urolithiasis in cats: recent updates and practice guidelines. Topeka (KS): Hill's Pet Nutrition Inc.; 2003. p. 26–8.

[58] Kruger JM, Osborne CA. The role of viruses in feline lower urinary tract disease. J Vet Intern Med 1990;4:71–8.

[59] Osborne CA, Kruger JM, Lulich JP, et al. Medical management of feline urethral obstruction. Vet Clin North Am Small Anim Pract 1996;26:483–98.

[60] Osborne CA, Caywood DD, Johnston GR, et al. Perineal urethrostomy versus dietary management in prevention of recurrent lower urinary tract disease. J Small Anim Pract 1991;32:296–305.

Vet Clin Small Anim 36 (2006) 1377–1384

VETERINARY CLINICS
SMALL ANIMAL PRACTICE

ELSEVIER
SAUNDERS

Nutritional Management of Chronic Renal Disease in Dogs and Cats

Denise A. Elliott, BVSc, PhD

Royal Canin USA, 500 Fountain Lakes Boulevard, Suite 100, St. Charles, MO, 63301, USA

D ietary therapy has remained the cornerstone of management of chronic renal failure for decades. The goals of dietary modification are to (1) meet the patient's nutrient and energy requirements, (2) alleviate clinical signs and consequences of the uremic intoxication, (3) minimize disturbances in fluid, electrolyte, vitamin, mineral, and acid–base balance, and (4) slow progression of the renal failure. Recommendations regarding dietary therapy and other components of conservative medical management must be individualized based on clinical and laboratory findings. Chronic renal failure is progressive and dynamic, and therefore serial clinical and laboratory assessment and modification of therapy in response to changes in the patient's condition are integral to successful therapy.

ENERGY

Sufficient energy must be provided to prevent endogenous protein catabolism, which results in malnutrition and exacerbation of azotemia. Although the energy requirements of dogs and cats that have chronic renal failure (CRF) are unknown, they are believed to be similar to those of healthy dogs and cats. Dogs should be fed $132 \times$ (body weight in kilograms)$^{0.75}$ per day and cats require 50 to 60 kcal/kg/d. Maintenance energy requirements may vary among individuals, and therefore energy intake should be customized based on serial determinations of body weight and body condition score. Carbohydrates and fats provide the nonprotein sources of energy in the diet. Typically diets designed for managing CRF are formulated with a high fat content because fat provides approximately twice the energy per gram than carbohydrate. This formulation results in an energy-dense diet that allows patients to obtain nutritional requirements from a smaller volume of food. A smaller volume of food minimizes gastric distention, which reduces the likelihood of nausea and vomiting.

E-mail address: Denise.elliott@royalcanin.us

0195-5616/06/$ – see front matter
doi:10.1016/j.cvsm.2006.08.011

PROTEIN

Azotemia and uremia are caused by the accumulation of nitrogenous metabolites derived from excessive dietary protein or degradation of endogenous protein. High protein intake exacerbates azotemia and the morbidity of CRF [1], whereas protein malnutrition is strongly correlated with morbidity and mortality. The rationale for formulating a diet that contains a reduced quantity of high-quality protein and adequate nonprotein calories is based on the premise that controlled reduction of nonessential protein results in decreased production of nitrogenous wastes, with consequent amelioration or elimination of clinical signs even though renal function may remain essentially unchanged. Studies have shown that modifying dietary protein intake can reduce blood urea nitrogen (BUN) and provide clinical benefits to dogs and cats with CRF [1–6].

Whether protein restriction alters progression of renal failure in dogs and cats is less uncertain [5,7,8,9–12]. Brown and colleagues [13,14] reported that protein restriction did not alleviate glomerular hypertension, hypertrophy, hyperfiltration, or progression in dogs with induced renal failure. Adams and colleagues [15] reported that protein and energy restriction had no effect on renal lesions or function in cats with induced renal failure. Similarly, Finco and colleagues [16] reported that protein restriction had no effect on the development of renal lesions or on renal function in cats with induced renal disease.

The minimal dietary protein requirements for dogs or cats with CRF are not known but are believed to be similar to the minimal protein requirements of healthy pets. However, this degree of restriction is necessary only in animals with profound renal failure, and more liberal prescriptions can be fed to dogs with greater renal function. The dietary protein intake should be adjusted to minimize excesses in azotemia while simultaneously avoiding excessive restriction of dietary protein because of the risk for protein malnutrition. If evidence of protein malnutrition occurs (hypoalbuminemia, anemia, weight loss, or loss of body tissue mass), dietary protein should be gradually increased until these abnormalities are corrected.

MINERALS AND ELECTROLYTES

Phosphate retention and hyperphosphatemia occur early in renal disease and play a primary role in the genesis and progression of renal secondary hyperparathyroidism, renal osteodystrophy, relative or absolute deficiency of 1,25-dihydroxyvitamin D, and soft tissue calcification. By minimizing hyperphosphatemia, secondary hyperparathyroidism and its sequela can be prevented. In addition, dietary phosphorus restriction has been shown to slow the progression of renal failure in dogs and cats. In one study of dogs with surgically induced reduced renal function, those fed a low phosphorous diet (0.44% dry matter [DM]) had a 75% survival versus a 33% survival in those fed a high phosphorous diet (1.44% DM) [17]. Renal function also deteriorated more rapidly in the high phosphorous group. Ross and colleagues [18] reported that cats with reduced renal mass fed a phosphorus-restricted diet (0.24% DM) showed little or no histologic change compared with those fed a normal phosphorus diet (1.56% DM), who showed mineralization, fibrosis, and mononuclear cell infiltration.

The goal of dietary therapy is to normalize the serum phosphate concentration, which may be achieved by limiting dietary phosphate intake. If normophosphatemia cannot been accomplished within 2 to 4 weeks of implementing dietary phosphate restriction, intestinal phosphate binders should be added to the treatment plan. Normalization of serum phosphate concentrations using these methods has been associated with a reduction in serum parathyroid hormone concentrations in cats with naturally occurring renal disease [19]. Parathyroid hormone concentrations may even return to the normal range [19].

Hypertension is common in dogs and cats with CRF [20–22], and has been implicated as a contributor to the progression of renal failure [21,22]. Jacob and colleagues [22] reported that dogs with naturally occurring chronic renal disease and systolic blood pressure higher than 180 mm Hg were more likely to develop a uremic crisis and die than dogs with normal systolic blood pressure. Furthermore, the risk for developing a uremic crisis and dying increased significantly as systolic blood pressure increased.

Sodium restriction has been recommended to alleviate hypertension associated with failure of the kidneys to excrete sodium. A report recently suggested that feeding more than 1.5 g of Na per 1000 kcal could promote progression of feline renal disease in its early stages [23]. However, altering sodium intake from 0.5 to 3.25 g Na per 1000 kcal did not influence development of hypertension or affect glomerular filtration rate in dogs with surgically induced renal reduction [24,25]. In addition, a recent study by Burankarl and colleagues [26] in cats with surgically induced moderate renal disease did not show any adverse effects associated with feeding 2 g Na per 1000 kcal [26]. These investigators also suggested that NaCl restriction (0.5 g Na per 1000 kcal) could activate neurohumoral axes that contribute to the progression of renal disease and exacerbate renal potassium wasting. A study of diet and lifestyle variables of cats with naturally occurring CRF suggested that increased dietary sodium intake was associated with decreased odds of developing CRF [27]. Therefore, the ideal dietary sodium concentrations for dogs and cats with CRF are not clearly defined. Current recommendations are for normal to mildly restricted sodium diets. As renal failure progresses, patients' ability to rapidly adjust sodium excretion in response to changes in intake becomes severely impaired. If sodium intake is rapidly reduced, dehydration and volume contraction may occur, with the potential to precipitate a renal crisis. Hence, a gradual change from the pet's previous diet to the salt-restricted diet is recommended.

Potassium deficiency has been identified in cats with CRF. This deficiency is caused by a combination of urinary potassium loss and decreased potassium intake [28]. However, not all cats are hypokalemic. One study reported that 13% of 116 cats with CRF were hyperkalemic, emphasizing the need to monitor potassium status and adjust intake with oral potassium gluconate on an individual basis [29].

ACID–BASE BALANCE

The kidneys excrete metabolically derived nonvolatile acid (sulfates, hydrogen ions) and are central to maintaining an acid–base balance. As renal function declines, the capacity to excrete hydrogen ions and reabsorb bicarbonate ions is reduced and metabolic acidosis ensues. Metabolic acidosis increases renal ammoniagenesis, which activates complement, contributing to the progression of renal failure. In addition, metabolic acidosis increases catabolism and degradation of skeletal muscle protein, disrupts intracellular metabolism, and promotes dissolution of bone mineral, exacerbating azotemia, loss of lean body mass, and renal osteodystrophy. Because dietary protein restriction results in the consumption of reduced quantities of protein-derived acid precursors, supplementation with additional alkalinizing agents, such as sodium bicarbonate, calcium carbonate, or potassium citrate, may be required.

LONG-CHAIN OMEGA-3 FATTY ACIDS

Long-chain omega-3 fatty acids compete with arachidonic acid and alter eicosanoid, thromboxane, and leukotriene production [30]. Remnant kidney studies in dogs have reported that omega-3 fatty acid supplementation (menhaden fish oil) reduces inflammation, lowers systemic arterial pressure, alters plasma lipid concentrations, and preserves renal function [31–34]. Because they cause an acute increase in glomerular filtration rate, omega-6 fatty acids (safflower oil) appear to be detrimental in dogs with naturally occurring renal disease [35]. Some commercially available diets have an adjusted omega-6:omega-3 ratio. However, focusing on the absolute concentrations of specific omega-3 fatty acids, rather than on ratios, would be more appropriate, but no studies have been reported. Studies of the effect of variation in dietary fatty acid composition in cats with renal disease have also not been reported.

FIBER

Fermentable fiber is a recent addition to the nutritional management of CRF. Experts hypothesize that fermentable fiber provides a source of carbohydrates for gastrointestinal bacteria, which consequently use blood urea as a source of nitrogen for growth. The increased bacterial cell mass increases fecal nitrogen excretion and has been suggested to decrease the BUN concentration and reduce the need for protein restriction. However, the major concern is that, unlike BUN, the molecular sizes of classical uremic toxins (middle-molecules) are too large to readily cross membrane barriers, and therefore the bacterial use of ammonia is unlikely to reduce these toxins. Furthermore, studies documenting these changes have not been reported. As a consequence, widespread application of fermentable fiber as a nitrogen trap currently cannot be recommended.

However, fermentable fibers have beneficial effects for modulating gastrointestinal health in patients who have CRF. New food supplements, including fiber-like polysaccharides derived from chitin and bacterial products, have recently been marketed as phosphate binders and agents that reduce azotemia, respectively. Although limited studies show a measurable reduction in phosphate, BUN, and creatinine with supplementation, maximal effects occur in combination with nutritional therapy [36–38].

ANTIOXIDANTS

Endogenous oxidative damage to protein, lipids, and DNA is believed to play an important role in the progression of renal disease in humans [39,40]. Nutrients such as vitamin E, vitamin C, taurine, carotenoids, and flavonols are effective antioxidants that trap free radical species. Humans who have CRF have been shown to have lower concentrations of vitamin E and vitamin C and high concentrations of markers of lipid peroxidation [41]. These studies suggest that humans who have CRF experience oxidative stress. Studies in rats have suggested that supplementation with vitamin E may modulate tubulointerstitial injury and glomerulosclerosis, suggesting that vitamin E may slow progression of renal damage [42,43]. Although no studies have evaluated oxidative stress or antioxidant status in dogs or cats that have renal disease, ensuring adequate antioxidant intake seems prudent to minimize oxidative stress.

FEEDING STRATEGY

Dietary therapy is only effective in ameliorating the clinical signs of uremia if it is administered appropriately. Patients who have CRF are often anorexic and have reduced appetites. Practical measures to improve intake include the use of highly odorous foods, warming the foods before feeding, and stimulating eating by positive reinforcement with petting and stroking. Although appetite stimulants, such as the benzodiazepam derivatives or serotonin antagonists, may be judiciously administered, more aggressive therapy, such as esophagostomy or gastrotomy tube feeding, is clinically indicated in these cases. Instituting dietary changes when patients are hospitalized is inadvisable because these patients have a high risk for developing food aversion. The renal support diet should instead be instituted at home when the pet is stable and in a comfortable environment.

CLINICAL STUDIES OF NATURALLY OCCURRING CHRONIC RENAL FAILURE

Elliott and colleagues [4] evaluated the effect of a modified protein, low phosphate diet on the outcome of 50 cats with stable, naturally occurring CRF. Of these, 29 received a modified protein, low phosphate diet, and the remaining 21 received their normal diets. The two groups had no significant differences in age, body weight, creatinine, phosphate, and parathyroid hormone concentrations at the start of the study. The median survival time of the cats fed the modified protein, low phosphate diet was significantly greater than that of those fed the normal diet (633 days vs. 264 days, $P < .0036$). Of the cats on the normal diet, 69% died of progressive renal failure. The median survival time for cats fed a renal diet was 2.4 times longer than for cats fed a maintenance diet. These results suggest that feeding a renal diet to cats with CRF doubles their life expectancy.

Ross and colleagues [44] evaluated the effect of a renal diet (modified in protein, phosphorus, sodium, and lipids) compared with an adult maintenance diet in 45 cats that had stage 2 or 3 kidney disease. Of the 23 cats fed the adult maintenance diet, 6 experienced an uremic crisis, whereas none of the 22 cats fed the renal diet experienced an uremic crisis. At the end of the study, 5 of the 23 cats fed the adult maintenance diet died from renal-related causes. No renal-related deaths occurred in the 22 cats fed the renal diet. The results of this study suggest that dietary modifications can reduce the number of uremic crises and the mortality in cats that have naturally occurring stage 2 or 3 renal disease.

The effect of a modified protein, low phosphate diet on the outcome of dogs that have stable, naturally occurring CRF has also recently been shown [2]. Dogs with mild to moderate CRF fed a renal diet experienced a 70% reduction in the relative risk for developing a uremic crisis, remained free of uremic signs almost 2.5 times longer, and had a median survival that was three times longer than those with CRF fed a maintenance diet. Renal function declined more slowly in the dogs fed the renal diet. In dogs fed the maintenance diet, the primary cause of death was renal-related.

MONITORING

Regular monitoring to ensure that dietary and medical management remain optimal for the needs of the patient is crucial for the well-being and long-term successful treatment of patients who have CRF. Frequent patient evaluation may also improve owner compliance. Patients should be reevaluated within 2 weeks of initiating nutritional therapy and then three to four times per year. A complete dietary history, physical examination, body weight, body condition score, and laboratory evaluation are indicated. The dietary history should include the type of diet (dry vs. wet), the amount eaten each day (eaten is more important than amount offered), and the method of feeding, and should also note all treats, snacks, and supplements. This information is invaluable for monitoring the response to dietary therapy.

SUMMARY

CRF is the clinical syndrome resulting from irreversible loss of the metabolic, endocrine, and excretory capacities of the kidney. Nutrition has been the cornerstone of management for decades. The goals of dietary modification are to meet the patient's nutrient and energy requirements; alleviate clinical signs and consequences of uremia; minimize disturbances in fluid, electrolyte, vitamin, mineral, and acid–base balance; and slow progression of renal failure. Regular monitoring to ensure that dietary and medical management remain optimal for the needs of the patient is crucial for the well-being and long-term successful treatment of patients who have CRF.

References
[1] Polzin DJ, Osborne CA, Stevens JB, et al. Influence of modified protein diets on the nutritional status of dogs with induced chronic renal failure. Am J Vet Res 1983;44:1694–702.

[2] Jacob F, Polzin DJ, Osborne CA, et al. Clinical evaluation of dietary modification for treatment of spontaneous chronic renal failure in dogs. J Am Vet Med Assoc 2002;220: 1163–70.

[3] Leibetseder JL, Neufeld KW. Effects of medium protein diets in dogs with chronic renal failure. J Nutr 1991;121:S145–9.

[4] Elliott J, Rawlings JM, Markwell PJ, et al. Survival of cats with naturally occurring chronic renal failure: effect of dietary management. J Small Anim Pract 2000;41:235–42.

[5] Finco DR, Crowell WA, Barsanti JA. Effects of three diets on dogs with induced chronic renal failure. Am J Vet Res 1985;46:646–53.

[6] Polzin DJ, Osborne CA. The importance of egg protein in reduced protein diets designed for dogs with renal failure. J Vet Intern Med 1988;2:15–21.

[7] Robertson JL, Goldschmidt M, Kronfeld DS, et al. Long-term renal responses to high dietary protein in dogs with 75% nephrectomy. Kidney Int 1986;29:511–9.

[8] Polzin DJ, Leininger JR, Osborne CA, et al. Development of renal lesions in dogs after 11/12 reduction of renal mass. Influences of dietary protein intake. Lab Invest 1988;58:172–83.

[9] Finco DR, Brown SA, Crowell WA, et al. Effects of dietary phosphorus and protein in dogs with chronic renal failure. Am J Vet Res 1992;53:2264–71.

[10] Finco DR, Brown SA, Crowell WA, et al. Effects of phosphorus/calcium-restricted and phosphorus/calcium-replete 32% protein diets in dogs with chronic renal failure. Am J Vet Res 1992;53:157–63.

[11] Finco DR, Brown SA, Crowell WA, et al. Effects of aging and dietary protein intake on uninephrectomized geriatric dogs. Am J Vet Res 1994;55:1282–90.

[12] Finco DR, Brown SA, Brown CA, et al. Progression of chronic renal disease in the dog. J Vet Intern Med 1999;13:516–28.

[13] Brown SA, Finco DR, Crowell WA, et al. Single-nephron adaptations to partial renal ablation in the dog. Am J Physiol 1990;258:F495–503.

[14] Brown SA, Finco DR, Crowell WA, et al. Dietary protein intake and the glomerular adaptations to partial nephrectomy in dogs. J Nutr 1991;121:S125–7.

[15] Adams LG, Polzin DJ, Osborne CA, et al. Influence of dietary protein/calorie intake on renal morphology and function in cats with 5/6 nephrectomy. Lab Invest 1994;70:347–57.

[16] Finco DR, Brown SA, Brown CA, et al. Protein and calorie effects on progression of induced chronic renal failure in cats. Am J Vet Res 1998;59:575–82.

[17] Brown SA, Crowell WA, Barsanti JA, et al. Beneficial effects of dietary mineral restriction in dogs with marked reduction of functional renal mass. J Am Soc Nephrol 1991;1:1169–79.

[18] Ross LA, Finco DR, Crowell WA. Effect of dietary phosphorus restriction on the kidneys of cats with reduced renal mass. Am J Vet Res 1982;43:1023–6.

[19] Barber PJ, Rawlings JM, Markwell PJ, et al. Effect of dietary phosphate restriction on renal secondary hyperparathyroidism in the cat. J Small Anim Pract 1999;40:62–70.

[20] Syme HM, Barber PJ, Markwell PJ, et al. Prevalence of systolic hypertension in cats with chronic renal failure at initial evaluation. J Am Vet Med Assoc 2002;220:1799–804.

[21] Elliott J, Barber PJ, Syme HM, et al. Feline hypertension: clinical findings and response to antihypertensive treatment in 30 cases. J Small Anim Pract 2001;42:122–9.

[22] Jacob F, Polzin DJ, Osborne CA, et al. Association between initial systolic blood pressure and risk of developing a uremic crisis or of dying in dogs with chronic renal failure. J Am Vet Med Assoc 2003;222:322–9.

[23] Kirk CA. Dietary salt and FLUTD: risk or benefit? Proceedings of the 20th Annual Forum American College of Veterinary Internal Medicine 2002;553–5.

[24] Greco DS, Lees GE, Dzendzel GS, et al. Effect of dietary sodium intake on glomerular filtration rate in partially nephrectomized dogs. Am J Vet Res 1994;55:152–9.

[25] Greco DS, Lees GE, Dzendzel G, et al. Effects of dietary sodium intake on blood pressure measurements in partially nephrectomized dogs. Am J Vet Res 1994;55:160–5.

[26] Burankarl C, Mathur S, Cartier L, et al. Effects of dietary sodium chloride (NaCl) supplementation on renal function and blood pressure (BP) in normal cats and in cats with induced renal

insufficiency. Presented at the 28th World Congress of the World Small Animal Veterinary Association. Bangkok, Thailand, October 24–28, 2003.

[27] Hughes KL, Slater MR, Geller S, et al. Diet and lifestyle variables as risk factors for chronic renal failure in pet cats. Prev Vet Med 2002;55:1–15.

[28] Dow SW, Fettman MJ, LeCouteur RA, et al. Potassium depletion in cats: renal and dietary influences. J Am Vet Med Assoc 1987;191:1569–75.

[29] Dow SW, Fettman MJ, Curtis CR, et al. Hypokalemia in cats: 186 cases 1984–1987. J Am Vet Med Assoc 1989;194:1604–8.

[30] Bauer JE, Markwell PJ, Rawlings JM, et al. Effects of dietary fat and polyunsaturated fatty acids in dogs with naturally developing chronic renal failure. J Am Vet Med Assoc 1999;215:1588–91.

[31] Brown SA. Dietary lipid composition alters the chronic course of canine renal disease. 1996.

[32] Brown SA, Finco DR, Brown CA. Is there a role for dietary polyunsaturated fatty acid supplementation in canine renal disease? J Nutr 1998;128:2765S–7S.

[33] Brown SA, Brown CA, Crowell WA, et al. Beneficial effects of chronic administration of dietary omega-3 polyunsaturated fatty acids in dogs with renal insufficiency. J Lab Clin Med 1998;131:447–55.

[34] Brown SA, Brown CA, Crowell WA, et al. Effects of dietary polyunsaturated fatty acid supplementation in early renal insufficiency in dogs. J Lab Clin Med 2000;135:275–86.

[35] Bauer J, Crocker R, Markwell PJ. Dietary n-6 fatty acid supplementation improves ultrafiltration in spontaneous canine chronic renal disease. J Vet Intern Med 1997;126:126.

[36] Ranganathan N, et al. Probiotics reduce azotemia in Gottingen minipigs. Poster presentation at the 3rd World Congress of Nephrology. Singapore, June 26–30, 2005.

[37] Palmquist R. A preliminary clinical evaluation of Kibow Biotics®, a probiotic agent, on feline azotemia. Journal of American Holistic Veterinary Medical Association 2006;24(4).

[38] Wagner E, Schwendenwein I, Zentek J. Effects of a dietary chitosan and calcium supplement on Ca and P metabolism in cats. Berl Munch Tierarztl Wochenschr 2004;117:310–5.

[39] Locatelli F, Canaud B, Eckardt KU, et al. Oxidative stress in end-stage renal disease: an emerging threat to patient outcome. Nephrol Dial Transplant 2003;18:1272–80.

[40] Cochrane AL, Ricardo SD. Oxidant stress and regulation of chemokines in the development of renal interstitial fibrosis. Contrib Nephrol 2003;139:102–19.

[41] Jackson P, Loughrey CM, Lightbody JH, et al. Effect of hemodialysis on total antioxidant capacity and serum antioxidants in patients with chronic renal failure. Clin Chem 1995;41:1135–8.

[42] Hahn S, Krieg RJ Jr, Hisano S, et al. Vitamin E suppresses oxidative stress and glomerulosclerosis in rat remnant kidney. Pediatr Nephrol 1999;13:195–8.

[43] Hahn S, Kuemmerle NB, Chan W, et al. Glomerulosclerosis in the remnant kidney rat is modulated by dietary alpha-tocopherol. J Am Soc Nephrol 1998;9:2089–95.

[44] Ross SJ, Osborne CA, Polzin DJ, et al. Clinical evaluation of dietary modification for treatment of spontaneous chronic kidney disease in cats. J Am Vet Med Assoc 2006;229:949–57.

Vet Clin Small Anim 36 (2006) 1385–1401

VETERINARY CLINICS
SMALL ANIMAL PRACTICE

Dietary Influences on Periodontal Health in Dogs and Cats

Ellen I. Logan, DVM, PhD[a,b,*]

[a]Hill's Pet Nutrition, PO Box 148, Topeka, KS 66601, USA
[b]Department of Clinical Sciences, Kansas State University, Manhattan, KS 66506, USA

O ral disease is common in dogs and cats, and factors related to oral health are the most common diagnoses in dogs and cats of all age categories. Oral diseases can be subdivided into conditions that affect the tooth, the periodontal apparatus, or other oral tissues. Nutrition, through nutrient composition and kibble esthetics, plays a key role in tooth development, gingival and oral tissue integrity, bone strength, and the prevention and management of oral and dental diseases. Periodontal disease is the principal cause of tooth loss in dogs and cats and is the focus of this article. The major oral health success story of the past 50 years is that periodontal disease can be prevented by a combination of individual and professional measures.

ORAL ANATOMY AND FUNCTION

Wild canids and felids depend on teeth for survival. Loss of teeth results in an inability of the animal to catch and prepare food and to defend itself. Although domesticated pets need not rely on capturing prey for survival, teeth serve a variety of functions and are important in eating, grooming, defense, and behavior. Different teeth provide different functions in dogs and cats. The incisor teeth are used for grasping and nibbling. The canine teeth are used for capturing and puncturing prey. The premolar and molar teeth are used for shearing, grinding, and chewing. The carnassial teeth, designated as the upper fourth premolar and the lower first molar, are the teeth primarily used for chewing [1].

Although the teeth of dogs and cats vary in size, shape, and function, the components and structure of all teeth are similar. A normal mature tooth has a crown and one to three roots. The junction of the crown and the root is termed the *cementoenamel junction* (CEJ). The crown is the portion of the tooth above the CEJ and is covered by dense smooth enamel.

The root or roots are the portion of the tooth below the CEJ and serve to anchor the tooth in the alveolar bone as well as to provide the neurovascular

*Hills Pet Nutrition, PO Box 148, Topeka, KS 66601. E-mail address: ellen_logan@hillspet.com

0195-5616/06/$ – see front matter
doi:10.1016/j.cvsm.2006.09.002

port (apical delta). A thin layer of cementum, the calcified structure in which the periodontal fibers are embedded, covers the root.

The dentin underlies the enamel and the cementum. Dentin is primarily collagen and inorganic hydroxyapatite. There are three types of dentin: primary, secondary, and tertiary. Primary dentin is present during formation of deciduous and permanent teeth. As the animal ages, primary dentin is replaced continuously by secondary dentin. Tertiary dentin is laid down as a reparative substance—a response by odontoblasts to trauma or excessive wear. The internal layer of the tooth, the pulp cavity, contains blood and lymphatic vessels, nerves, and odontoblasts supported in a connective tissue matrix. The tissues that support and protect the tooth comprise the periodontium, including the gingiva, periodontal ligament, cementum, and alveolar bone [2].

The gingiva is an extension of the oral mucosa and consists of keratinized epithelial tissue that attaches to the alveolar process and extends to the neck of the tooth. The gingivae are divided into the attached gingiva and the free gingiva. Normal attached gingiva extends from the mucogingival line to the CEJ. Normal free gingiva surrounds the neck of the tooth without attachment. The coronal edge of the free gingiva is termed the *marginal gingiva*. The space between the free gingiva and the tooth surface is the gingival sulcus or crevice [3].

The periodontal ligament is composed of collagenous connective tissue fibers that attach the teeth to the alveolar bone. The periodontal ligament acts as a cushion, allowing slight movement of teeth during mastication to prevent trauma to teeth from occlusal and root-to-alveolar bone contact.

Thin dense alveolar bone lines the tooth socket (lamina dura) and surrounds the root, providing attachment for the periodontal ligament and passage of blood and lymphatic vessels. Alveolar bone is surrounded and supported by trabecular and compact bone, which varies in thickness depending on the anatomic location. The alveolar process is a relatively active tissue that responds to external forces and systemic influences by resorption and remodeling [4].

DENTAL FORMULAS

Dogs and cats are diphyodont, erupting two dentitions termed *deciduous* (primary or baby) teeth and *permanent* teeth. Deciduous teeth begin erupting at approximately 3 weeks of age in dogs and cats. Breed, environment, nutrition, hormones, and season may influence eruption times.

Puppies have 28 teeth, and adult dogs have 42 teeth. Normal dental formulas for dogs are as follows [5]: deciduous: 2 (I3/3, C1/1, and P3/3) and permanent: 2 (I3/3, C1/1, P4/4, and M2/3).

Kittens have 26 teeth, and adult cats have 30 teeth. Normal dental formulas for cats are as follows: deciduous: 2 (I3/3, C1/1, and P3/2) and permanent: 2 (I3/3, C1/1, P3/2, and M1/1).

Dental formulas represent teeth that should normally be present in all dogs and cats. Anatomically, the maxillary first premolars and the mandibular first and second premolars are absent in cats. Thus, feline premolars are identified as the maxillary second, third, and fourth premolars and the mandibular third and fourth premolars [6,7].

Individual dogs and cats may have abnormal numbers of teeth. Oligodontia and supernumerary teeth occur commonly in dogs and less frequently in cats. Missing teeth may predispose to soft tissue trauma from occluding teeth and may reduce the effect of oral cleansing, particularly in the carnassial area. Extra teeth may lead to overcrowding, which affects anatomic positioning and may increase plaque retention, decrease effectiveness of dietary cleansing, and require more aggressive oral hygiene to maintain gingival health.

NUTRITION AND TOOTH DEVELOPMENT

Puppies and kittens are born edentulous; however, the nutrition that the bitch or queen receives during gestation and lactation is critical to tooth development in the offspring. Maternal nutrients must supply the pre-eruptive teeth with the appropriate building blocks for proper development and formation. After eruption, nutrient intake continues to affect tooth development and mineralization, enamel strength, and the eruption patterns of remaining teeth. Local nutritional effects influence bacterial composition and dental substrate accumulation. Throughout life, nutritional intake and dietary form affect tooth, bone, and mucosal integrity; resistance to infection; and tooth longevity. Food texture and nutritional composition can affect the oral environment through maintenance of tissue integrity, metabolism of plaque bacteria, stimulation of salivary flow, salivary composition, and contact with tooth and oral surfaces.

NUTRITION AND PERIODONTAL DISEASE

Etiopathogenesis

As the gateway to the body, the mouth is challenged by a constant barrage of invaders—bacteria, viruses, parasites, and fungi. Periodontal diseases are infections caused by bacteria in the biofilm (dental plaque) that forms on oral surfaces. Periodontal disease occurs in all mammals and is a common and potentially serious condition. Periodontal disease has been observed in adult dogs and cats of various breeds and ages. Surveys representing data from several countries report prevalence rates of periodontal disease that range from 60% to more than 80% of dogs and cats examined [8–20]. As early as 1899, Eugene Talbot [114] described "interstitial gingivitis or so-called pyorrhea alveolaris" found in dogs at necropsy. A decade later, Lund and colleagues [21] reported that dental calculus and gingivitis were the most commonly diagnosed disorders in an epidemiologic survey of 31,484 dogs and 15,226 cats across 54 veterinary practices in the United States. It is commonly reported that most adult dogs and cats older than the age of 5 years demonstrate some degree of periodontitis. Perhaps more relevant is the statement that all dogs and cats need preventive or therapeutic periodontal care.

Periodontal diseases comprise a variety of conditions affecting the health of the periodontium, the tissues that surround and support the tooth. Periodontal disease commonly refers to gingivitis and periodontitis. Gingivitis is the reversible stage of periodontal disease and can be appropriately treated and largely prevented with thorough plaque removal and effective supragingival plaque control. Periodontitis is more severe and requires advanced therapy and meticulous plaque control to prevent progression of the disease. Periodontal disease is a "silent" disease, often progressing without overt clinical signs to the pet or the pet owner. Left untreated, periodontal disease leads to oral pain and dysfunction and eventual tooth loss. The discomfort and effect on tooth function associated with the disease may lead to many behavior changes, ranging from changes in eating habits to general behavioral changes, such as reluctance to groom and socialization or subtle signs of "depression." Emerging evidence in people and in dogs supports the critical relation between oral health and systemic health. In people, an association has been demonstrated between periodontal diseases and diabetes, cardiovascular disease, stroke, and adverse pregnancy outcomes [22–25]. In dogs, it has been reported that increased periodontal disease severity is positively correlated with histopathologic changes in the myocardium and renal interstitium [26]. It is often reported that pets "act younger" or are "more energetic" after periodontal therapy. Periodontal disease may not be considered immediately life threatening; however, there are clinically significant effects that warrant preventive and therapeutic care.

There are many risk factors associated with the prevalence and severity of periodontal disease. The primary cause results from bacterial colonization and subsequent inflammation and infection. Several materials accumulate on tooth surfaces and participate in the pathophysiology of dental and periodontal disease. These substances are commonly referred to as tooth-accumulated materials or dental substrates and include enamel pellicle, plaque, materia alba, calculus, and stain. These substrates accumulate in a dynamic process, and the influence of nutrition and diet for maintaining oral health is best understood by appreciating this continuum of periodontal disease.

Enamel pellicle is a thin film or cuticle composed of proteins and glycoproteins deposited from salivary and gingival crevicular fluids. Pellicle begins formation immediately on a cleaned tooth surface and initially provides a protective and lubricating layer. Studies have demonstrated that within minutes after polishing, approximately 1 million organisms are deposited per square millimeter of enamel surface [27]. As pellicle ages, modifications occur and additional bacterial components are incorporated, which provides a framework for bacterial colonization. The bacteria colonizing the mouth are known as the oral flora. They form a complex community that adheres to tooth surfaces in a gelatinous mat, or biofilm, commonly called dental plaque. Aggregates of bacteria combine with salivary glycoproteins, extracellular polysaccharides, and occasional epithelial and inflammatory cells to form a soft adherent plaque that covers tooth surfaces. Plaque deposits begin within 24 hours of a prophylaxis procedure. Dental plaque is a biofilm and has a specific microbial composition and structure that changes with time [28]. Supragingival plaque and subgingival plaque are distinct compositional masses that influence the inflammatory reaction of gingival tissues. There is an organized progression of microbial colonization and growth that leads to the development of mature pathogenic dental plaque. Hundreds of bacterial species have been identified in normal and infected mouths of dogs and cats [29]. Supragingival plaque, which forms above and along the gingival margin, is composed primarily of gram-positive aerobic organisms. Growth and maturation of supragingival plaque is necessary for subsequent colonization of subgingival plaque [30]. Subgingival plaque, which forms within the gingival sulcus, is composed of gram-negative anaerobic organisms. The inflammation and destruction that accompany periodontal disease result from the direct action of bacteria and their byproducts on periodontal tissues as well as from the indirect activation of the host immune response. Bacterial plaque is the most important substrate in the development of periodontal disease [31–33]. Other soft accumulations, termed *material alba*, occur on and between the teeth and do not demonstrate the organized structure or the adherence of dental plaque. Materia alba is a soft mixture of salivary proteins, bacteria, desquamated epithelial cells, and leukocyte fragments. Additionally, dogs and cats (particularly dogs) are prone to deposition of oral debris, including impacted hair, food, and foreign materials related to chewing behaviors. Any foreign body impacted in the oral tissues provides a nidus for bacterial accumulation and incites an inflammatory reaction by the host.

Dental calculus, or tartar, is a hard mineralized shell of plaque. Existing plaque is exposed to salivary and crevicular calcium and phosphate ions and undergoes mineralization. Calculus can occur within 48 hours of plaque deposition and is also located supragingivally and subgingivally. Calculus formation is influenced by the alkalinity of the oral environment and dietary composition [34]. It has been reported that in the presence of plaque control, calculus deposits are primarily cosmetic. Although plaque bacteria are the primary cause of periodontal disease, calculus has a contributory role because of its roughened surface, which enhances bacterial attachment and further plaque development and also irritates gingival tissues. Dental stain refers to a discoloration of the tooth surface and may be extrinsic, which is discoloration of any of the previously described substrates, or intrinsic, which is discoloration of dentin or enamel because of some influence during tooth development or posteruption injury. Dietary factors and chewing behaviors may affect dental stain. Stain is nonpathologic but is often a key signal to the pet owner of a tooth abnormality.

Bacterial-laden plaque induces inflammation in adjacent gingival tissues. Without plaque removal or control, gingivitis progresses in severity and local changes occur, allowing subsequent bacterial colonization of subgingival sites. Inflammatory mediators damage the integrity of the gingival margin and sulcular epithelium, allowing further infiltration of bacteria. The immune response of the host attempts to localize the invasion of the periodontal tissues; the result may be further destruction of local tissues because of cytokines released from inflammatory cells [35–37]. Although progression and severity are dependent on a variety of factors, periodontal disease, left untreated, leads to increased destruction of the periodontal apparatus, resulting in tooth mobility and eventual tooth loss.

Nutrients

Nutritional factors have the potential to affect all the various oral tissues during development, maturation, and maintenance. Mature enamel is a static tissue, but nutrition may affect its growth and maturation. The periodontal apparatus surrounds, protects, and supports teeth. Any negative influences affecting these structures may progress to tooth mobility and exfoliation. Oral mucosa has a high turnover rate; adequate nutrition is necessary to maintain tissue integrity. Table 1 provides general nutrient guidelines for foods designed to prevent periodontal disease.

The role of nutrients in periodontal disease is a topic that has not received extensive or recent attention in human or veterinary medicine. Periodontal disease develops slowly, and it is likely that studies investigating the influence of nutrients on various components of periodontal disease do not reflect lifetime nutritional status. Although the amount of available information is small and dated, the following information reviews specific nutrients of concern in the occurrence and management of periodontal disease.

Specific nutrients that have been investigated, at least in part, include water, protein, soluble carbohydrates, fiber, minerals, and vitamins. Most commercial foods provide adequate levels of nutrients to prevent deficiency diseases provided that the food meets levels recommended by the Association of American Feed Control Officials (AAFCO) and adequate amounts are fed to meet daily energy requirements [38,39].

PROTEIN

Protein deficiencies cause degenerative changes in the periodontium, specifically the gingivae, periodontal ligament, and alveolar bone in laboratory animals [40]. In 1962, Ruben and coworkers [41] investigated the effects of a soft-consistency protein-deficient food on the periodontium of 22 dogs over a 1-year period. Results included inflammatory and dystrophic changes in the gingivae, periodontal ligament, and alveolar bone. The study did not

Table 1
Key nutritional factors in foods designed to promote dental health

Nutritional factor	Adult dogs	Adult cats
Protein[a]	16%–35%	30%–50%
Digestibility	>80%	>80%
Calcium[a]	0.5%–1.5%	0.5%–1.5%
Phosphorus[a]	0.4%–1.3%	0.4%–1.3%
Texture	Fiber	Fiber
Kibble size	Increased	Increased

[a]Avoid deficiency or excess.

quantify the individual effects of food consistency and protein content. Protein deficiency, however, occurs rarely in dogs and cats and is not a practical consideration as a typical cause of periodontal disease in these species.

The role of soluble carbohydrates (sugars) in the development of dental caries has been well documented in people and rodents [42]. Dental caries, however, occurs infrequently in dogs and cats. One study demonstrated that dogs do not develop carious lesions even after long periods of consuming carbohydrate-rich foods [43]. Carlsson and Egelberg [44] reported that the addition of sucrose to a soft food resulted in no difference in plaque accumulation and gingival inflammation in a group of 12 mongrel dogs. Human studies have demonstrated that larger amounts of plaque were formed when sucrose was the primary sugar consumed [45,46]. Commercial and homemade pet foods typically contain large quantities of soluble carbohydrates, usually in the form of starch.

Fiber-containing foods have long been viewed as "nature's toothbrush." It is theorized that fibrous foods (1) exercise the gums, (2) promote gingival keratinization, and (3) clean the teeth. Fiber in foods, especially as it relates to texture, has been shown to affect plaque and calculus accumulation and gingival health in dogs and cats and is discussed in this article in relation to maintaining periodontal health [47–49].

MINERALS

Foods deficient in calcium and excessive in phosphorus may lead to secondary nutritional hyperparathyroidism and significant loss of alveolar bone [50,51].

Experiments in dogs have demonstrated resorption of alveolar bone after consumption of a low-calcium high-phosphorus food [52]. It has been proposed that periodontal disease results from a nutritional deficiency of calcium, an excess of phosphorus, or both [53,54]. Svanberg and colleagues [55] reported that nutritional secondary hyperparathyroidism occurred in a group of Beagles fed a food deficient in calcium. The food did not have any effect on the initiation or rate of progression of periodontal disease when compared with findings in a control group fed a nutritionally adequate food. Although secondary nutritional hyperparathyroidism may contribute to bone loss, and thus affect the progression of periodontal disease, there is little evidence to support the theory that it is the primary cause. Calcium deficiency is essentially unheard of in dogs and cats that consume commercial pet foods containing calcium levels that meet AAFCO allowances.

A more realistic concern is the excessive levels of calcium and phosphorus present in many commercial pet foods. High levels of calcium and phosphorus are calculogenic in rats [56]. In people, the plaque deposits of heavy calculus formers contain significantly higher levels of calcium and phosphorus compared with deposits of slow calculus formers. Further research to define the role of dietary calcium and phosphorus is warranted; however, the role that these minerals have in calculus formation should be kept in mind when recommending a food as part of an oral care regimen.

Polyphosphates, such as hexametaphosphate (HMP), are sequestrants that bind salivary calcium, making it unavailable for incorporation into the plaque biofilm to form calculus [57,58]. HMP is delivered as a coating on various treats, dental chews, and foods. The purported benefits of polyphosphates are that they are released during chewing and remain in the oral cavity for prolonged periods. It has been demonstrated that the addition of HMP to the surface of baked biscuit treats, rawhide chews, and dry foods results in reduced calculus accumulation [57,59,60]. There is also evidence to support no significant differences in plaque or calculus accumulation in dogs fed dry foods plus HMP-coated biscuits [61]. Polyphosphates have no known direct effect on oral microflora populations or plaque accumulation, and an effective plaque control regimen should always be the primary recommendation for prevention or post-therapeutic care of periodontal disease. Zinc ascorbate, zinc gluconate, and other soluble zinc salts are found in a variety of oral cleansing gels, rinses, and denti-frices and have been reported to help control plaque accumulation because of their antimicrobial activity [62,63].

VITAMINS

Vitamins that have been studied in relation to periodontal disease include vitamins A, B, C, and D. Deficiencies in vitamin A have been reported to cause marginal gingivitis, gingival hypoplasia, and resorption of alveolar bone [64]. B-complex vitamin (including folic acid, niacin, pantothenic acid, and riboflavin) deficiencies have been associated with gingival inflammation, epithelial necrosis, and resorption of alveolar bone [65]. Vitamin C plays a key role in collagen synthesis. Ascorbic acid deficiencies have been reported to affect periodontal tissues adversely in people [66]. Vitamin D helps to regulate serum calcium concentrations. Vitamin D deficiencies affect calcium homeostasis and reportedly affect the gingivae, periodontal ligament, and alveolar bone [67]. Almost all commercial pet foods contain adequate levels of these vitamins. Furthermore, cats and dogs do not have a dietary vitamin C requirement because it is synthesized within the liver.

SUPPLEMENTAL INGREDIENTS

There are a variety of supplemental ingredients that have purported antibacterial or anti-inflammatory characteristics, and there are a variety of oral rinses, sprays, and additives marketed for use in pets. Many of these agents have demonstrated variable efficacy in reducing plaque bacteria and gingival inflammation when used as oral hygiene aids in people; however, comparable studies in pets are lacking. Dietary antioxidants have been reported to have beneficial effects in people with chronic inflammatory periodontal disease [68,69]. Essential oils, such as thymol, eugenol, menthol, and eucalyptol, have demonstrated efficacy in reducing plaque and gingival inflammation in human beings [70]. Chlorhexidine gluconate, a cationic bisbiguanide, has been shown to be effective in reducing plaque accumulation and gingival inflammation [71–77]. One study in dogs evaluated the addition of chlorhexidine to a dental hygiene chew and demonstrated no significant difference in gingivitis or calculus accumulation but did report a significant reduction in plaque accumulation [78]. Xylitol, a sugar alcohol, has been associated with reduced salivary bacterial count and plaque accumulation in people [79]. Polyphenols and herbals, such as green tea, magnolol, and honokiol, have been evaluated for antimicrobial activity against caries and periodontal pathogens in people [80]. The evidence for efficacy as part of a nutritional regimen for these supplemental ingredients is lacking in dogs and cats. It is important to evaluate critically whether the addition of these agents is at a level that is safe and efficacious to provide the needed dental benefit and support the marketed claim or if the ingredients are added primarily as label dressing.

FOOD TEXTURE

Food texture and composition can directly affect the oral environment through (1) maintenance of tissue integrity, (2) alteration of the metabolism of plaque bacteria, (3) stimulation of salivary flow, and (4) cleansing of tooth and oral surfaces by appropriate physical contact. The physical consistency, or texture, of foods has long been thought to affect the oral health of dogs and cats. Historically, several studies have demonstrated that animals eating soft foods develop more plaque and gingivitis than animals fed fibrous foods [81,82]. The studies traditionally cited to substantiate those claims are old reports that used small numbers of animals, had varying evaluation methods, and did not report data analysis, making study comparison difficult. It has been considered conventional wisdom that typical dry crunchy commercial foods provide a dental benefit to cats and dogs. Many of the recommendations made about the effect of food texture on oral health are unsubstantiated, and several have turned out to be untrue when exposed to rigorous study. Although consumption of soft foods may promote plaque accumulation, the general belief that dry foods provide significant oral cleansing should be regarded with skepticism. It has been reported that a canned food performed similar to a dry food in the degree of plaque and calculus accumulation in dogs (Table 2) [83]. A large epidemiologic survey reported that in dogs, consumption of dry food alone did not consistently demonstrate improved periodontal health [84]. Plain baked biscuits have long been considered to have dental benefits. Studies in dogs have shown that plain baked biscuit treats provide little additional plaque and calculus reduction when compared with feeding dry dog food alone [82]. More recent research has clearly demonstrated that pet foods

Table 2
Comparison of moist versus dry foods on dental substrate accumulation in dogs

	Plaque index	Calculus index	Stain index
Canned A	10.12	6.28	4.37
Canned B	9.77	7.82	5.30
Dry A	10.19	6.90	5.63

can be specifically formulated and processed to provide an effective means of plaque and calculus control (Fig. 1) [89].

Many dry treats and chew aids have offered dental claims for many years, such as "promotes clean teeth, fresh breath, and healthy gums," "cleans teeth, freshens breath," or "scrubs away tartar buildup to help clean teeth and freshens breath." The AAFCO supports and recommends guidelines developed by the Center for Veterinary Medicine (CVM) of the US Food and Drug Administration for dental health claims [85]. These guidelines state that food products bearing claims to cleanse, freshen, or whiten teeth by virtue of their abrasive or mechanical action are not objectionable. Food products bearing claims for plaque or calculus reduction or for prevention or control of breath odor may be misbranded. Enforcement is a low priority for CVM and state regulatory agencies if these claims are made only with respect to the product's abrasive action, however. This has led to a wide availability of products that make some type of plaque or calculus control claim with little or no evidence to document their effectiveness. There is no single system for establishing quality evidence supporting dental claims. One method of recognizing effective products is through identification of the Veterinary Oral Health Council (VOHC) seal of acceptance. The VOHC recognizes products with proven efficacy for mechanical control of plaque or mechanical or chemical control of calculus through a data review system. Products approved by VOHC can display the VOHC seal for tartar control or plaque control on packaging and promotional materials. More information about the VOHC and a listing of products that carry the VOHC seal is available through the VOHC web site [86,87].

DENTAL FOODS

Most dogs and cats eat something everyday; thus, use of foods that provide dental benefits seems appropriate. Food texture can be an effective means of controlling dental plaque and, ultimately, periodontal disease. As a tooth penetrates a typical kibble or biscuit, the initial contact causes the food to shatter

Oral health 25 weeks post-prophylaxis

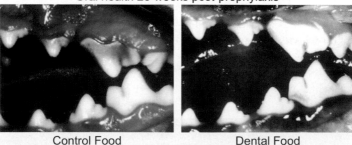

Control Food   Dental Food

Fig. 1. Comparison of dental plaque and tartar in dogs fed a control food (Purina Dog Chow, Ralston Purina Co.) compared with a dental food (Prescription t/d Canine, Hill's Pet Nutrition, Inc.) for 6 months after dental prophylaxis. Note the extensive accumulation of plaque, tartar, and gingivitis in the oral cavity of dogs fed a control diet.

and crumble with contact only at the coronal tip of the tooth surface. To provide effective mechanical cleansing, a food should promote chewing and maintain contact with the tooth surface.

Several complete and balanced adult pet foods are available that provide significant oral cleansing compared with typical dry, moist, or snack foods. The mechanism of action for these dental foods is based on the enhanced textural characteristics and kibble size that provide mechanical cleansing of the teeth. Combining increased fiber content with a size and pattern (texture) that promotes chewing and maximizes contact with teeth is critical to obtaining a dental benefit. Numerous short-term and long-term (6-month) studies have demonstrated that dental foods with enhanced textural characteristics provide significant plaque, calculus, and stain control in cats and dogs when used after dental prophylaxis [88–95].

NATURAL DIETS

Early literature reported that the natural diets of wild canids and felids had a plaque-retardant effect and that those wild canids and felids were not afflicted with the generalized form of periodontal disease seen in domesticated pets [96]. Pet food commercialization is often implicated as a contributing factor to the increased prevalence and severity of periodontal disease in domestic dogs and cats [97]. There are no published data that compare controlled populations of domestic dogs or cats consuming a natural diet with those consuming a commercial food. Reports have demonstrated that dogs and cats fed a natural diet had varying signs of periodontal disease as well as a high rate of tooth fractures [98–100]. Anecdotal reports suggest that feeding raw meaty bones improves oral health in cats and dogs [101]. Several potential health problems exist with feeding raw foods to cats and dogs, including increased dental fractures (Fig. 2) and nutritional and public health concerns associated with exposure to bacterial pathogens [102–106].

DENTAL TREATS AND CHEW AIDS

Studies suggest that dental treats and chew aids can be used as an adjunct to other dental home care techniques. It has been reported that dogs with access to chewing materials had less calculus accumulation, gingivitis, and periodontitis than those without any enhanced chewing activity. The study did not

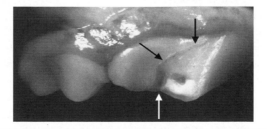

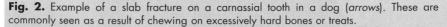

Fig. 2. Example of a slab fracture on a carnassial tooth in a dog (*arrows*). These are commonly seen as a result of chewing on excessively hard bones or treats.

measure how often or how long dogs chewed on their respective materials, however [107]. Consumption of cartilaginous materials, rawhide chew strips, and dental hygiene chews has been reported to reduce plaque and calculus accumulation and gingival inflammation [108]. Some veterinary dentists have expressed concern that hard dental treats may increase the risk for dental fractures (see **Fig. 2**) [109], whereas anecdotal reports of esophageal and intestinal obstruction have been associated with compressed vegetable protein chews.

DENTAL HOME CARE

Oral health is achieved through a combination of professional periodontal care as well as appropriate and effective client-provided dental home care. The primary goal of dental home care is effective plaque control that maintains oral hygiene and prevents the development of gingivitis and periodontal disease [110]. Appropriate home care recommendations that address the degree of oral pathologic change present and the ability of the client to provide frequent oral hygiene are critical. The key to effective home treatment is compliance. Compliance is a significant issue in veterinary medicine. A comprehensive study of compliance revealed that in the approximately 15.5 million dogs and cats with stage 2, 3, or 4 periodontal diseases, appropriate care was not received [111]. Reported compliance through pet owner surveys indicated that compliance with dental home care recommendations is 30% to 50% [112]. Although mechanical cleansing through frequent tooth brushing is an effective means of plaque control, compliance remains an issue. The simpler the required behavior, the more likely it is to be performed. If the complexity of the pet owner behavioral response is high, it is likely that the long-term effective compliance rate is going to be low [113]. These findings, coupled with evidence-based research, support the use of dental foods with textural characteristics as an appropriate effective means of daily plaque control and gingival health maintenance in dogs and cats.

SUMMARY

A pet cannot be healthy without oral health. Periodontal disease is a significant disease that has local and systemic ramifications. It has been stated earlier that effective plaque control prevents gingivitis. In human beings, 90% of periodontitis occurs as the result of progression of gingivitis, and this type of periodontitis can be completely prevented by plaque control. It is reasonable that dogs and cats react similarly and that effective plaque control could prevent a large percentage of periodontitis cases. Proper nutrition and effective oral hygiene are necessary components of oral health and should be jointly promoted in the management of oral disease in dogs and cats.

References

[1] Harvey CE. Function and formation of the oral cavity. In: Veterinary dentistry. Philadelphia: WB Saunders; 1985. p. 5–22.

[2] Grove TK. Periodontal disease. In: Harvey CE, editor. Veterinary dentistry. Philadelphia: WB Saunders; 1985. p. 59–78.

[3] Löe H, Listgarten MA, Terranova VP. The gingiva. In: Genco RJ, Goldman HM, Cohen DW, editors. Contemporary periodontics. St. Louis (MO): CV Mosby; 1990. p. 3–32.

[4] Terranova VP, Goldman HM, Listgarten MA. The periodontal attachment apparatus. In: Genco RJ, Goldman HM, Cohen DW, editors. Contemporary periodontics. St. Louis (MO): CV Mosby; 1990. p. 33–54.

[5] Hale FA. Juvenile veterinary dentistry. Vet Clin North Am Small Anim Pract 2005;35: 789–817.

[6] Colyer F. Variation in number, size and shape. In: Miles AEW, Grigson C, editors. Variations and diseases of the teeth of animals. New York: Cambridge University Press; 1990. p. 62–4.

[7] Gioso MA, Carvalho VGG. Oral anatomy of the dog and cat in veterinary dentistry practice. Vet Clin North Am Small Anim Pract 2005;35:763–80.

[8] Gray H. Pyorrhoea in the dog. Vet Rec 1923;10:167–9.

[9] Bell AF. Dental disease in the dog. J Small Anim Pract 1965;6:421–8.

[10] Rosenberg HM, Rehfeld CE, Emmering TE. A method for the epidemiologic assessment of periodontal health-disease state in a beagle hound colony. J Periodontol 1966;37: 208–13.

[11] Saxe SR, Greene JC, Bohann HM, et al. Oral debris, calculus and periodontal disease in the beagle dog. Periodontics 1967;5:217–25.

[12] Gad T. Periodontal disease in dogs. J Periodont Res 1968;3:268–72.

[13] Hamp SV, Viklands P, Farso-Madsen K, et al. Prevalence of periodontal disease in dogs [abstract]. J Dent Res 1975;(SIA):19.

[14] Hamp SV, Lindberg R. Histopathology of spontaneous periodontitis in dogs. J Periodont Res 1971;6:266–77.

[15] Sorensen WP, Löe H, Ramfjord SP. Periodontal disease in the beagle dog. J Periodont Res 1980;15:380–9.

[16] Page RC, Schroeder HE. Spontaneous chronic periodontitis in adult dogs. J Periodontol 1979;52:60–73.

[17] Golden AL, Stoller N, Harvey CE. A survey of oral and dental diseases in dogs anesthetized at a veterinary hospital. J Am Anim Hosp Assoc 1982;18:891–9.

[18] Reichart PA, Dürr UM, Triadan H, et al. Periodontal disease in the domestic cat. J Periodont Res 1984;19:67–75.

[19] Isogai H, Isogai E, Okamoto H, et al. Epidemiological study on periodontal diseases and some other dental disorders in dogs. Jpn J Vet Sci 1989;51:1151–62.

[20] Hoffman TH, Gaengler P. Epidemiology of periodontal disease in poodles. J Small Anim Pract 1996;37:309–16.

[21] Lund EM, Armstrong PJ, Kirk CA, et al. Health status and population characteristics of dogs and cats examined at private veterinary practices in the United States. J Am Vet Med Assoc 1999;214:1336–41.

[22] Beck JD, Offenbacher S. The association between periodontal diseases and cardiovascular diseases: a state-of-the-science review. Ann Periodontol 2001;6(1):9–15.

[23] Soskolne WA, Klinger A. The relationship between periodontal diseases and diabetes: an overview. Ann Periodontol 2001;6(1):91–8.

[24] Jeffcoat MK, Geurs NC, Reddy MS, et al. Current evidence regarding periodontal disease as a risk factor in preterm birth. Ann Periodontol 2001;6(1):183–8.

[25] DeBowes LJ. The effects of dental disease on systemic disease. Vet Clin North Am Small Anim Pract 1998;28(5):1057–62.

[26] DeBowes LJ, Mosier D, Logan EI, et al. Association of periodontal disease and histologic lesions in multiple organs from 45 dogs. J Vet Dent 1996;13:57–60.

[27] Lindhe J. Pathogenesis of plaque-associated periodontal disease. In: Textbook of clinical periodontology. 2nd edition. Copenhagen (Denmark): WB Saunders; 1989. p. 189–205.

[28] DuPont G. Understanding plaque: biofilm dynamics. J Vet Dent 1997;14:91–4.

[29] Harvey CE, Thornsberry C, Miller BR. Subgingival bacteria—comparison of culture results in dogs and cats with gingivitis. J Vet Dent 1995;12:147–50.

[30] Kornman KS. The role of supragingival plaque in the prevention and treatment of periodontal diseases. J Periodont Res 1986;5–22.

[31] Fedi PF. Etiology of periodontal disease. In: The periodontic syllabus. Philadelphia: Lea & Febiger; 1985. p. 13–8.

[32] Logan EI, Wiggs RB, Zetner K, et al. Dental disease. In: Hand MS, Thatcher CD, Remillard RL, et al, editors. Small animal clinical nutrition. 4th edition. Topeka (KS): Mark Morris Institute; 2000. p. 475–92.

[33] Harvey CE. Management of periodontal disease: understanding the options. Vet Clin North Am Small Anim Pract 2005;35(4):819–36.

[34] Loux JJ, Alioto R, Yankell SL. Effects of glucose and urea on dental deposit pH in dogs. J Dent Res 1972;51:1610–3.

[35] Fedi PF. Etiology of periodontal disease. In: The periodontic syllabus. Philadelphia: Lea & Febiger; 1985. p. 13–8.

[36] Genco RJ. Pathogenesis and host responses in periodontal disease. In: Genco RJ, Goldman HM, Cohen DW, editors. Contemporary periodontics. St. Louis (MO): CV Mosby; 1990. p. 184–93.

[37] DeBowes LJ. Dentistry: periodontal aspects. In: Ettinger SJ, Feldman EC, editors. Textbook of veterinary internal medicine. 5th edition. Philadelphia: WB Saunders; 2000. p. 1127–34.

[38] Association of American Feed Control Officials. Official publication. 2004. p. 126–7.

[39] Dzanis DA. The AAFCO dog and cat food nutrient profiles. In: Bonagura JD, editor. Current veterinary therapy XII. Philadelphia: WB Saunders; 1995. p. 1418–21.

[40] Chawla TN, Glickman I. Protein deprivation and the periodontal structures of the albino rat. Oral Surg Oral Med Oral Pathol 1951;4:578–602.

[41] Ruben MP, McCoy J, Person P, et al. Effects of soft dietary consistency and protein deprivation on the periodontium of the dog. Oral Surg Oral Med Oral Pathol 1962;15:1061–70.

[42] DePaola D, Faine MP, Vogel RI. Nutrition in relation to dental medicine. In: Shils ME, Olson JA, Shike M, editors. Modern nutrition in health and disease. 8th edition. Philadelphia: Lea & Febiger; 1994. p. 1007–28.

[43] Lewis TM. Resistance of dogs to dental caries: a two-year study. J Dent Res 1965;44:1354–7.

[44] Carlsson J, Egelberg J. Local effect of diet on plaque formation and development of gingivitis in dogs. II. Effect of high carbohydrate versus high protein-fat diets. Odontologisk Revy 1965;16:42–9.

[45] Carlsson J, Egelberg J. Effect of diet on early plaque formation in man. Odontologisk Revy 1965;16:112–25.

[46] Makinen KK, Scheinin A. Turku sugar studies VII; principal biochemical findings on whole saliva and plaque. Acta Odontol Scand 1975;33:129–71.

[47] Watson ADJ. Diet and periodontal disease in dogs and cats. Aust Vet J 1994;71:313–8.

[48] Boyce EN, Logan EI. Oral health assessment in dogs: study design and results. J Vet Dent 1994;11:64–74.

[49] Logan EI, Finney O, Hefferren JJ. Effects of a dental food on plaque accumulation and gingival health in dogs. J Vet Dent 2002;19:15–8.

[50] Bawden JW, Anderson JJB, Garner SC. Calcium and phosphorus nutrition in health and disease: Dental tissues. In: Wolinsky I, Hickson JF, editors. Modern nutrition. Boca Raton (FL): CRC Press; 1995. p. 119–26.

[51] Becks H, Weber M. The influence of diet on the bone system with special reference to the alveolar process and labyrinthine capsule. J Am Dent Assoc 1931;18:197–264.

[52] Henrikson PA. Periodontal disease and calcium deficiency. An experimental study in the dog. Acta Odontol Scand 1968;26(Suppl 50):1–132.

[53] Krook L, Lutwak L, Whalen JP, et al. Human periodontal disease. Morphology and response to calcium therapy. Cornell Vet 1972;62:32–53.

[54] Krook L, Whalen JP, Less GV, et al. Human periodontal disease and osteoporosis. Cornell Vet 1972;62:371–81.

[55] Svanberg G, Lindhe J, Hugoson A, et al. Effect of nutritional hyperparathyroidism on experimental periodontitis in the dog. Scand J Dent Res 1973;81:155–62.

[56] Navia JM. Experimental oral calculus. In: Animal models in dental research. Tuscaloosa (AL): University of Alabama Press; 1977. p. 298–311.

[57] Stookey GK, Warrick JM, Miller LL, et al. Hexametaphosphate-coated snack biscuits significantly reduce calculus formation in dogs. J Vet Dent 1996;13:27–30.

[58] White DJ, Gerlach RW. Anticalculus effects of a novel, dual-phase polyphosphate dentifrice: chemical basis, mechanism and clinical response. J Contemp Dent Pract 2000;1: 1–19.

[59] Stookey GK, Warrick JM, Miller LL. Sodium hexametaphosphate reduces calculus formation in dogs. Am J Vet Res 1995;56:913–8.

[60] Warrick JM, Stookey GK, Inskeep GA, et al. Reducing calculus accumulation in dogs using an innovative rawhide treat system coated with hexametaphosphate. In: Proceedings of the 15th Veterinary Dental Forum; 2001. p. 379–82.

[61] Roudebush P, Logan EI, Hale FA. Evidence-based veterinary dentistry: a systematic review of homecare for prevention of periodontal disease in dogs and cats. J Vet Dent 2005;22(1):6–15.

[62] Clarke DE. Clinical and microbiological effects of oral zinc ascorbate gel in cats. J Vet Dent 2001;18:177–83.

[63] Wolinsky LE, Cuomo J, Quesada K, et al. A comparative pilot study of the effects of a dentifrice containing green tea bioflavonoids, sanguinarine or triclosan on oral bacterial biofilm formation. J Clin Dent 2000;11:535–59.

[64] King JD. Abnormalities in the gingival and subgingival tissues due to diets deficient in vitamin A and carotene. Br Dent J 1940;68:349–60.

[65] Becks H, Wainwright WW, Morgan AF. Comparative study of oral changes in dogs due to deficiencies of pantothenic acid, nicotinic acid and an unknown of the B vitamin complex. Am J Orthodontol Oral Surg 1943;29:183–207.

[66] Ismail AI. Relation between ascorbic acid intake and periodontal disease in the United States. J Am Dent Assoc 1983;107:927–31.

[67] Becks H, Weber M. The influence of diet on the bone system with special reference to the alveolar process and labyrinthine capsule. J Am Dent Assoc 1931;18:197–264.

[68] Battino M, Bullon P, Wilson M, et al. Oxidative injury and inflammatory and periodontal disease: the challenge of antioxidants to free radicals and reactive oxygen species. Crit Rev Oral Biol Med 1999;10:458–76.

[69] Neiva RF, Steigenga J, Al-Shammari KF, et al. Effects of specific nutrients on periodontal disease onset, progression and treatment. J Clin Peridontol 2003;30:579–89.

[70] DePaola LG, Overholser CD, Meiller TF, et al. Chemotherapeutic inhibition of supragingival dental plaque and gingivitis development. J Clin Periodontol 1989;16:311–5.

[71] Lamster IB, Alfano MC, Seiger MC, et al. The effect of Listerine antiseptic on reduction of existing plaque and gingivitis. Clin Prev Dent 1983;5:112–5.

[72] Hamp SE, Emilson CG. Some effects of chlorhexidine on the plaque flora of the beagle dog. J Periodontal Res 1973;12:28–35.

[73] Hull PS, Davis RM. The effect of a chlorhexidine gel on tooth deposits in beagle dogs. J Small Anim Pract 1972;13:207–12.

[74] Hamp SE, Lindhe J, Loe H. Long-term effects of chlorhexidine on developing gingivitis in the beagle dog. J Peridont Res 1973;8:63–70.

[75] Tepe JH, Leonard GJ, Singer RE, et al. The long term effect of chlorhexidine on plaque, gingivitis, sulcul depth, gingival recession and loss of attachment in beagle dogs. J Peridontal Res 1983;18:452–8.

[76] Gruet P, Gaillard C, Boisrame B, et al. Use of an oral antiseptic bioadhesive tablet in dogs. J Vet Dent 1995;12:87–91.

[77] Hennet P. Effectiveness of a dental gel to reduce plaque in beagle dogs. J Vet Dent 2002;19:11–4.

[78] Rawlings JM, Gorrel C, Markwell PJ. Effect on canine oral health of adding chlorhexidine to a dental hygiene chew. J Vet Dent 1998;15(3):129–34.

[79] Jannesson L, Renvert S, Kjellsdotter P, et al. Effect of a triclosan-containing toothpaste supplemented with 10% xylitol on mutans streptococci in saliva and dental plaque. A 6-month clinical study. Caries Res 2002;36:36–9.

[80] Ciancio SG. Chemical agents: plaque control, calculus reduction and treatment of dentin hypersensitivity. In: Periodontology 2000: mechanical and chemical supragingival plaque control. Cambridge (MA): Munksgaard International Publishers Ltd.; 1995. p. 75–86.

[81] Watson ADJ. Diet and periodontal disease in dogs and cats. Aust Vet J 1994;71:313–8.

[82] Logan EI, Wiggs RB, Zetner K, et al. Dental disease. In: Hand MS, Thatcher CD, Remillard RL, et al, editors. Small animal clinical nutrition. 4th edition. Topeka (KS): Mark Morris Institute; 2000. p. 475–92.

[83] Boyce EN, Logan EI. Oral health assessment in dogs: study design and results. J Vet Dent 1994;11:64–74.

[84] Harvey CE, Shofer FS, Laster L. Correlation of diet, other chewing activities and periodontal disease in North American client-owned dogs. J Vet Dent 1996;3:101–5.

[85] Association of American Feed Control Officials. Official publication; 2004.

[86] Veterinary Oral Health Council. Available at: http://www.vohc.org. Accessed March 2006.

[87] Harvey CE. Establishment of a veterinary oral health center proposed to AVMA. J Vet Dent 1995;12:115–7.

[88] Logan EI, Finney O, Heffərren JJ. Effects of a dental food on plaque accumulation and gingival health in dogs. J Vet Dent 2002;19:15–8.

[89] Logan EI. Oral cleansing by dietary means: results of six-month studies. In: Logan EI, Heffernen JJ, editors. Proceedings of the Companion Animal Oral Health Conference. Topeka (KS); 1996. p. 11–5.

[90] Logan EI. Oral cleansing by dietary means: feline methodology and study results. In: Logan EI, Heffernen JJ, editors. Proceedings of the Companion Animal Oral Health Conference. Topeka (KS); 1996. p. 31–4.

[91] Jensen L, Logan EI, Finney O, et al. Reduction in accumulation of plaque, stain and calculus in dogs by dietary means. J Vet Dent 1995;12:161–3.

[92] Cupp CJ, Gerheart LA, Pinnick DV, et al. Reduction of plaque and tartar accumulation in cats and its role in a feline dental health program. In: Friskies product technology center bulletin; 2000.

[93] Boyce EN, Logan EI. Oral health assessment in dogs: study design and results. J Vet Dent 1994;11:64–74.

[94] Boyce EN. Feline experimental models for control of periodontal disease. Vet Clin North Am Small Anim Pract 1992;22:1309–21.

[95] Theyse LFH, Drieling HE, Dijkshoorn NA, et al. A comparative study of 4 dental home care regiments in client owned cats. In: Debraekeleer J, Meyer H, editors. Proceedings of the Hill's European Symposium on Oral Care. Watford, UK; 2003. p. 60–3.

[96] Colyer F. Dental disease in animals. Br Dent J 1947;82:31–5.

[97] Harvey CE, Emily PP. Periodontal disease. In: Ladig D, editor. Small animal dentistry. St. Louis (MO): Mosby–Year Book; 1993. p. 89–144.

[98] Clarke DE. Clinical and microbiological effects of oral zinc ascorbate gel in cats. J Vet Dent 2001;18:177–83.

[99] Robinson JGA, Gorrel C. The oral status of a pack of foxhounds fed a "natural" diet. In: Proceedings of the Fifth World Veterinary Dental Congress; 1997. WVDC. p. 35–7.

[100] DuPont G. Prevention of periodontal disease. Vet Clin North Am Small Anim Pract 1998;28(5):1129–45.

[101] Billinghurst I. Give your dog a bone. Alexandria (Australia): Bridgge Printery; 1993.

[102] Joffe DJ, Schlesinger DP. Preliminary assessment of the risk of *Salmonella* infection in dogs fed raw chicken diets. Can Vet J 2002;43:441–2.

[103] LeJeune JT, Hancock DD. Public health concerns associated with feeding raw meat diets to dogs. J Am Vet Med Assoc 2001;219:1222–5.

[104] Freeman LM, Michel KE. Evaluation of raw food diets for dogs. J Am Vet Med Assoc 2001;218:705–9, 1716.

[105] Miller EP, Cullor JS. Food safety. In: Hand MS, Thatcher CD, Remillard RL, et al, editors. Small animal clinical nutrition. 4th edition. Topeka (KS): Mark Morris Institute; 2000. p. 183–98.

[106] Chengappa MM, Staats J, Oberst RD, et al. Prevalence of *Salmonella* in raw meat used in diets of racing greyhounds. J Vet Diag Invest 1993;5:372–7.

[107] Harvey CE, Shofer FS, Laster L. Correlation of diet, other chewing activities and periodontal disease in North American client owned dogs. J Vet Dent 1996;13:101–5.

[108] Roudebush P, Logan EI, Hale FA. Evidence-based veterinary dentistry: a systematic review of homecare for prevention of periodontal disease in dogs and cats. J Vet Dent 2005; 22(1):6–15.

[109] Hale FA. Home care for the dental patient. In: Debraekeleer J, Meyer H, editors. Proceedings of the Hill's European Symposium on Oral Care. Watford, UK; 2003. p. 50–9.

[110] Hale FA. The owner-animal-environment triad in the treatment of canine periodontal disease. J Vet Dent 2003;20:118–22.

[111] American Animal Hospital Association. The path to high-quality care. Lakewood (CO): American Animal Hospital Association; 2003.

[112] Miller BR, Harvey CE. Compliance with oral hygiene recommendations following periodontal treatment in client-owned dogs. J Vet Dent 1994;11(1):18–9.

[113] Wilson TG Jr. How patient compliance to suggested oral hygiene and maintenance affect periodontal therapy. Dent Clin North Am 1998;42(2):389–403.

[114] Talbot E. Interstitial gingivitis or so-called pyorrhoea alveolaris. Philadelphia: SS White Dental Manufacturing; 1899.

ELSEVIER
SAUNDERS

INDEX

Note: Page numbers of article titles are in **boldface** type.

0195-5616/06/$ – see front matter
doi:10.1016/S0195-5616(06)00128-8

Moving?

Make sure your subscription moves with you!

To notify us of your new address, find your **Clinics Account Number** (located on your mailing label above your name), and contact customer service at:

E-mail: elspcs@elsevier.com

800-654-2452 (subscribers in the U.S. & Canada)
407-345-4000 (subscribers outside of the U.S. & Canada)

Fax number: 407-363-9661

Elsevier Periodicals Customer Service
6277 Sea Harbor Drive
Orlando, FL 32887-4800

*To ensure uninterrupted delivery of your subscription, please notify us at least 4 weeks in advance of move.

ELSEVIER

United States Postal Service
Statement of Ownership, Management, and Circulation

1. Publication Title	2. Publication Number	3. Filing Date
Veterinary Clinics of North America:		
Small Animal Practice	0 0 3 - 1 5 0	9/15/06

4. Issue Frequency	5. Number of Issues Published Annually	6. Annual Subscription Price
Jan, Mar, May, Jul, Sep, Nov	6	$170.00

7. Complete Mailing Address of Known Office of Publication (Not printer) (Street, city, county, state, and ZIP+4)

Contact Person
Sarah Carmichael

Elsevier Inc.
360 Park Avenue South
New York, NY 10010-1710

Telephone
(215) 239-3681

8. Complete Mailing Address of Headquarters or General Business Office of Publisher (Not printer)

Elsevier Inc., 360 Park Avenue South, New York, NY 10010-1710

9. Full Names and Complete Mailing Addresses of Publisher, Editor, and Managing Editor (Do not leave blank)

Publisher (Name and complete mailing address)

John Schrefer, Elsevier Inc., 1600 John F. Kennedy Blvd., Suite 1800, Philadelphia, PA 19103-2899

Editor (Name and complete mailing address)

John Vassallo, Elsevier Inc., 1600 John F. Kennedy Blvd., Suite 1800, Philadelphia, PA 19103-2899

Managing Editor (Name and complete mailing address)

Catherine Bewick, Elsevier Inc., 1600 John F. Kennedy Blvd., Suite 1800, Philadelphia, PA 19103-2899

10. Owner (Do not leave blank. If the publication is owned by a corporation, give the name and address of the corporation immediately followed by the names and addresses of all stockholders owning or holding 1 percent or more of the total amount of stock. If not owned by a corporation, give the names and addresses of the individual owners. If owned by a partnership or other unincorporated firm, give its name and address as well as those of each individual owner. If the publication is published by a nonprofit organization, give its name and address.)

Full Name	Complete Mailing Address
Wholly owned subsidiary of	4520 East-West Highway
Reed/Elsevier Inc., US holdings	Bethesda, MD 20814

11. Known Bondholders, Mortgagees, and Other Security Holders Owning or Holding 1 Percent or More of Total Amount of Bonds, Mortgages, or Other Securities. If none, check box ▸ None

Full Name	Complete Mailing Address
N/A	

12. Tax Status (For completion by nonprofit organizations authorized to mail at nonprofit rates) (Check one)
The purpose, function, and nonprofit status of this organization and the exempt status for federal income tax purposes:
☐ Has Not Changed During Preceding 12 Months
☐ Has Changed During Preceding 12 Months (Publisher must submit explanation of change with this statement)

(See Instructions on Reverse)

PS Form **3526**, October 1999

---

13. Publication Title	14. Issue Date for Circulation Data Below
Veterinary Clinics of North America: Small Animal Practice	July, 2006

15. Extent and Nature of Circulation		Average No. Copies Each Issue During Preceding 12 Months	No. Copies of Single Issue Published Nearest to Filing Date
a. Total Number of Copies (Net press run)		4,250	4,000
b. Paid and/or Requested Circulation	(1) Paid/Requested Outside-County Mail Subscriptions Stated on Form 3541. (Include advertiser's proof and exchange copies)	2,627	2,549
	(2) Paid In-County Subscriptions Stated on Form 3541 (Include advertiser's proof and exchange copies)		
	(3) Sales Through Dealers and Carriers, Street Vendors, Counter Sales, and Other Non-USPS Paid Distribution	575	597
	(4) Other Classes Mailed Through the USPS		
c. Total Paid and/or Requested Circulation [Sum of 15b. (1), (2), (3), and (4)]	▸	3,202	3,146
d. Free Distribution by Mail (Samples, complimentary, and other free)	(1) Outside-County as Stated on Form 3541	129	106
	(2) In-County as Stated on Form 3541		
	(3) Other Classes Mailed Through the USPS		
e. Free Distribution Outside the Mail (Carriers or other means)			
f. Total Free Distribution (Sum of 15d. and 15e.)	▸	129	106
g. Total Distribution (Sum of 15c. and 15f.)	▸	3,331	3,252
h. Copies not Distributed		919	748
i. Total (Sum of 15g. and h.)	▸	4,250	4,000
j. Percent Paid and/or Requested Circulation (15c. divided by 15g. times 100)		96.13%	96.74%

16. Publication of Statement of Ownership
☐ Publication required. Will be printed in the **November 2006** issue of this publication. ☐ Publication not required

17. Signature and Title of Editor, Publisher, Business Manager, or Owner

[signature] Date 9/15/06

Jeffrey Pancici – Executive Director of Subscription Services

I certify that all information furnished on this form is true and complete. I understand that anyone who furnishes false or misleading information on this form or who omits material or information requested on the form may be subject to criminal sanctions (including fines and imprisonment) and/or civil sanctions (including civil penalties).

Instructions to Publishers

1. Complete and file one copy of this form with your postmaster annually on or before October 1. Keep a copy of the completed form for your records.
2. In cases where the stockholder or security holder is a trustee, include in items 10 and 11 the name of the person or corporation for whom the trustee is acting. Also include the names and addresses of individuals who are stockholders who own or hold 1 percent or more of the total amount of bonds, mortgages, or other securities of the publishing corporation. In item 11, if none, check the box. Use blank sheets if more space is required.
3. Be sure to furnish all circulation information called for in item 15. Free circulation must be shown in items 15d, e, and f.
4. Item 15h., Copies not Distributed, must include (1) newsstand copies originally stated on Form 3541, and returned to the publisher, (2) estimated returns from news agents, and (3), copies for office use, leftovers, spoiled, and all other copies not distributed.
5. If the publication had Periodicals authorization as a general or requester publication, this Statement of Ownership, Management, and Circulation must be published; it must be printed in any issue in October or, if the publication is not published during October, the first issue printed after October.
6. In item 16, indicate the date of the issue in which this Statement of Ownership will be published.
7. Item 17 must be signed.
Failure to file or publish a statement of ownership may lead to suspension of Periodicals authorization.

PS Form **3526**, October 1999 (Reverse)